AF694979

PAP flap computer-animated video is available at MediaCenter.thieme.com – use the code below to access it!

Simply visit MediaCenter.thieme.com and, when prompted during the registration process, enter the code below to get started today.

6H2B-CHX3-2K24-Y25H

	WINDOWS	MAC	TABLET
Recommended Browser(s)*	Microsoft Internet Explorer 8.0 or later, Firefox 3.x	Firefox 3.x, Safari 4.x	HTML5 mobile browser. iPad — Safari. Opera Mobile — Tablet PCs referred.
	** all browsers should have JavaScript enabled*		
Flash Player Plug-in	Flash Player 9 or Higher** *** Mac users: ATI Rage 128 GPU does not support full-screen mode with hardware scaling*		Tablet PCs with Android OS support Flash 10.1
Minimum Hardware Configurations	Intel® Pentium® II 450 MHz, AMD Athlon™ 600 MHz or faster processor (or equivalent) 512 MB of RAM	PowerPC® G3 500 MHz or faster processor Intel Core™ Duo 1.33 GHz or faster processor 512MB of RAM	Minimum CPU powered at 800MHz 256MB DDR2 of RAM
Recommended for optimal usage experience	Monitor resolutions: • Normal (4:3) 1024×768 or Higher • Widescreen (16:9) 1280×720 or Higher • Widescreen (16:10) 1440×900 or Higher DSL/Cable internet connection at a minimum speed of 384.0 Kbps or faster WiFi 802.11 b/g preferred.		7-inch and 10-inch tablets on maximum resolution. WiFi connection is required.

Thieme

Perforator Flaps for Breast Reconstruction

Joshua L. Levine, MD
Chief of Surgical Services
Department of Plastic Surgery
Center for the Advancement of Breast Reconstruction
at New York Eye and Ear Infirmary of Mt. Sinai
New York, New York

Julie V. Vasile, MD, FACS
Division of Plastic and Reconstructive Surgery
Northern Westchester Hospital
Mt. Kisco, New York
New York Eye and Ear Infirmary of Mt. Sinai
New York, New York

Constance M. Chen, MD, MPH, FACS
Director of Microsurgery
Department of Plastic and Reconstructive Surgery
New York Eye and Ear Infirmary of Mt. Sinai
Lenox Hill Hospital
New York-Presbyterian Hospital
New York, New York

Robert J. Allen, Sr., MD, FACS
Clinical Professor of Plastic Surgery
New York University Langone Medical Center
New York, New York
Medical University of South Carolina
Charleston, South Carolina
Louisiana State University Health Sciences Center
New Orleans, Louisiana

257 illustrations

Thieme
New York • Suttgart • Delhi • Rio de Janeiro

Executive Editor: Timothy Hiscock
Managing Editor: Elizabeth Palumbo
Director, Editorial Services: Mary Jo Casey
Editorial Assistant: Haley Paskalides
Production Editor: Barbara A. Chernow
Consulting Editor: Charles Herman, MD
International Production Director: Andreas Schabert
Vice President, Editorial and E-Product Development: Vera Spillner
International Marketing Director: Fiona Henderson
International Sales Director: Louisa Turrell
Director of Sales, North America: Mike Roseman
Senior Vice President and Chief Operating Officer: Sarah Vanderbilt
President: Brian D. Scanlan
Typesetting by Carol Pierson, Chernow Editorial Services, Inc.

Library of Congress Cataloging-in-Publication Data

Perforator flaps for breast reconstruction / [edited by] Joshua L. Levine, Julie V. Vasile, Constance M. Chen, Robert J. Allen, Sr.
p. ; cm.
Includes bibliographical references and index.
ISBN 978-1-62623-094-1 (alk. paper)
I. Levine, Joshua L., editor. II. Vasile, Julie V., editor. III. Chen, Constance M., editor. IV. Allen, Robert J. (Robert Johnson), 1951– , editor.
[DNLM: 1. Mammaplasty–instrumentation. 2. Perforator Flap–surgery. 3. Mammaplasty–methods. WP 910]
RD539.8
618.1'90592–dc23 2015031874

333 Seventh Avenue, New York, NY 10001 USA
+1 800 782 3488, customerservice@thieme.com
Thieme Publishers Stuttgart
Rüdigerstrasse 14, 70469 Stuttgart, Germany
+49 [0]711 8931 421, customerservice@thieme.de

Thieme Publishers Delhi
A-12, Second Floor, Sector-2, Noida-201301
Uttar Pradesh, India
+91 120 45 566 00, customerservice@thieme.in

Thieme Publishers Rio de Janeiro, Thieme Publicações
Ltda. Edifício Rodolpho de Paoli, 25º andar
Av. Nilo Peçanha, 50 – Sala 2508
Rio de Janeiro 20020-906, Brasil
+55 21 3172 2297

Printed in China by Everbest Printing Ltd 5 4 3 2 1

ISBN 978-1-62623-094-1

Also available as an e-book:
eISBN 978-1-62623-095-8

Contents

Preface

Stuart Milton, working in Bert Myers's research lab at Louisiana State University Medical Center in the 1960s, proved that skin flaps survive to the same length regardless of width as long as the vascular pedicle is included in the flap. Although this set the stage for the evolution of perforator flaps, popularization of muscle and myocutaneous flaps in the 1970s overshadowed this breakthrough and became a detour that I regard as the "Dark Ages" of plastic surgery.

Beginning in the late 1980s and early 1990s, plastic surgeons working independently around the world, including Isao Koshima in Japan and Claudio Angrigiani in Argentina, redirected their efforts back to skin flaps by dissecting musculocutaneous perforators through the muscle, thereby creating less bulky, more elegant skin flaps without muscle sacrifice.

As a microsurgeon with an interest in autogenous breast reconstruction, I realized that the available options of the latissimus dorsi, rectus abdominis, and gluteus maximus myocutaneous flaps needed to be expanded. By doing vascular injection studies on fresh abdominoplasty specimens, I discovered that a large skin–fat flap would survive on either the superficial inferior epigastric artery (SIEA) or a single paraumbilical deep inferior epigastric perforator (DIEP). Working at Charity Hospital in New Orleans, the first SIEA and DIEP flaps for breast reconstruction were performed in 1989 and 1992, respectively.

Ian Taylor and others have done extensive anatomic studies of perforators all over the body. With this key understanding, an ever-expanding armamentarium of perforator flaps for breast reconstruction have been developed, including the gluteal artery perforator (GAP), thoracodorsal artery perforator (TDAP), lateral thigh perforator (LTP), and profunda artery perforator (PAP) flaps.

A 10-year review of DIEP breast reconstruction at Louisiana State University Medical Center from 1992 to 2002 published in the *Journal of Plastic and Reconstructive Surgery* reported a counterintuitive finding: The incidence of fat necrosis was inversely proportional to the number of perforators in the flap. The least fat necrosis occurred in flaps with only one perforator. To explain this, we go back to 1838 when Jean Leonard Marie Poiseuille derived the equation now known as Poiseuille's law, which states that the blood flow is directly proportional to the pressure to the fourth power of the radius. Doubling the radius increases the blood supply to the flap sixteen times! This means that the diameter of the perforator trumps everything. Preoperative imaging of the donor-site vessels has become routine. The identification of the largest perforator enables most flaps to be based on one perforator, thus ensuring excellent flap perfusion and decreasing donor site morbidity.

The editors and contributors of this book invite you on the exciting and ever-evolving journey of perforator flap breast reconstruction.

Robert J. Allen, Sr.

Contributors

Robert J. Allen, Sr., MD, FACS
Clinical Professor of Plastic Surgery
New York University Langone Medical Center
New York, New York
Medical University of South Carolina
Charleston, South Carolina
Louisiana State University Health Sciences Center
New Orleans, Louisiana

Sarah E. Appleton, MD, MSc
Senior Resident
Department of Plastic and Reconstructive Surgery
Dalhousie University
Halifax, Nova Scotia, Canada

Edward Buchel, MD, BSc, FACS
Associate Professor and Section Head
Faculty of Medicine Plastic Surgery
University of Manitoba
Health Sciences Centre
Winnipeg, Manitoba, Canada

Constance M. Chen, MD, MPH, FACS
Director of Microsurgery
Department of Plastic and Reconstructive Surgery
New York Eye and Ear Infirmary of Mt. Sinai
Lenox Hill Hospital
New York-Presbyterian Hospital
New York, New York

Ming-Huei Cheng, MD
Division of Reconstructive Microsurgery
Department of Plastic and Reconstructive Surgery
Chang Gung Memorial Hospital
Kweishan, Taoyuan, Taiwan

Thomas Constantinescu, MD, CM, FRCSC
Fellow in Reconstructive Microsurgery
Division of Reconstructive Microsurgery
Department of Plastic Reconstructive Surgery
Chang Gung Memorial Hospital
Chang Gung College of Medicine
Chang Gung University
Kweishan, Taoyuan, Taiwan

James Ernest Craigie, MD
Co-director
Center for Natural Breast Reconstruction
Mt. Pleasant, South Carolina

David Greenspun, MD, MSc, FACS
Plastic, Reconstructive, and Microvascular Surgery
Greenwich Hospital
Greenwich, Connecticut
Private Practice
New York, New York

Moustapha Hamdi, MD, PhD
Chief, Department of Plastic and Reconstructive Surgery
University Hospital of Brussels
Brussels, Belgium

Rene Remmelt Willie Johan van der Hulst, MD, PhD
University Hospital Maastricht
Maastricht, The Netherlands

Richard Mahlon Kline, Jr., MD
Center for Natural Breast Reconstruction
Mt. Pleasant, South Carolina

Arno Lataster, MD
Associate Professor
Department of Anatomy and Embryology
Faculty of Health, Medicine and Life Sciences
Maastricht University
Maastricht, The Netherlands

Bernard T. Lee, MD, MBA, FACS
Chief, Division of Plastic and Reconstructive Surgery
Department of Surgery
Beth Israel Deaconess Medical Center
Associate Professor of Surgery
Harvard Medical School
Editor-in-Chief
Journal of Reconstructive Microsurgery
Boston, Massachusetts

Joshua L. Levine, MD
Chief of Surgical Services
Department of Plastic Surgery
Center for the Advancement of Breast Reconstruction
at New York Eye and Ear Infirmary of Mt. Sinai
New York, New York

Maria M. LoTiempo, MD
Assistant Professorship
Mt. Sinai Weill Cornell Medical Center
New York, New York
Medical University at South Carolina
Charleston, South Carolina

James L. Mayo, MD
Microsurgery Fellow
Institute for Reconstructive Plastic Surgery
New York University Langone Medical Center
New York, New York

Steven F. Morris, MD, MSc, FRCSC
Professor
Department of Surgery
Dalhousie University
Haligan, Nova Scotia

Aldona J. Spiegel, MD
Associate Professor
Weill Cornell Medical College
Director, Center for Breast Restoration
Center for Breast Restoration at Institute for Reconstructive Surgery
Houston Methodist Hospital
Houston Texas

Stephania Tuinder, MD, PhD
University Hospital Maastricht
Maastricht, The Netherlands

Koenraad Van Landuyt, MD
University Hospital
Ghent Department of Plastic Surgery
Universitair Ziekenhuis Gent Dienst Plastische Heelkunde
De Pintelaan, Gent, Belgium

Christina R. Vargas, MD
Resident in General Surgery
Beth Israel Deaconess Medical Center
Boston, Massachusetts

Julie V. Vasile, MD, FACS
Division of Plastic and Reconstructive Surgery
Northern Westchester Hospital
Mt. Kisco, New York
New York Eye and Ear Infirmary of Mt. Sinai
New York, New York

Assaf Zeltzer, MD
Clinique du Parc Léopold–Chirec
Etterbeek, Belgium

Michael R. Zenn, MD, MBA, FACS
Professor and Vice Chief
Plastic and Reconstructive Surgery
Duke University Medical Center
Durham, North Carolina

1

The History of the Use of Perforator Flaps for Microsurgical Breast Reconstruction

Sarah E. Appleton and Steven F. Morris

The quest to perfect postmastectomy breast reconstruction has been accelerating for the past few decades. Results have steadily improved, and expectations have continued to mount as surgical techniques for autologous breast reconstruction have evolved. Although plastic surgeons have been performing surgery to improve breast aesthetics for centuries, postmastectomy breast reconstruction did not become widely accepted until the mid-1900s. Today, breast reconstruction is an essential part of the overall treatment plan and recovery of the patient with breast cancer. The psychological benefits of postmastectomy breast reconstruction are improved overall satisfaction, body image, self-esteem, and quality of life, as well as decreased anxiety and depression.[1,2] Thus, breast reconstruction is popular among patients. In the United States, support for breast reconstruction was written into law in 1998 when President Bill Clinton signed the federal Breast Cancer Reconstruction Law as part of the Women's Health and Cancer Rights Act that requires group health plans and individual insurance policies to cover the costs of reconstructive breast surgery.[3,4]

Plastic surgeons now have a large variety of alloplastic and autologous breast reconstruction options to perform breast reconstruction.[5] Improved understanding of flap physiology and anatomy has yielded an increasing number of flap options. Advances in the field of microsurgery have provided surgeons with the ability to reconstruct a breast mound using autologous tissue that both looks and feels like the native breast with minimal donor-site morbidity. Cosmetic results of the reconstructed breast have steadily improved, which has led to increasing demand among breast cancer patients for breast reconstruction postmastectomy and postlumpectomy.[6] The skill required to balance patient expectations and technical challenges and to produce an excellent cosmetic outcome has proven breast reconstruction to be a rewarding field within plastic surgery.

Cancer and Mastectomy

For over a century, surgeons have used autologous tissue to reconstruct the breast. Breast reconstruction after mastectomy, however, did not become popularized until the mid–20th century in part due to the widely publicized work of the famous American surgeon, Dr. William Stewart Halsted. Halsted, who was known for his radical mastectomy technique **(Fig. 1.1)**, was concerned that closure of the chest "might conceal tumour recurrence and increase the chance of tumour dissemination."[7] Therefore, it was common practice to allow mastectomy wounds to heal by secondary intention or to close primarily under high tension, resulting in significant morbidities including chest wall deformities and restricted shoulder movement.[8] This erroneous belief led to a highly disfiguring cosmetic result and devastating psychological effects.[1]

The early 20th century women's right movement began to question radical breast surgeries, and this prompted the development of breast conservation techniques.[9] In 1948, Patey and Dyson[10] introduced the modified radical mastectomy, which has since replaced Halsted's mastectomy as the standard of care. Over the past 30 years, breast cancer surgery has steadily become less invasive.[11] Breast conservation surgery techniques such as the lumpectomy, the skin-sparing mastectomy, and the nipple-sparing mastectomy have been shown in prospective randomized controlled trials to be safe, reliable, and effective options for the treatment of breast cancer in selected patients.[12,13] These breast conservation methods treat the breast cancer effectively and yet preserve the skin, which improves the overall aesthetic result of breast reconstruction. When combined with immediate breast reconstruction, a skin-sparing mastectomy can reduce operating room costs, preserve the breast pocket, limit the anesthetic risk, and improve the overall aesthetic results.[11,14,15]

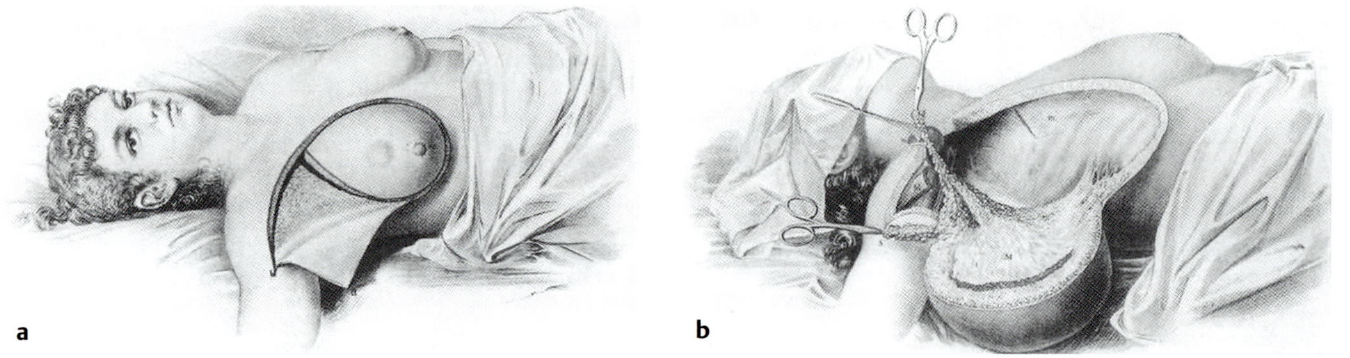

Fig. 1.1 The Halsted radical mastectomy. **(a)** Halsted mastectomy incision and triangular flap. **(b)** mastectomy specimen just before amputation. (From Cotlar AM, Dubose JJ, Rose DM. History of surgery for breast cancer: radical to the sublime. Curr Surg 2003;60:329–337.)

Early Flap Surgery

The word *flap* is derived from the Dutch "*flappe*," defined as something "to hang broadly and loosely, fastened only by one side."[9] Skin flaps have been used since ancient times to reconstruct defects throughout the body. According to translations by Bhishagratna, the earliest evidence of a pedicled forehead flap for nasal reconstruction comes from Sushruta in 700 A.D., who used a skin graft from the cheek to complete his reconstruction.[16,17] In 1440 A.D., the Kanghiara family from India also described the forehead flap for nasal reconstruction.[18] Joseph Constantine Carpue in England later popularized the same ancient Indian forehead flap for nasal reconstruction, which was widely adopted by surgeons in Germany, France, and Italy in the early 19th century.[19] In 1597, Gaspare Tagliacozzi classically described a successful distally based tubed upper arm flap for nasal reconstruction.[19,20]

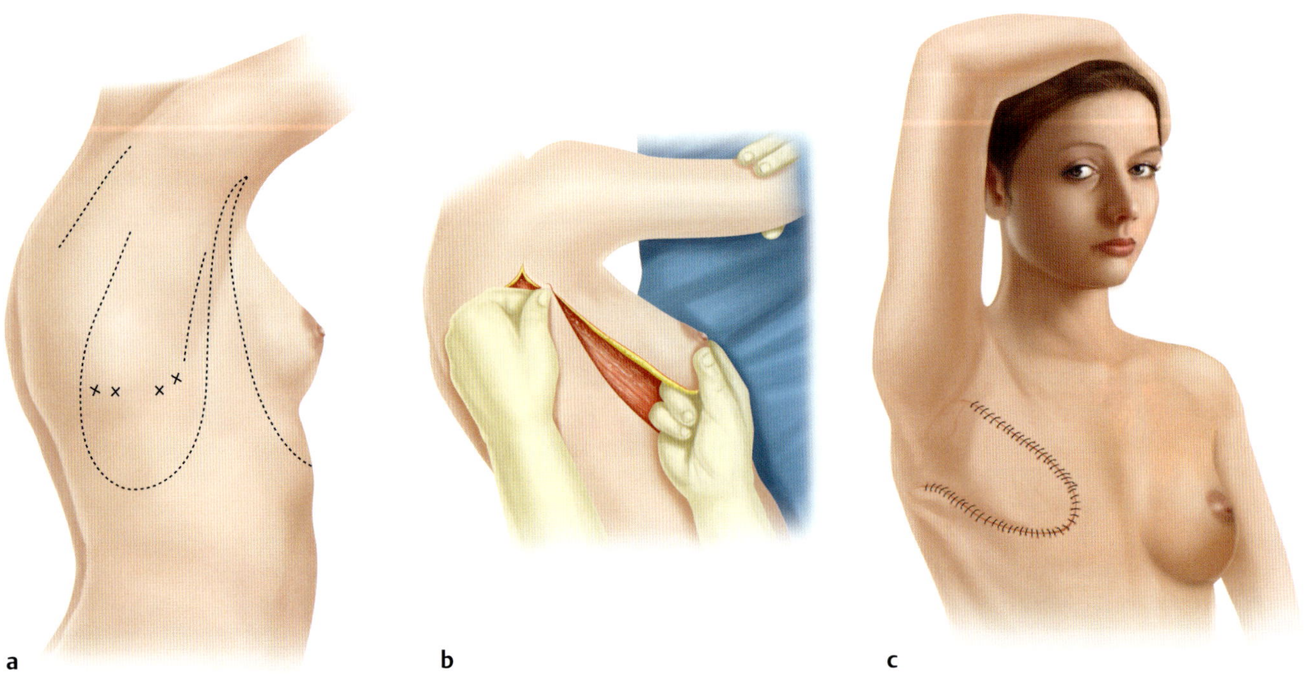

Fig. 1.2 The latissimus dorsi musculocutaneous flap according to Tansini. **(a)** Flap outlined. **(b)** Flap transposition. **(c)** Final result.

French surgeon Aristide Verneuil[21] was the first to describe the use of autologous tissue to reconstruct the breast in 1887, when he transferred breast tissue on a pedicle to reconstruct the contralateral breast. However, it was the German surgeon Vincent Czerny[22] who is credited with the first successful postmastectomy breast reconstruction in 1895, when he transferred a large lipoma from the lumbar region to fill a mastectomy defect. Shortly thereafter in 1896, the first documented muscle flap was performed by Iginio Tansini,[23,24] when he described the successful application of the latissimus dorsi myocutaneous flap for postmastectomy breast reconstruction[25] **(Fig. 1.2)**.

For the first half of the 20th century, randomly designed tubed flaps dominated all forms of reconstruction, including breast reconstruction. Over the next half-century, multiple attempts at breast reconstruction using local tissue transfers in the form of tubed pedicle flaps harvested from the contralateral breast, abdomen, or extended thoracoabdominal region were attempted. Ombredanne[26] described the tubed axilloabdominal flap in 1924.

World War II stimulated a period of great innovation in the field of plastic and reconstructive surgery. Battlefield injuries, in particular difficult ballistic wounds and facial burns, proved to be significant reconstructive challenges for surgeons at the time. Innovative local flaps were developed and widely used to reconstruct these difficult defects. Conceptually, these flaps were all of a random pattern because they lacked any significant recognized orientation to its vascular blood supply.

Tubed Flaps

In 1942, Sir Harold Gillies[27] successfully marched a tubed pedicle flap from the lower half of the contralateral breast, abdomen, and chest along the torso in multiple stages to re-create a breast mound. In 1950, Yannilos[28] successfully performed a composite tubed pedicled contralateral breast flap to reconstruct the breast. In 1956, Holdsworth[29] described his four-stage tube flap technique for breast reconstruction with a fairly good aesthetic result **(Fig. 1.3)**. Tubed flaps were eventually abandoned due to poor design and donor-site morbidity, and were replaced by flaps based on known blood supply **(Fig. 1.4)**.

Axial Pattern Skin Flaps

In 1918, Esser[30] made the astute observation that skin overlying a vascular pedicle could be dispensed with as long as the feeding and draining vessels remained intact. In 1969, Milton[31] confirmed Esser's work. These observations are the earliest evidence of the axial pattern flap in the literature. McGregor and Jackson's[32] groin flap was the one of the first known axial pattern flaps. In 1973, McGregor and Morgan[33] described differences between random and axial pattern flaps. Axial pattern flaps are characterized by the vascular pedicle situated along the flap long axis. The earliest axial pattern flaps described in the literature were the hypogastric flap,[34] the deltopectoral flap,[35] and the groin flap.[32]

Musculocutaneous Flaps

Shortly after Tansini's[24] ground-breaking work on musculocutaneous flaps, Morax[36] described in 1908 the use of a platysma musculocutaneous flap for head and neck reconstruction. In the 1970s, McGraw,[37] Mathes and Nahai,[38,39] and others revisited and popularized musculocutaneous flaps recognizing their reliable vascularity from the large source vessel supplying the muscle. The increased activity and focus on muscle flaps led to the Mathes and Nahai[38] classification of muscle and musculocutaneous flaps in 1981,[38] which helped introduce these flaps to all reconstructive surgeons, including those performing breast reconstruction. Musculocutaneous flaps were readily adopted because a large skin flap could be reliably transferred based on a large source vessel supplying the muscle. The pedicled transverse rectus abdominis musculocutaneous (TRAM) flap revolutionized breast reconstructive surgery and was widely accepted worldwide.[40] However, musculocutaneous flaps were often bulky and often needlessly sacrificed the donor muscle, which was not required for the reconstruction.

Fasciocutaneous Flaps

Although musculocutaneous flaps have been in use since the early 20th century, septocutaneous perforators and their importance in flap design were not recognized until later. Septocutaneous perforators are vessels that follow the intermuscular septum and travel along the fascia to eventually supply the skin. Pontén[41] first introduced the concept of fasciocutaneous flaps in 1981 with his work on lower leg reconstruction. Haertsch[42] and Barclay and colleagues[43] further developed the vascular basis of the fasciocutaneous flap. The major advantage of fasciocutaneous flaps over random skin flaps is the inclusion of fascia, which may contain a source vessel and its cutaneous branches. Cormack and Lamberty[44] described in even greater detail the fascial structures throughout the body, and classified four main types of fasciocutaneous flaps.

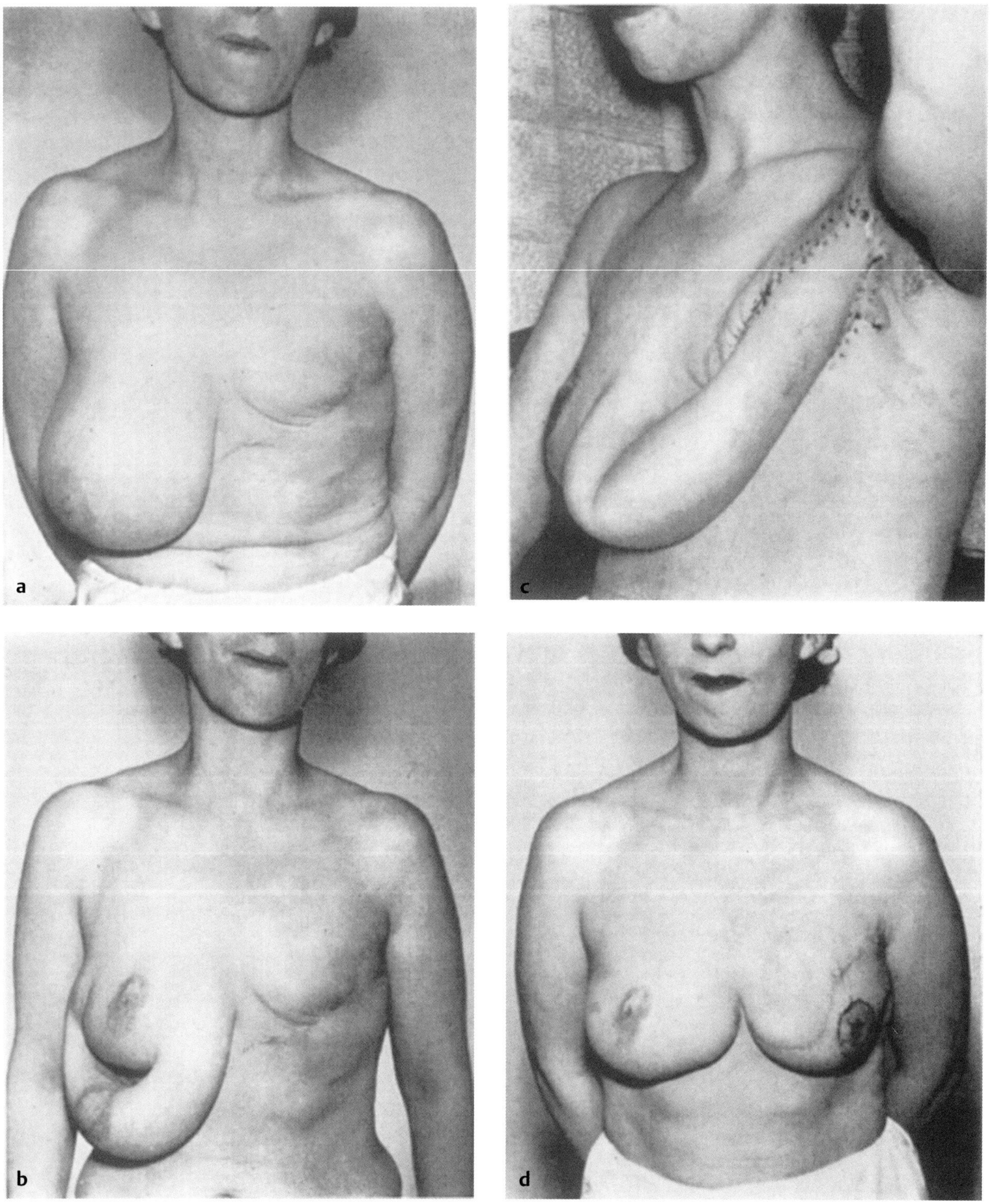

Fig. 1.3 (a) A 36-year-old patient 1 year after a left breast mastectomy. **(b)** A tube flap was created from the inferior portion of the right breast and attached to the sternum and axilla. The nipple was transplanted superiorly on the new breast mound. **(c)** The tube flap was divided from the right axilla and inset to an incision positioned high in the anterior left axilla. **(d)** Final division of the tube flap with areola and nipple reconstruction using a free graft. (From Holdsworth WG. A method of reconstructing the breast. Br J Plast Surg 1956;9:161–162.)

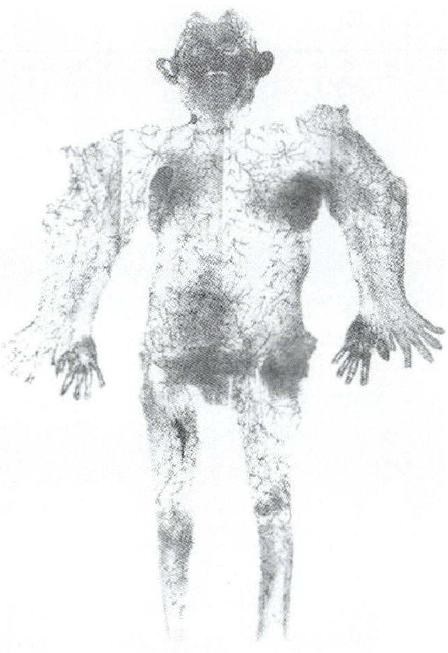

Fig. 1.4 Montage of the cutaneous arteries of the body. This is a cadaver specimen from which skin has been incised along the ulnar border in the upper extremities, and the integument has been removed with the deep fascia intact on the left side and without it on the right side. The direction, size, and density of perforators can be appreciated as well the reduced-caliber (choke) anastomotic arteries, linking the perforators into a continuous network. (From Taylor GI, Palmer JH. The vascular territories (angiosomes) of the body: experimental study and clinical applications. Br J Plast Surg 1987;40:113–141.)

Perforator Flaps

The advances in our knowledge of the anatomic characteristics of the musculocutaneous perforators eventually led to the evolution of the musculocutaneous perforator flap. Strictly defined, a perforator flap is a skin flap based on a musculocutaneous perforator, which is dissected through the muscle, preserving muscle function. A major advancement in this field was the discovery that the inclusion of a source vessel did not require the harvest of an entire muscle, and perforators could be dissected through the muscle. Perforator flaps require the incision of the desired skin paddle for transfer, followed by the identification of the perforating vessels that supply the skin and dissection of the perforators down to source artery. Practically, a perforator flap may be defined as a vascularized tissue transfer nourished by an adequate cutaneous perforator, which may be a musculocutaneous, septocutaneous, or direct perforator. Perforator flaps have enabled surgeons to tailor flaps to specific defects and minimize donor-site morbidity. For breast reconstruction in particular, perforator flaps have been widely adopted due to the close similarity between the skin and adipose tissue of a perforator flap and the native breast tissue lost after a lumpectomy or mastectomy. In particular, the following flaps have been used extensively for breast reconstruction: deep inferior epigastric perforator (DIEP), superior gluteal artery perforator (SGAP), superficial inferior epigastric artery (SIEA), thoracodorsal artery perforator (TDAP), and profunda artery perforator (PAP).

Microsurgery

Perhaps the most significant advancement in reconstructive surgery has been the development and refinement of microvascular techniques in the late 1960s and early 1970s. The introduction of the operating microscope for small-vessel anastomosis revolutionized microsurgery and opened the door to the era of free tissue transfer.[45–47] In 1960, vascular surgeon Jules Jacobson[48] performed the first microsurgical anastomosis of a 1.4-mm vessel under surgical magnification. Harry Buncke,[49] the "father of microsurgery," performed the first successful microvascular replantation of a rabbit's ear in 1964 with vessels measuring 1 mm in size. In 1969, McLean and Buncke[50] performed the first successful microvascular transplant using omentum to fill a large scalp defect. Taylor and Daniel[51–53] performed the first successful skin free flap transfer of an iliofemoral island flap to reconstruct a lower limb defect in 1973. These refinements in microsurgical instrumentation and technique laid the groundwork for the field of microsurgery and free flap reconstruction.

After Taylor and Daniel's[52,53] 1973 report of a successful free microvascular skin flap, the landscape of breast reconstruction was forever changed. In 1975, Toyomi Fujino[54,55] performed the first successful microvascular reconstruction of a congenital breast aplasia defect with a "dermal-fat–muscle" free flap harvested from the buttocks and anastomosed to the thoracoacromial artery. Hans Holmström[56] performed the first abdominal free flap called the "abdominoplasty flap" based on the deep inferior epigastric artery, including the rectus abdominus muscle in the flap. Other free flaps proposed for breast reconstruction over the years include the deep circumflex iliac artery (groin) flap (Rubens flap),[57,58] lateral thigh (tensor fascia lata) flaps,[59] anterior thigh flap,[60] superior and inferior gluteal musculocutaneous flaps,[61–63] gracilis flaps,[64] triceps flaps,[65] and others.

In 1987, Taylor[66] published his landmark paper describing the angiosome theory of the vascular anatomy of the skin and integument, which he later elaborated on[67,68] **(Fig. 1.4)**. This work has provided a roadmap to the vasculature of the integument for the reconstructive surgeon. The angiosome theory was greatly influenced by Manchot's[69] and Salmon's[70] earlier descriptions of human vascular anatomy and vascular territories. Taylor's angiosome concept depicts the body as a mosaic of 40 three-dimensional (3D) composite units of tissue supplied by named source arteries. An angiosome can further be broken down into smaller territories that are linked by reduced-caliber choke anastomotic vessels. The angiosome concept and understanding of the overall vascular anatomy of the skin has led to a more sophisticated surgical planning of free tissue transfers.[65–67]

Imaging

Taylor and colleagues[71] used a handheld Doppler probe to outline the perforating vessels intraoperatively for flap planning. Preoperative imaging with Doppler flowmetry or Doppler sonography and color duplex imaging are commonly used for perforator flap planning.[72,73] Masia et al[74] introduced the preoperative computed tomography (CT) angiography for perforator mapping. Since that time, advances in the field of vascular imaging have led to the use of multidetector row CT, 3D CT, as well as magnetic resonance imaging (MRI) for preoperative perforator imaging and flap planning.[75–79] Preoperative imaging can significantly reduce operative time. These new techniques have improved spatial resolution images, enabling the detection of stenotic or diseased peripheral vessels.[80] Recently, several laser-assisted fluorescence angiography systems have been developed. For instance, the SPY laser-assisted fluorescence angiography system (Novadaq, Bonita Springs, FL) has been employed for intraoperative real-time flap perfusion mapping. This technology uses indocyanine green fluorescence angiography and enables the reconstructive surgeon to confirm intraoperatively whether a perforator will provide adequate flap perfusion. This technology is able to predict postoperative mastectomy flap necrosis with great accuracy.[81,82]

Evolution of Breast Reconstruction

Breast reconstruction has a history that spans nearly 130 years, beginning with the late 19th-century work discussed earlier in the chapter. Over the next half-century, multiple attempts at breast reconstruction using local tissue transfers in the form of tubed pedicle flaps harvested from the contralateral breast, abdomen, or extended thoracoabdominal region were attempted. Tubed flaps were largely abandoned due to poor design, donor-site morbidity, and poor cancer survival rates. With an improved understanding of abdominal wall anatomy and advances in the abdominoplasty technique, efforts to use the abdomen as a donor site subsequently dominated the field.

Autologous flap reconstruction of the breast has used the abdomen as a donor site since the mid–20th century, when Gillies (discussed earlier) and D.R. Millard, Jr.[83] transposed a racquet-shaped abdominal flap to the mastectomy defect. In 1977, Stephen Mathes and John Bostwick[84] described the rectus abdominis musculocutaneous flap to reconstruct abdominal wall defects and later for use in breast reconstruction. In 1979, Robbins[85,86] first reported the use of the rectus abdominis musculocutaneous flap for breast reconstruction. In 1977, Drever[87] first described the vertically orientated epigastric island flap now commonly known as the vertical rectus abdominis musculocutaneous (VRAM) flap for use in breast reconstruction. By the end of the 1970s, the rectus abdominis musculocutaneous flap became the workhorse of autologous breast reconstruction in many centers.

In 1982, Carl Hartrampf[88] first described and performed the pedicled TRAM flap, an abdominal island flap composed of a transverse ellipse of skin and subcutaneous tissue isolated on its superior epigastric vascular pedicle **(Fig. 1.5)**. The pedicled TRAM flap has the advantages of being a well-vascularized flap, with an adequate large arc of rotation and volume to reconstruct an aesthetic breast

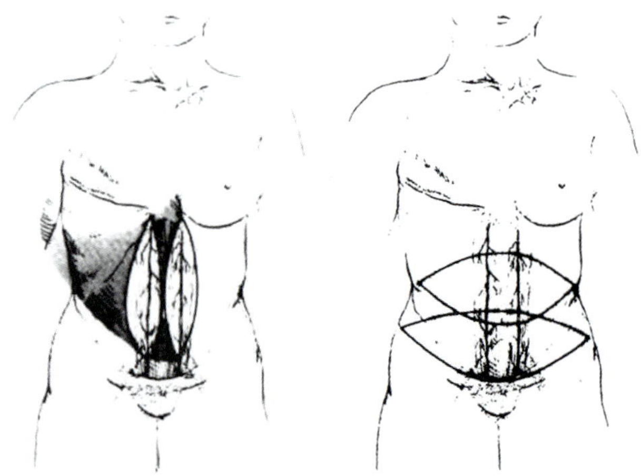

Fig. 1.5 Horizontal and vertical designs of Hartrampf's rectus abdominis musculocutaneous flap based superiorly on either the ipsilateral or contralateral rectus abdominis muscle and its underlying deep epigastric pedicle. (From Hartrampf CR, Scheflan M, Black PW. Breast reconstruction with a transverse abdominal island flap. Plast Reconstr Surg 1982;69:216–224.)

mound without the need for microsurgical anastomosis. Furthermore, the donor-site scar was cosmetically hidden in the lower abdomen.

However, it was quickly recognized that the pedicled TRAM was associated with significant donor-site morbidity in the form of abdominal wall hernias and weakness. Abdominal wall fascial defects were commonly repaired by synthetic mesh and were associated with significant long-term complications.[89] The field gradually focused on the generation of a muscle-sparing technique for the elevation of the rectus abdominis flap. In 1989, Grotting[90,91] started to use the free microvascular TRAM (free TRAM) flap for primary breast reconstruction, with good results. The advantages of the free TRAM over the pedicled TRAM include the use of the dominant inferior epigastric pedicle (which is larger in diameter), the avoidance of a bulge in the epigastrium, reduced partial flap necrosis, and reduced donor-site morbidity. Both free and pedicled TRAM flaps remain widely used for breast reconstruction today, despite the risk of donor-site morbidity. The concept of muscle-sparing TRAM flaps evolved as surgeons reduced the amount of rectus abdominis muscle and fascia harvested with the flap to lessen the insult to the abdominal wall, while preserving the all-important periumbilical perforators.

Perforator Flap Breast Reconstruction

With improved understanding of the abdominal wall anatomy, it was recognized that the sacrifice of the rectus abdominis muscle was not required for the successful harvest of a lower abdominal wall flap. Furthermore, the pedicled TRAM flap was associated with skin and fat necrosis and flap loss in zone 4, the region of poorest flap perfusion. An alternative to the TRAM flap with improved flap perfusion and muscle sparing was sought for breast reconstruction. In 1983, G. Ian Taylor[92] described a variation on the TRAM flap: the extended deep inferior epigastric perforator (DIEP) flap, which is composed of the lower half of the rectus abdominis muscle and a superolateral fasciocutaneous extension based on periumbilical deep inferior epigastric artery perforators **(Fig. 1.6)**. In 1986, Onishi and Maruyama[93] published a small study that provided the anatomic basis for a perforator-based fasciocutaneous flap of the lower abdominal wall integument. In 1989, Japanese surgeons Isao Koshima and Shugo Soeda[94] described the superthin paraumbilical perforator (PUP) flap based on the paraumbilical perforator of the deep inferior epigastric artery for the reconstruction of a contralateral groin flap and an oral floor defect, respectively **(Fig. 1.7)**.

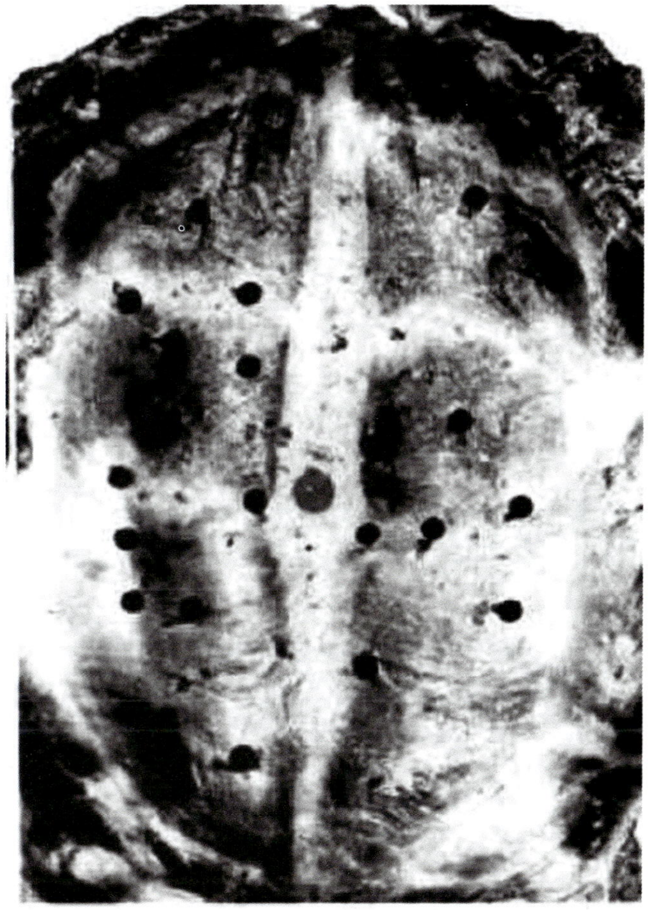

Fig. 1.6 Boyd and Taylor's original work on the vascular anatomy of the superior epigastric and deep inferior epigastric system. Anterior abdominal wall from a cadaver specimen after removal of fat and perforator mapping. Large perforators greater than 0.5 cm in diameter are identified with a marking pen. Note the paraumbilical perforator distribution. (From Boyd JB, Taylor GI, Corlett R. The vascular territories of the superior epigastric and deep inferior epigastric systems. Plast Reconstr Surg 1984;73:1–14.)

In 1992, Robert J. Allen[95] introduced the now well-known DIEP flap for breast reconstruction **(Fig. 1.8)**, In a presentation at the American Society of Plastic and Reconstructive Surgery (ASPRS) meeting in New Orleans in September 1993, Phillip Blondeel, a plastic surgery resident from Belgium, heard the presentation and convinced his chief to begin the DIEP flap in Belgium. Blondeel was responsible for popularizing the procedure in Europe. In January 1994, Allen and Treece[95] reported on breast reconstruction with the DIEP flap. Later in 1994, Blondeel[96] reported on refinements in the technique. Since that time, Blondeel[97–99] has reported on his extensive personal experience with DIEP flap breast reconstruction **(Fig. 1.9)**.

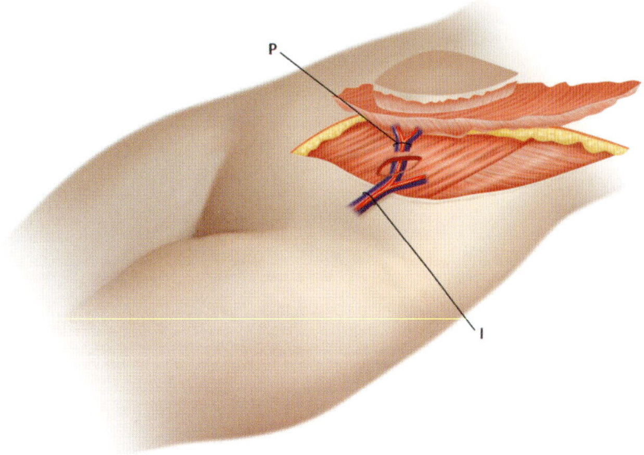

Fig. 1.7 A paraumbilical adipofascial perforator flap with muscle perforators sparing the deep inferior epigastric vessels and muscle. P, muscle perforator; I, deep inferior epigastric vessel.

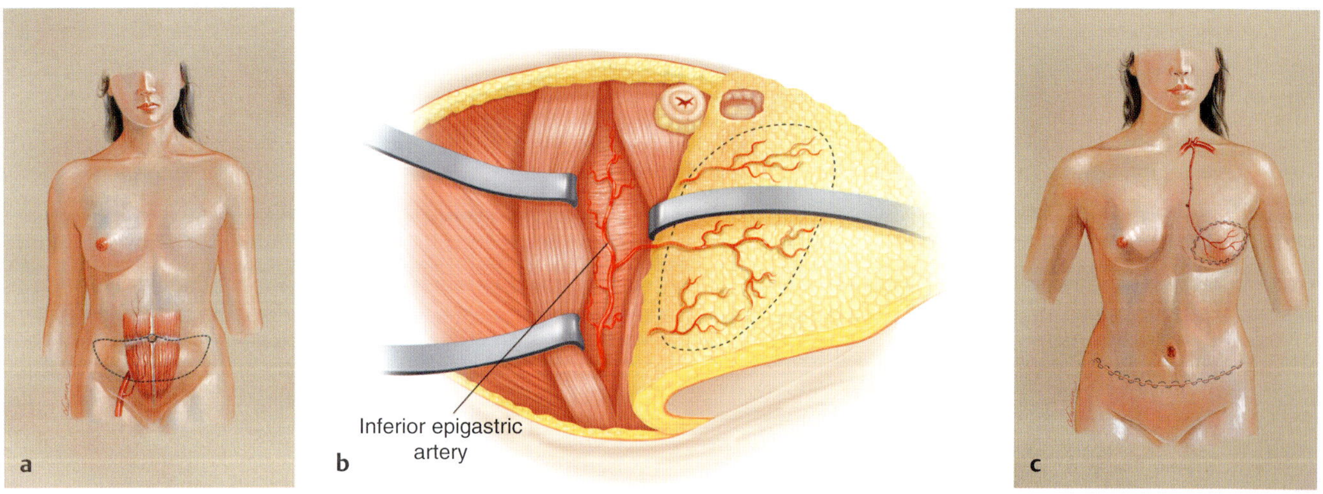

Fig. 1.8 A deep inferior epigastric perforator (DIEP) flap for breast reconstruction depicting **(a)** preoperative markings, **(b)** intraoperative dissection, and **(c)** anastomosis to the internal mammary artery. (Parts a and c from Allen RJ, Treece P. Deep inferior epigastric artery perforator flap for breast reconstruction. Ann Plast Surg 1994;32:32–38.)

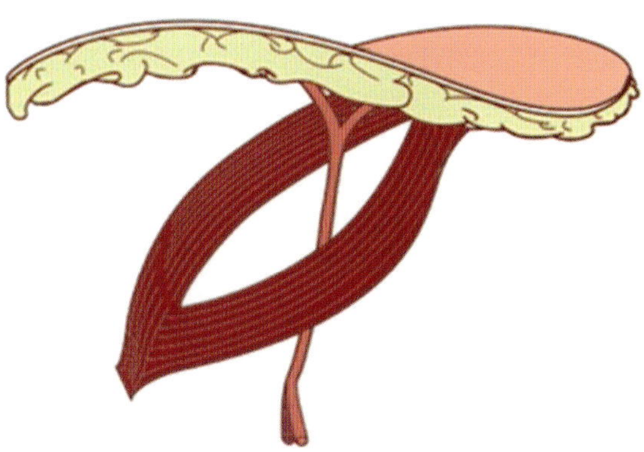

Fig. 1.9 Logo of the International Perforator Society, designed by Dr. Phil Blondeel.

Other Abdominal Perforator Flaps

Two additional flaps from the abdomen have been used for autologous breast reconstruction. The first is the superficial inferior epigastric artery (SIEA) flap. After first performing the SIEA flap for breast reconstruction in 1989, Allen presented his first seven cases at the Southeastern Society of Plastic and Reconstructive Surgeons annual meeting in 1990. Grotting[91] reported a case report of the SIEA in 1991, followed by Arnez et al[100] in 1999. The SIEA flap can be harvested without an incision through the anterior rectus sheath, as with a DIEP flap, or with an excision of the rectus muscle or sheath as with a pedicled or free TRAM flap, thereby reducing donor-site morbidity. It offers a regional reconstruction with a large volume of tissue. Unfortunately, the SIEA is not as consistent anatomically as the DIEP flap, and the pedicle length is shorter and the vessel diameter is smaller.[101,102] Based on 100 cadaver dissections performed by Taylor and Daniel,[101] a complete absence of the SIEA is present in 35% of patients (**Fig. 1.10**).

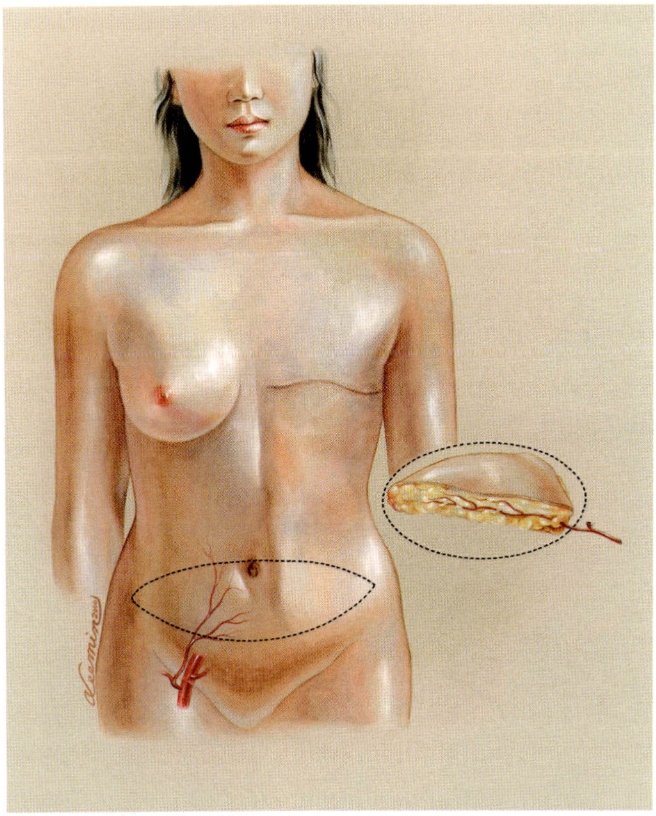

Fig. 1.10 The superficial inferior epigastric artery (SIEA) flap preoperative markings and anatomy. (From Arnez ZM, Khan U, Pogorelec D, Planinsek F. Breast reconstruction using free superficial epigastric artery SIEA flaps. Br J Plast Surg 1999;52:276.)

Elliott and Hartrampf[57,103] described the Rubens flap, referring to the redundant peri-iliac fat pad of the upper thigh and iliac crest region. This flap is based on the deep circumflex iliac artery (DCIA) and offers an autologous breast reconstruction option from the abdomen in women who had previous abdominoplasty or TRAM flap harvest. The harvest is more tedious and still presents the risk of abdominal-site morbidity and hernia. The DCIA perforator flap can be combined with the DIEP flap to supply a larger flap based on the DCIA perforator and the DIEP perforator(s) and their pedicles.[104]

Latissimus Dorsi Flap, Thoracodorsal Artery Perforator Flap, and Intercostal Artery Perforator Flap

First described in 1906 by Tansini[24] for chest wall reconstruction, the latissimus dorsi flap based on the thoracodorsal vessels is a reliable and widely used pedicled flap option for breast reconstruction. In 1912, d'Este[105] first proposed the use of the pedicled latissimus dorsi flap for the reconstruction of a breast mastectomy defect. In 1939, Hutchins[106] recommended the use of the latissimus dorsi flap to both reconstruct the breast mound and to reduce lymphedema in postmastectomy patients. In 1976, Nevin Olivari[107] rediscovered the latissimus dorsi flap for breast reconstruction and recommended its use in patients with skin and chest wall radiation damage. Hokin[108] described the use of an extended latissimus flap in 1987 with the incorporation of lumbar fat to increase the volume of reconstruction. However, the use of the latissimus dorsi flap sacrifices a large and important functioning muscle. Three perforator flaps harvested in the lateral chest area have been described that are considered superior because there is no need to sacrifice the latissimus dorsi muscle.

In 1985 Holmström and Lossing[109] described a fasciocutaneous lateral thoracodorsal transposition flap based on the same thoracodorsal pedicle for late breast reconstruction with a prosthesis. More recently the lateral thoracodorsal flap has been demonstrated to be a reliable option for immediate partial breast reconstruction of defects of the lateral breast.[110,111] In 1995, Angrigiani[112] used cadaver latex injection studies to describe the elevation of a latissimus dorsi musculocutaneous flap without muscle now known as the TDAP flap (**Fig. 1.11**). The vascular anatomy was further clarified by Thomas et al.[113] In 2004, Hamdi and colleagues[114] used an intraoperative Doppler probe to identify more perforator flap options based on the intercostal artery system. Both the TDAP

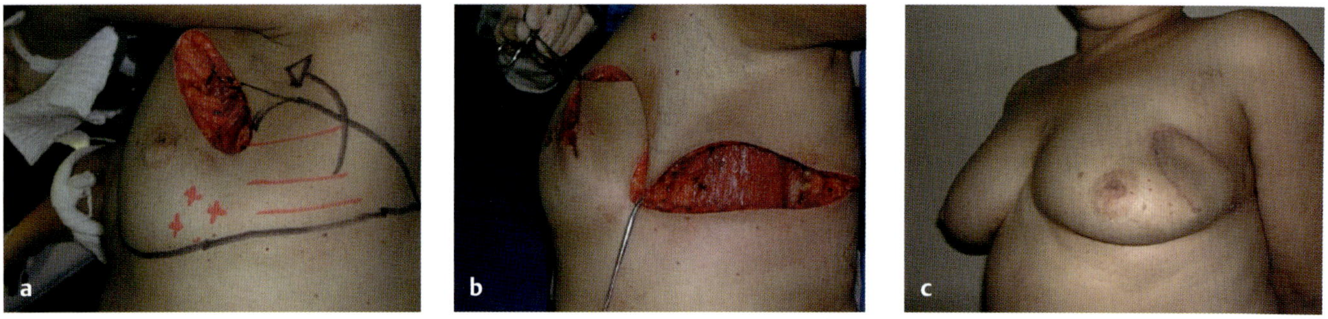

Fig. 1.11 The thoracodorsal artery perforator (TDAP) flap for partial breast reconstruction. A 59-year-old patient with invasive ductal carcinoma of the breast in the upper outer quadrant after lateral quadrantectomy and a total axillary dissection through the same incision. **(a)** Preoperative markings of a large TDAP fasciocutaneous flap. **(b)** TDAP flap dissected and rotated into lateral breast defect. **(c)** Six months postoperative appearance after radiation. (From Munhoz AM, Montag E, Arrunda EG, Aldrighi C, Gemperli R, Aldrighi JM, Ferreira MC. The role of the lateral thoracodorsal fasciocutaneous flap in immediate conservative breast surgery reconstruction. Plast Reconstr Surg 2006;117:1699–1710.)

and the intercostal artery perforator (ICAP) flaps are large and reliable pedicled fasciocutaneous flap options from the lateral chest for breast reconstruction in addition to the musculocutaneous latissimus dorsi flap. In 2008, Hamdi et al[115] presented the lateral intercostal artery perforator (LICAP) flap based on the posterior neurovascular bundle as a reliable option for reconstruction of complex deformities of the lateral breast that preserves the thoracodorsal pedicle **(Fig. 1.12).** There are two additional variants of the ICAP flap based on the dorsal cutaneous branch of the posterior intercostal artery (DICAP) and the anterior intercostal artery perforator (AICAP).[116,117] However, these flaps have a more limited arch of rotation compared with the LICAP due to their shorter pedicle lengths and may be less useful for breast reconstruction.[117]

Gluteal Flaps

In 1973, Orticochea[118] utilized the buttock region as a donor site when he performed a pedicled, multistage gluteal musculocutaneous flap. In 1975, Fujino[61] performed a free superior gluteal artery musculocutaneous flap for primary postmastectomy breast reconstruction. In 1989, Paletta, Bostwick, and Nahai[62] described the inferior gluteal musculocutaneous free flap for breast reconstruction. In 1993, Allen[63] introduced the gluteal artery perforator (GAP) flaps for breast reconstruction. The GAP flap is ideal for women with more skin and fat available in the gluteal region than in the abdominal area, or when the abdominal region is not available. The adipose tissue in the flap tends to be quite firm, and the harvested flaps tend to be smaller than the DIEP flaps. Similar to the DIEP and

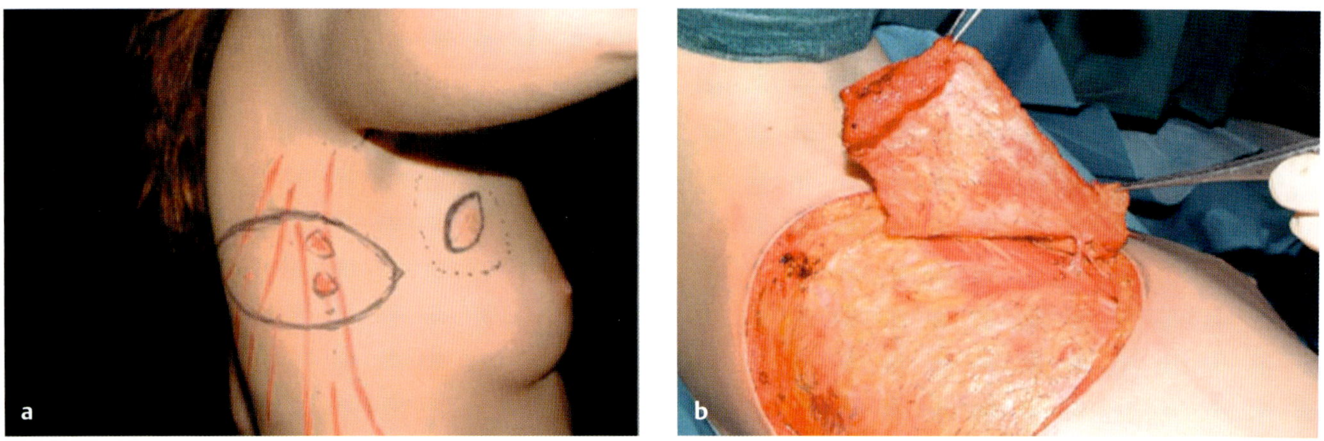

Fig. 1.12 The lateral intercostal artery perforator (LICAP) flap for partial breast reconstruction. **(a)** LICAP flap designed based on two intercostal artery perforators to reconstruct a partial breast defect as outlined. **(b)** Flap elevated on a single intercostal artery perforator and nerve. (From Hamdi M, Van Landuyt K, de Frene B, Roche N, Blondeel P, Monstrey S. The versatility of the inter-costal artery perforator ICAP flaps. J Plast Reconstr Aesthet Surg 2006;59:644–652.)

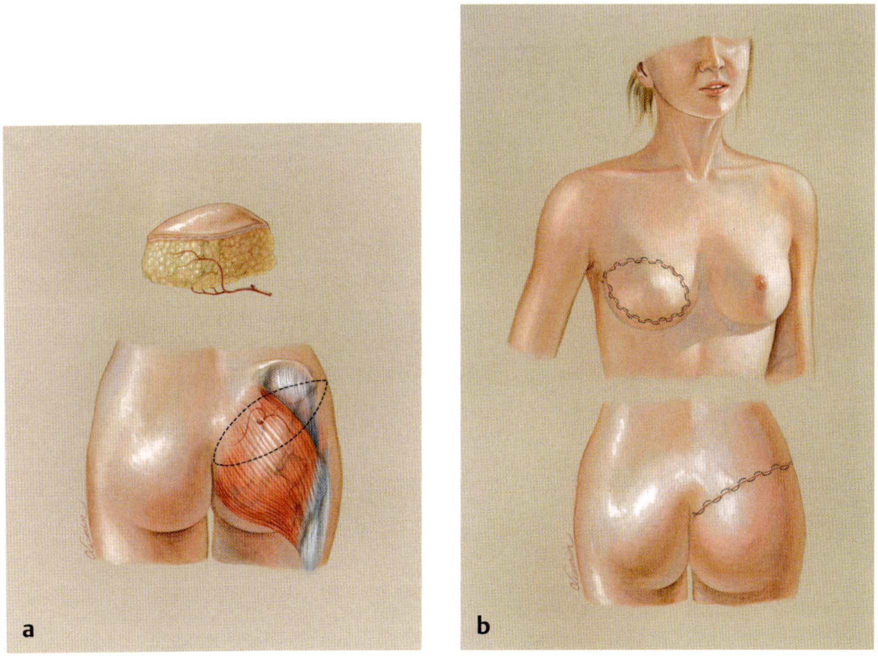

Fig. 1.13 The superior gluteal artery perforator (SGAP) flap for breast reconstruction. **(a)** SGAP preoperative markings. **(b)** Buttock donor-site scar and flap inset. (From Allen RJ, Tucker C. Superior gluteal artery perforator flap for breast reconstruction. Plast Reconstr Surg 1995;95(7): 1207–1212.)

the superficial inferior epigastric artery (SIEA) flaps, donor-site morbidity is minimal and no muscle is sacrificed.

The GAP flaps can be based on either the superior gluteal artery perforator (SGAP) or the inferior gluteal artery perforator (IGAP).[119] The skin paddle for the SGAP flap harvest has been proposed to mimic the tissue removed during a buttock lift **(Fig. 1.13).** Some proponents believe it elevates the buttock in a more natural shape, but it may leave a thick scar and dent in the buttock contour.[120] The IGAP has the advantage of a camouflaged scar hidden within the gluteal crease[120–123] **(Fig. 1.14).** However, both the SGAP and IGAP flaps can result in contour irregularities that are noticeable if too large a flap is harvested. In 2011, Tuinder and colleagues[124] performed a septocutaneous gluteal artery perforator (sc-GAP) for postmastectomy breast reconstruction in a small group of ideal patients, with good results. This flap is based on septocutaneous perforators between the gluteus maximus and medius muscles and has the advantage of avoiding intramuscular dissection and resulting in increased pedicle length. All

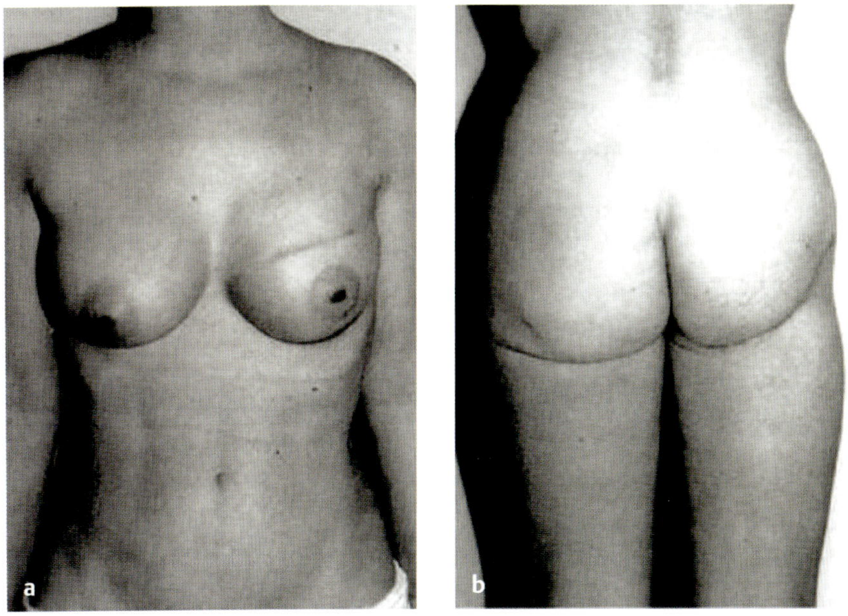

Fig. 1.14 The inferior gluteal artery perforator (IGAP) flap for breast reconstruction. **(a)** A 32-year-old woman with a mastectomy defect secondary to breast cancer reconstructed with a IGAP flap. **(b)** The donor-site defect. (From Paletta CE, Bostwick J III, Nahai F. The inferior gluteal free flap in breast reconstruction. Plast Reconstr Surg 1989;84:875–883).

flaps harvested from the gluteal region have the disadvantage of patient repositioning for breast reconstruction.

Lumbar Artery Perforator Flaps

In one of the original descriptions of perforator flaps, Kroll and Rosenfield[125] in 1988 described the lumbar artery perforator (LAP) flap based on unnamed perforators near the midline of the lower back **(Fig. 1.15)**. The LAP flap is a fasciocutaneous flap based on the lumbar artery perforators that supply a large cutaneous region extending from the posterior midline to the anterior rectus sheath and extending 10 cm above the anterior superior iliac spine (ASIS).[126] The LAP flap is usually positioned along the ASIS and offers an alternative to autologous breast reconstruction in patients who are not candidates for a DIEP flap[126,127] **(Fig. 1.16)**. This flap has the advantage of a well-hidden scar and a donor site where adequate fat for breast recon-

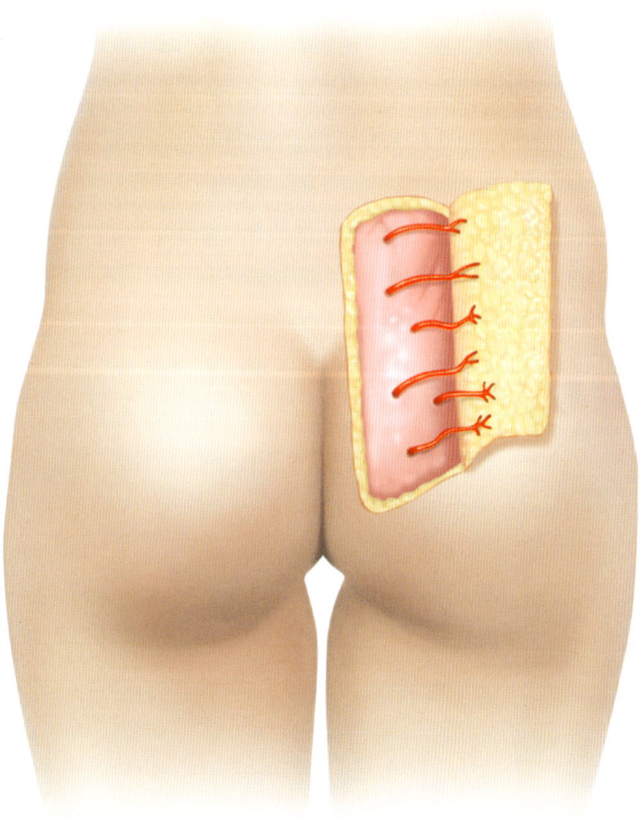

Fig. 1.15 Gluteal and lumbar perforators, described originally as "random parasacral perforators."

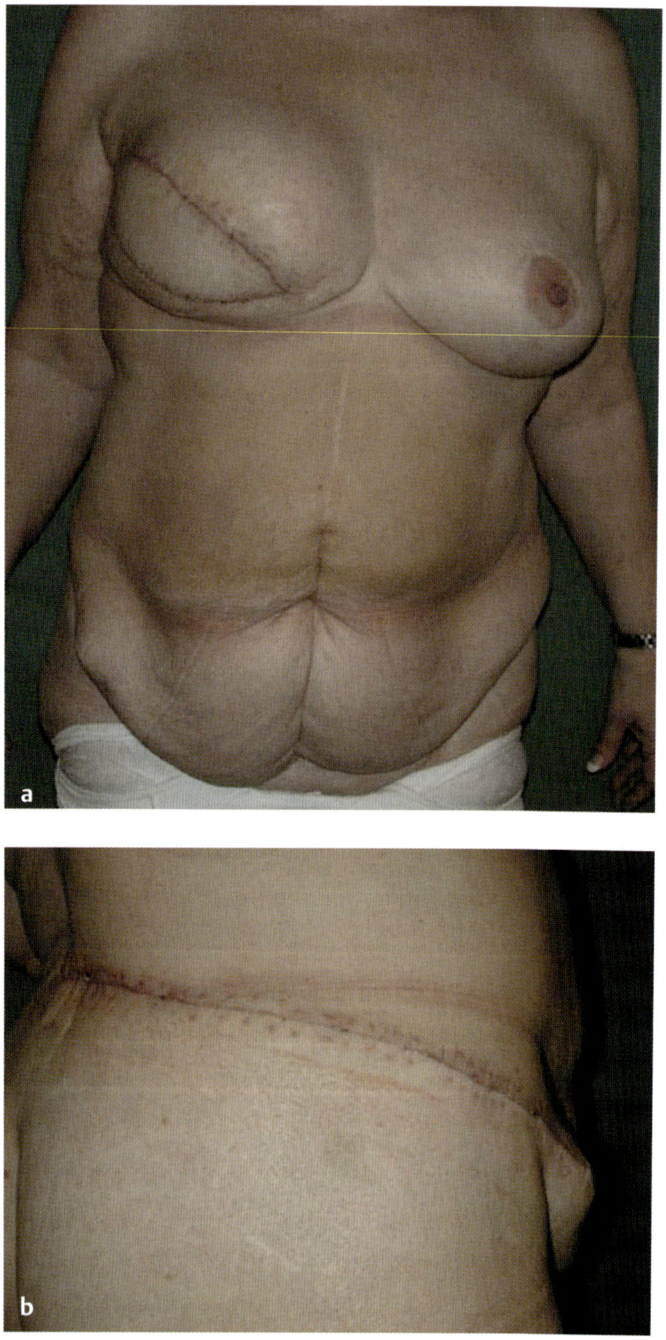

Fig. 1.16 The lumbar artery perforator (LAP) flap for breast reconstruction. **(a)** Delayed right breast reconstruction in a 51-year-old woman with a LAP flap at 3 weeks postoperatively. **(b)** Donor site at 3 weeks postoperatively. (From De Weerde L, Elvenes OP, Strandenes E, Weum S. Autologous breast reconstruction study and case reports. Br J Plast Surg 2003;56(2):180–183.)

struction is present. The disadvantage is a short vascular pedicle length that often requires vein grafts.[128]

Thigh Flaps

Hurwitz[129,130] described in 1980 the first posterior thigh flap when he used a musculocutaneous flap based on the inferior gluteal artery and documented the anatomy of the posterior thigh 1 year later. Hurteau et al[131] described a musculocutaneous flap based on branches of the profunda femoris artery for coverage of ischial decubitus ulcers. In 1983, Baek[132] first reported the lateral thigh flap based on the third perforator of the profunda femoral vessels.

Profunda Artery Perforator Flap

In 1984, Song and colleagues[133] first described the posterior thigh free flap. In 2001, Angrigiani and colleagues[134] described the adductor flap raised from the posterior and medial thigh skin based on a musculocutaneous perforator from the first medial branch of the profunda femoris artery. Cadaver studies performed in 2007 identified the source vessel as the profunda femoris artery[135] **(Fig. 1.17).** The first profunda artery perforator (PAP) flap for breast reconstruction was performed at the 13th International Course on Perforator Flaps in Mexico City in 2010 by Robert J. Allen.[136] In 2011, Allen and colleagues[137,138] presented their work using the PAP flap for autologous breast reconstruction **(Fig. 1.18).** This flap has the advantage of a donor site composed of dispensable significant fatty tissue and a well-hidden scar. It has a long pedicle, preserves muscle function, and is easily coned into a breast shape. As well, the flap can be harvested in the frog leg position so that the vessel preparation can be done concurrently.

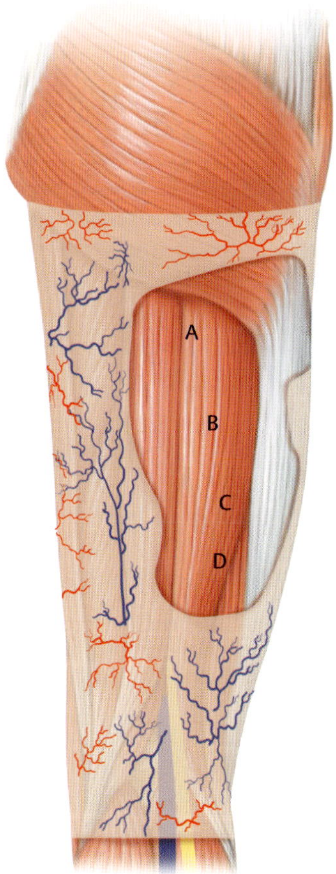

Fig. 1.17 The vascular anatomy of the profunda artery perforator (PAP) flap demonstrating both musculocutaneous (*A* and *B*) and septocutaneous (*C* and *D*) perforator arteries.

Evolving Fields In Breast Reconstruction

The goal of breast reconstruction remains the creation of an aesthetically pleasing breast that matches the size, shape, and feel of the previous or contralateral breast. Autologous fat injection has been used increasingly to correct and improve contour deformities of the reconstructed breast.[139] Recent technical advances of fat harvesting and handling methods have improved the survival of the injected autologous fat grafts. Roger Khouri[140] has obtained impressive results with his nonsurgical Brava megavolume autologous fat grafting technique for breast augmentation, with excellent long-term fat retention. At this time, however, autologous fat grafting alone generally remains unsuitable for the reconstruction of an entire breast due to the number of stages required but may be possible for the reconstruction of some partial breast defects.[141]

The field of tissue regeneration and stem cells research is popular across multiple disciplines. In 2011, Morrison's group[142] published their work with adipose tissue-engineering animal models and the generation of large-volume adipose tissue for breast reconstruction. The generation of a stem cell–derived adipose tissue for the creation of a new breast tissue could be the new frontier of breast reconstruction.

Upper extremity lymphedema is one of the most debilitating complications related to breast cancer treatment. Originally thought to have no cure, new microsurgical techniques are showing promise for the surgical treatment of lymphedema. In particular, the technique of supermicrosurgery (anastomosis of very small vessels ranging

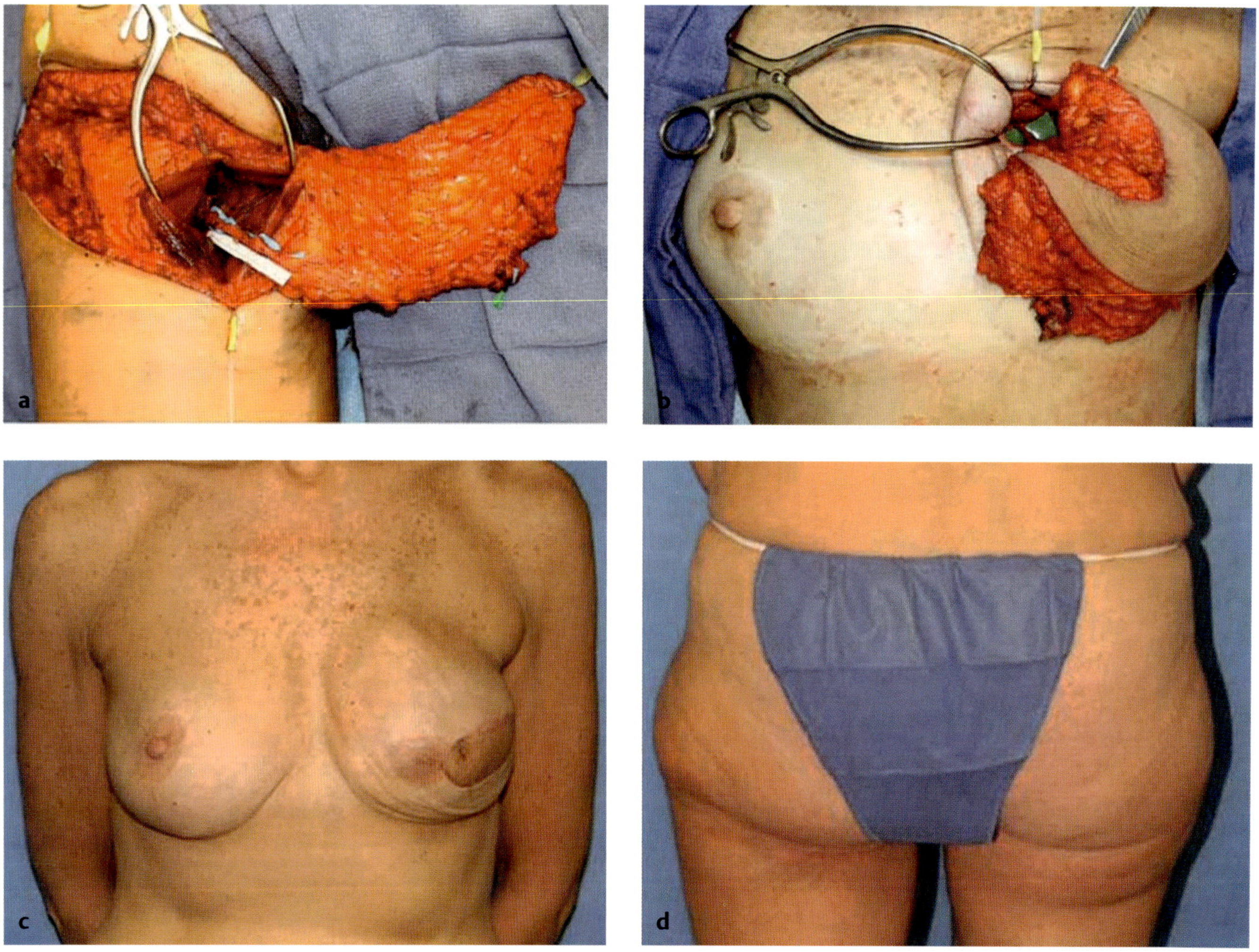

Fig. 1.18 The PAP flap for breast reconstruction. **(a)** The PAP flap harvested with the patient in the prone position. **(b)** The PAP flap inset provides ideal shape for creating a natural cone-shaped breast. **(c)** Four months after left breast reconstruction with the PAP flap. **(d)** Donor-site 4 months postoperatively concealed within the gluteal fold. (From Allen RJ, Haddock NT, Ahn CY, Sadeghi A. Breast reconstruction with the profunda artery perforator flap. Plast Reconstr Surg 2012;129:16e–23e.)

in size from 0.8 to 0.5 mm in diameter) has been employed for the lymphaticovenular micro anastomoses.[143] This technique has shown impressive 10-year results exceeding those of traditional lymphaticovenous anastomosis for the surgical treatment of lymphedema.[144] Several clinical studies have shown that the autologous microvascular transfer of groin lymph nodes to the axilla and wrist in postmastectomy patients with lymphedema can improve the lymphatic drainage in the affected limb.[145,146]

The concept of total breast anatomy restoration (TBAR) was introduced by Jaume Masia[147,148] and is characterized by autologous breast reconstructions in combination with an inguinal flap of lymphatic tissue from the superficial circumflex vascular pedicle. TBAR has been proposed to reconstruct both the breast mound and the lymphatic drainage to the upper limb that may have been damaged as a result of the original oncological resection or axillary node dissection.[149] These clinical studies, along with an improved understanding of lymphangiogenesis at the molecular level, are promising new advances in the field of lymphedema, which was originally thought to be incurable.

Conclusion

Microvascular perforator flap breast reconstruction is a sophisticated surgical procedure to restore breast aesthetics following lumpectomy or mastectomy for malignant or premalignant disease or to correct congenital abnormalities. The techniques highlighted in this chapter evolved over decades based on an increasing appreciation of the anatomic basis of the tissue transfers available and a greater drive to reduce donor-site morbidity. This evolution is ongoing, and the quest continues to be to optimize the reconstruction for each patient who requests breast reconstruction.

References

1. Wilkins EG, Cederna PS, Lowery JC, et al. Prospective analysis of psychosocial outcomes in breast reconstruction: one-year postoperative results from the Michigan Breast Reconstruction Outcome Study. Plast Reconstr Surg 2000;106:1014–1025, discussion 1026–1027
2. Al-Ghazal SK, Fallowfield L, Blamey RW, Blarney RW. Comparison of psychological aspects and patient satisfaction following breast conserving surgery, simple mastectomy and breast reconstruction. Eur J Cancer 2000;36:1938–1943
3. U.S. Department of Labor, Employee Benefits Security Administration. Your Rights After a Mastectomy: Women's Health and Cancer Rights Act of 1998. www.dol.gov/ebsa/Publications/whcra.html. Accessed on January 16, 2014
4. Hait P. History of the American Society of Plastic and Reconstructive Surgeons, Inc. 1931–1994. Plast Reconstr Surg 1994;94:1A–109A
5. Ballard TN, Momoh AO. Advances in breast reconstruction of mastectomy and lumpectomy defects. Surg Oncol Clin N Am 2014;23:525–548
6. Jagsi R, Jiang J, Momoh AO, et al. Trends and variation in use of breast reconstruction in patients with breast cancer undergoing mastectomy in the United States. J Clin Oncol 2014;32:919–926
7. Halsted WS. The results of operations for the cure of cancer of the breast performed at the Johns Hopkins Hospital from June, 1889 to January 1894. Ann Surg 1894;20:497–555
8. De Cholnoky T. Late adverse results following breast reconstructions. Plast Reconstr Surg 1963;31:445–452
9. Champaneria MC, Wong WW, Hill ME, Gupta SC. The evolution of breast reconstruction: a historical perspective. World J Surg 2012;36:730–742
10. Patey DH, Dyson WH. The prognosis of carcinoma of the breast in relation to the type of operation performed. Br J Cancer 1948;2:7–13
11. Toth BA, Forley BG, Calabria R. Retrospective study of the skin-sparing mastectomy in breast reconstruction. Plast Reconstr Surg 1999;104:77–84
12. Fisher B, Anderson S, Bryant J, et al. Twenty-year follow-up of a randomized trial comparing total mastectomy, lumpectomy, and lumpectomy plus irradiation for the treatment of invasive breast cancer. N Engl J Med 2002;347:1233–1241
13. Veronesi U, Cascinelli N, Mariani L, et al. Twenty-year follow-up of a randomized study comparing breast-conserving surgery with radical mastectomy for early breast cancer. N Engl J Med 2002;347:1227–1232
14. Carlson GW. Skin sparing mastectomy: anatomic and technical considerations. Am Surg 1996;62:151–155
15. Patani N, Mokbel K. Oncological and aesthetic considerations of skin-sparing mastectomy. Breast Cancer Res Treat 2008;111:391–403
16. Sushruta S. Sushruta Samhita. Calcutta: Bose; 1916
17. Bhishagratna KK. An English translation of Sushruta Samhita Base on the Original Sanskrit text, vols 1–3. Calcutta: Bose; 1916:107
18. Morris SF, Miller BJ, Taylor GI. Vascular anatomy of the integument. In: Blondeel PN, Hallock GG, Morris SF, Neligan PC, eds. Perforator Flaps: Anatomy Technique and Clinical Applications. St. Louis: QMP; 2006:12–36
19. Tagliacozzi D. De curtorum Chirurgia per Insitionem. Venetiis: G. Bindonus; 1597
20. Tolhurst DE, Hallock GG. History of flap surgery. In: Blondeel PN, Hallock GG, Morris SF, Neligan PC, eds. Perforator Flaps: Anatomy Technique and Clinical Applications. St. Louis: QMP; 2006:3–9
21. Verneuil AA. Memoires de Chirurgie. Paris: G. Masson; 1887
22. Czerny V. Plasticher ersatz der brustdrusse durch ein limpm. Zentralbl Chir 1895;27:72
23. Tansini I. Nuovo processo per l'amputazione della mammaella per cancre. Riforma Med 1896;12:3
24. Tansini I. Sopra il mio nuovo processo di amputazione della mammella. [Coverage of the anterior chest wall following mastectomy] Gazz Med Ital 1906;57:141
25. Maxwell GP. Iginio Tansini and the origin of the latissimus dorsi musculocutaneous flap. Plast Reconstr Surg 1980;65:686–692
26. Ombredanne L. Titres et Travaux Scientifiques. Paris: Masson; 1924
27. Gillies H. Surgical replacement of the breast. Proc R Soc Med 1959;52:597–602
28. Yannilos HG. The use of composite tube pedicle in the reconstruction of breast defect with subsequent cosmetic repair of the donor breast. Plast Reconstr Surg (1946) 1950;6:396–399
29. Holdsworth WG. A method of reconstructing the breast. Br J Plast Surg 1956;9:161–162
30. Esser JFS. Schwerer Verschluss einer Brustwand perforation. Berl Klin Wochenschr 1918;55:1197
31. Milton SH. The tubed pedicle flap. Br J Plast Surg 1969;22:53–59
32. McGregor IA, Jackson IT. The groin flap. Br J Plast Surg 1972;25:3–16
33. McGregor IA, Morgan G. Axial and random pattern flaps. Br J Plast Surg 1973;26:202–213
34. Shaw DT. Open abdominal flaps for repair off surface defects of the upper extremity. Surg Clin North Am 1944;24:293–308
35. Bakamjian VY. A two stage method of pharyngo-oesophageal reconstruction with a primary pectoral skin flap. Plast Reconstr Surg 1965;36:173–184
36. Morax V. L'autoplastic palpebrale ou faciale l'aide de lambeau pedicules emprunte a la region cervicale (procede de Snydacker) et de l-autoplastie en deux temps avec utilization pedicule. Annales Oculist 1908;89:14
37. McCraw JB, Dibbell DG. Experimental definition of independent myocutaneous vascular territories. Plast Reconstr Surg 1977;60:212–220

38. Mathes SJ, Nahai F. Classification of the vascular anatomy of muscles: experimental and clinical correlation. Plast Reconstr Surg 1981;67:177–187
39. Mathes SJ, Nahai F. Clinical Applications for Muscle Musculocutaneous Flaps. St Louis: Mosby; 1982
40. Holmström H. The free abdominoplasty flap and its use in breast reconstruction. An experimental study and clinical case report. Scand J Plast Reconstr Surg 1979;13:423–427
41. Pontén B. The fasciocutaneous flap: its use in soft tissue defects of the lower leg. Br J Plast Surg 1981;34:215–220
42. Haertsch PA. The blood supply to the skin of the leg: a post-mortem investigation. Br J Plast Surg 1981;34:470–477
43. Barclay TL, Cardoso E, Sharpe DT, Crockett DJ. Repair of lower leg injuries with fascio-cutaneous flaps. Br J Plast Surg 1982;35:127–132
44. Cormack GC, Lamberty BGH. A classification of fascio-cutaneous flaps according to their patterns of vascularisation. Br J Plast Surg 1984;37:80–87
45. Hoerenz P. The operating microscope. IV. Documentation. J Microsurg 1980;2:126–139
46. Tamai S. History of microsurgery—from the beginning until the end of the 1970s. Microsurgery 1993;14:6–13
47. Buncke HJ. Microsurgery—retrospective. Clin Plast Surg 1986;13:315–318
48. Jacobson JH, Suarez EL. Microsurgery in anatomosis of small vessels. Surg Forum 1960;11:243–245
49. Buncke HJ Jr, Schulz WP. Total ear reimplantation in the rabbit utilising microminiature vascular anastomoses. Br J Plast Surg 1966;19:15–22
50. McLean DH, Buncke HJ Jr. Autotransplant of omentum to a large scalp defect, with microsurgical revascularization. Plast Reconstr Surg 1972;49:268–274
51. Daniel RK, Williams HB. The free transfer of skin flaps by microvascular anastomoses. An experimental study and a reappraisal. Plast Reconstr Surg 1973;52:16–31
52. Daniel RK, Taylor GI. Distant transfer of an island flap by microvascular anastomoses. A clinical technique. Plast Reconstr Surg 1973;52:111–117
53. Taylor GI, Daniel RK. The free flap: composite tissue transfer by vascular anastomosis. Aust N Z J Surg 1973;43:1–3
54. Fujino T, Harasina T, Aoyagi F. Reconstruction for aplasia of the breast and pectoral region by microvascular transfer of a free flap from the buttock. Plast Reconstr Surg 1975;56:178–181
55. Fujino T, Harashina T, Enomoto K. Primary breast reconstruction after a standard radical mastectomy by a free flap transfer. Case report. Plast Reconstr Surg 1976;58:371–374
56. Holmström H. The free abdominoplasty flap and its use in breast reconstruction. An experimental study and clinical case report. Scand J Plast Reconstr Surg 1979;13:423–427
57. Hartrampf CR Jr, Noel RT, Drazan L, Elliott FL, Bennett GK, Beegle PH. Ruben's fat pad for breast reconstruction: a peri-iliac soft-tissue free flap. Plast Reconstr Surg 1994;93:402–407
58. Taylor GI, Townsend P, Corlett R. Superiority of the deep circumflex iliac vessels as the supply for free groin flaps. Clinical work. Plast Reconstr Surg 1979;64:745–759
59. Elliott LF, Beegle PH, Hartrampf CR Jr. The lateral transverse thigh free flap: an alternative for autogenous-tissue breast reconstruction. Plast Reconstr Surg 1990;85:169–178, discussion 179–181
60. Wei FC, Suominen S, Cheng MH, Celik N, Lai YL. Anterolateral thigh flap for postmastectomy breast reconstruction. Plast Reconstr Surg 2002;110:82–88
61. Fujino T, Abe O, Enomoto K. Primary reconstruction of the breast by free myocutaneous gluteal flap. Int Adv Surg Oncol 1981;4:127–143
62. Paletta CE, Bostwick J III, Nahai F. The inferior gluteal free flap in breast reconstruction. Plast Reconstr Surg 1989;84:875–883, discussion 884–885
63. Allen RJ, Tucker C Jr. Superior gluteal artery perforator free flap for breast reconstruction. Plast Reconstr Surg 1995;95:1207–1212
64. Peek A, Müller M, Exner K. [The free gracilis perforator flap for autologous breast reconstruction]. Handchir Mikrochir Plast Chir 2002;34:245–250
65. Hartrampf CR Jr, Elliott LF, Feldman S. A triceps musculocutaneous flap for chest-wall defects. Plast Reconstr Surg 1990;86:502–509
66. Taylor GI, Palmer JH. The vascular territories (angiosomes) of the body: experimental study and clinical applications. Br J Plast Surg 1987;40:113–141
67. Taylor GI, Palmer JH, McManamay D. The vascular territories of the body (angiosomes) and their clinical applications. In: McCarthy J, ed. Plastic Surgery. Philadelphia: WB Saunders; 1990
68. Taylor GI. The angiosomes of the body and their supply to perforator flaps. Clin Plast Surg 2003;30:331–342, v
69. Manchot C. The Cutaneous Arteries of the Human Body. New York: Springer-Verlag; 1982
70. Salmon M, Taylor GI, Tempest MN, eds. Arteries of the Skin. London: Churchill Livingstone; 1988
71. Taylor GI, Doyle M, McCarten G. The Doppler probe for planning flaps: anatomical study and clinical applications. Br J Plast Surg 1990;43:1–16
72. Blondeel PN, Beyens G, Verhaeghe R, et al. Doppler flowmetry in the planning of perforator flaps. Br J Plast Surg 1998;51: 202–209
73. Hallock GG. Doppler sonography and color duplex imaging for planning a perforator flap. Clin Plast Surg 2003;30:347–357, v–vi
74. Masia J, Kosutic D, Clavero JA, Larranaga J, Vives L, Pons G. Preoperative computed tomographic angiogram for deep inferior epigastric artery perforator flap breast reconstruction. J Reconstr Microsurg 2010;26:21–28
75. Masia J, Clavero JA, Larrañaga JR, Alomar X, Pons G, Serret P. Multidetector-row computed tomography in the planning of abdominal perforator flaps. J Plast Reconstr Aesthet Surg 2006;59:594–599
76. Mathes DW, Neligan PC. Current techniques in preoperative imaging for abdomen-based perforator flap microsurgical breast reconstruction. J Reconstr Microsurg 2010;26:3–10
77. Rosson GD, Williams CG, Fishman EK, Singh NK. 3D CT angiography of abdominal wall vascular perforators to plan DIEAP flaps. Microsurgery 2007;27:641–646

78. Newman TM, Vasile J, Levine JL, et al. Perforator flap magnetic resonance angiography for reconstructive breast surgery: a review of 25 deep inferior epigastric and gluteal perforator artery flap patients. J Magn Reson Imaging 2010;31:1176–1184
79. Masia J, Navarro C, Clavero JA, Alomar X. Noncontrast magnetic resonance imaging for preoperative perforator mapping. Clin Plast Surg 2011;38:253–261
80. Jakobs TF, Wintersperger BJ, Becker CR. MDCT-imaging of peripheral arterial disease. Semin Ultrasound CT MR 2004;25:145–155
81. Pestana IA, Coan B, Erdmann D, Marcus J, Levin LS, Zenn MR. Early experience with fluorescent angiography in free-tissue transfer reconstruction. Plast Reconstr Surg 2009;123:1239–1244
82. Munabi NC, Olorunnipa OB, Goltsman D, Rohde CH, Ascherman JA. The ability of intra-operative perfusion mapping with laser-assisted indocyanine green angiography to predict mastectomy flap necrosis in breast reconstruction: a prospective trial. J Plast Reconstr Aesthet Surg 2014;67:449–455
83. Gillies HD, Millard DR Jr. The Principles and Art of Plastic Surgery. Boston: Brown & Company; 1957
84. Mathes SJ, Bostwick J III. A rectus abdominis myocutaneous flap to reconstruct abdominal wall defects. Br J Plast Surg 1977; 30:282–283
85. Robbins TH. Rectus abdominis myocutaneous flap for breast reconstruction. Aust N Z J Surg 1979;49:527–530
86. Robbins TH. Post-mastectomy breast reconstruction using a rectus abdominis musculocutaneous island flap. Br J Plast Surg 1981;34:286–290
87. Drever JM. The epigastric island flap. Plast Reconstr Surg 1977;59:343–346
88. Hartrampf CR, Scheflan M, Black PW. Breast reconstruction with a transverse abdominal island flap. Plast Reconstr Surg 1982;69:216–225
89. Bucky LP, May JW Jr. Synthetic mesh. Its use in abdominal wall reconstruction after the TRAM. Clin Plast Surg 1994;21:273–277
90. Grotting JC, Urist MM, Maddox WA, Vasconez LO. Conventional TRAM flap versus free microsurgical TRAM flap for immediate breast reconstruction. Plast Reconstr Surg 1989;83:828–841, discussion 842–844
91. Grotting JC. The free abdominoplasty flap for immediate breast reconstruction. Ann Plast Surg 1991;27:351–354
92. Taylor GI, Corlett R, Boyd JB. The extended deep inferior epigastric flap: a clinical technique. Plast Reconstr Surg 1983;72:751–765
93. Onishi K, Maruyama Y. Cutaneous and fascial vasculature around the rectus abdominis muscle: anatomic basis of abdominal fasciocutaneous flaps. J Reconstr Microsurg 1986;2:247–253
94. Koshima I, Soeda S. Inferior epigastric artery skin flaps without rectus abdominis muscle. Br J Plast Surg 1989;42:645–648
95. Allen RJ, Treece P. Deep inferior epigastric perforator flap for breast reconstruction. Ann Plast Surg 1994;32:32–38
96. Blondeel PN, Boeckx WD. Refinements in free flap breast reconstruction: the free bilateral deep inferior epigastric perforator flap anastomosed to the internal mammary artery. Br J Plast Surg 1994;47:495–501
97. Blondeel N, Vanderstraeten GG, Monstrey SJ, et al. The donor site morbidity of free DIEP flaps and free TRAM flaps for breast reconstruction. Br J Plast Surg 1997;50:322–330
98. Blondeel PN. One hundred free DIEP flap breast reconstructions: a personal experience. Br J Plast Surg 1999;52:104–111
99. Blondeel PN, Arnstein M, Verstraete K, et al. Venous congestion and blood flow in free transverse rectus abdominis myocutaneous and deep inferior epigastric perforator flaps. Plast Reconstr Surg 2000;106:1295–1299
100. Arnez ZM, Khan U, Pogorelec D, Planinsek F. Breast reconstruction using the free superficial inferior epigastric artery (SIEA) flap. Br J Plast Surg 1999;52:276–279
101. Taylor GI, Daniel RK. The anatomy of several free flap donor sites. Plast Reconstr Surg 1975;56:243–253
102. Chevray PM. Breast reconstruction with superficial inferior epigastric artery flaps: a prospective comparison with TRAM and DIEP flaps. Plast Reconstr Surg 2004;114:1077–1083, discussion 1084–1085
103. Elliott LF, Hartrampf CR Jr. The Rubens flap. The deep circumflex iliac artery flap. Clin Plast Surg 1998;25:283–291
104. Bergeron L, Tang M, Morris SF. The anatomical basis of the deep circumflex iliac artery perforator flap with iliac crest. Plast Reconstr Surg 2007;120:252–258
105. D'Este S. La technique de l'amputation de al mamelle pour carcinoma mammary. Rev Chir (Paris) 1912;45:164–210
106. Hutchins EH. A method for the prevention of elephantiasis. Surg Gynecol Obstet 1939;69:795
107. Olivari N. The latissimus flap. Br J Plast Surg 1976;29:126–128
108. Hokin JA, Silfverskiold KL. Breast reconstruction without an implant: results and complications using an extended latissimus dorsi flap. Plast Reconstr Surg 1987;79:58–66
109. Holmström H, Lossing C. The lateral thoracodorsal flap in breast reconstruction. Plast Reconstr Surg 1985;77:933–941
110. Munhoz AM, Montag E, Arruda EG, et al. The role of the lateral thoracodorsal fasciocutaneous flap in immediate conservative breast surgery reconstruction. Plast Reconstr Surg 2006;117: 1699–1710
111. Yang JD, Ryu DW, Lee JW, et al. Usefulness of a lateral thoracodorsal flap after breast conserving surgery in laterally located breast cancer. Arch Plast Surg 2013;40:367–373
112. Angrigiani C, Grilli D, Siebert J. Latissimus dorsi musculocutaneous flap without muscle. Plast Reconstr Surg 1995;96:1608–1614
113. Thomas BP, Geddes CR, Tang M, Williams J, Morris SF. The vascular basis of the thoracodorsal artery perforator flap. Plast Reconstr Surg 2005;116:818–822
114. Hamdi M, Van Landuyt K, Monstrey S, Blondeel P. Pedicled perforator flaps in breast reconstruction: a new concept. Br J Plast Surg 2004;57:531–539
115. Hamdi M, Spano A, Van Landuyt K, D'Herde K, Blondeel P, Monstrey S. The lateral intercostal artery perforators: anatomical study and clinical application in breast surgery. Plast Reconstr Surg 2008;121:389–396

116. Hamdi M. Anterior thorax: lateral intercostals artery perforator (LICAP) flap. In: Zenn MR, Jones G, eds. Reconstructive Surgery: Anatomy, Technique, and Clinical Application. St. Louis: QMP; 2012:474–491
117. Hamdi M, Van Landuyt K, de Frene B, Roche N, Blondeel P, Monstrey S. The versatility of the inter-costal artery perforator (ICAP) flaps. J Plast Reconstr Aesthet Surg 2006;59:644–652
118. Orticochea M. Use of the buttock to reconstruct the breast. Br J Plast Surg 1973;26:304–309
119. Ahmadzadeh R, Bergeron L, Tang M, Morris SF. The superior and inferior gluteal artery perforator flaps. Plast Reconstr Surg 2007;120:1551–1556
120. Zenn MR. Gluteus maximus and IGAP/SCAP flaps. In: Zenn MR, Jones G, eds. Reconstructive Surgery: Anatomy, Technique, and Clinical Application. St. Louis: QMP; 2012:584–619
121. Allen RJ, Levine JL, Granzow JW. The in-the-crease inferior gluteal artery perforator flap for breast reconstruction. Plast Reconstr Surg 2006;118:333–339
122. Babineaux K, Granzow JG, Bardin E, et al. Gluteal artery perforator flap for breast reconstruction: The preferred buttock scar and shape. Plast Reconstr Surg 2005;116(3, Suppl):174–176
123. Guerra AB, Metzinger SE, Bidros RS, Gill PS, Dupin CL, Allen RJ. Breast reconstruction with gluteal artery perforator (GAP) flaps: a critical analysis of 142 cases. Ann Plast Surg 2004;52:118–125
124. Tuinder S, Chen CM, Massey MF, Allen RJ Sr, Van der Huist R. Introducing the septocutaneous gluteal artery perforator flap: a simplified approach to microsurgical breast reconstruction. Plast Reconstr Surg 2011;127:489–495
125. Kroll SS, Rosenfield L. Perforator-based flaps for low posterior midline defects. Plast Reconstr Surg 1988;81:561–566
126. Kato H, Hasegawa M, Takada T, Torii S. The lumbar artery perforator based island flap: anatomical study and case reports. Br J Plast Surg 1999;52:541–546
127. de Weerd L, Elvenes OP, Strandenes E, Weum S. Autologous breast reconstruction with a free lumbar artery perforator flap. Br J Plast Surg 2003;56:180–183
128. Ao M, Mae O, Namba Y, Asagoe K. Perforator-based flap for coverage of lumbosacral defects. Plast Reconstr Surg 1998;101:987–991
129. Hurwitz DJ. Closure of a large defect of the pelvic cavity by an extended compound myocutaneous flap based on the inferior gluteal artery. Br J Plast Surg 1980;33:256–261
130. Hurwitz DJ, Swartz WM, Mathes SJ. The gluteal thigh flap: a reliable, sensate flap for the closure of buttock and perineal wounds. Plast Reconstr Surg 1981;68:521–532
131. Hurteau JE, Bostwick J, Nahai F, Hester R, Jurkiewicz MJ. V-Y advancement of hamstring musculocutaneous flap for coverage of ischial pressure sores. Plast Reconstr Surg 1981;68:539–542
132. Baek SM. Two new cutaneous free flaps: the medial and lateral thigh flaps. Plast Reconstr Surg 1983;71:354–365
133. Song YG, Chen GZ, Song YL. The free thigh flap: a new free flap concept based on the septocutaneous artery. Br J Plast Surg 1984;37:149–159
134. Angrigiani C, Grilli D, Thorne CH. The adductor flap: a new method for transferring posterior and medial thigh skin. Plast Reconstr Surg 2001;107:1725–1731
135. Ahmadzadeh R, Bergeron L, Tang M, Geddes CR, Morris SF. The posterior thigh perforator flap or profunda femoris artery perforator flap. Plast Reconstr Surg 2007;119:194–200, discussion 201–202
136. Chen MC, LoTempio M, Allen RJ. Profunda artery perforator (PAP) flap for breast reconstruction. In: Spiegel AJ, ed. Breast reconstruction: Current Perspectives and State of the Art Techniques. InTech; 2013
137. Allen RJ, Haddock NT, Ahn CY, Sadeghi A. Breast reconstruction with the profunda artery perforator flap. Plast Reconstr Surg 2011;129:16e–23e
138. Chen CM, Lotempio MT, Allen RJ. Our first 101 profunda artery perforator (PAP) flaps for breast reconstruction. Poster presentation at the American Association of Plastic Surgeons 92nd annual meeting, New Orleans, April 20–23, 2013
139. Weichman KE, Broer PN, Tanna N, et al. The role of autologous fat grafting in secondary microsurgical breast reconstruction. Ann Plast Surg 2013;71:24–30
140. Khouri RK, Rigotti G, Cardoso E, Khouri RK Jr, Biggs TM. Megavolume autologous fat transfer: part I. Theory and principles. Plast Reconstr Surg 2014;133:550–557
141. Uda H, Sugawara Y, Sarukawa S, Sunaga A. Brava and autologous fat grafting for breast reconstruction after cancer surgery. Plast Reconstr Surg 2014;133:203–213
142. Findlay MW, Dolderer JH, Trost N, et al. Tissue-engineered breast reconstruction: bridging the gap toward large-volume tissue engineering in humans. Plast Reconstr Surg 2011;128:1206–1215
143. Koshima I, Inagawa K, Urushibara K, Moriguchi T. Supermicrosurgical lymphaticovenular anastomosis for the treatment of lymphedema in the upper extremities. J Reconstr Microsurg 2000;16:437–442
144. Koshima I, Nanba Y, Tsutsui T, Takahashi Y, Itoh S. Long-term follow-up after lymphaticovenular anastomosis for lymphedema in the leg. J Reconstr Microsurg 2003;19:209–215
145. Becker C, Assouad J, Riquet M, Hidden G. Postmastectomy lymphedema: long-term results following microsurgical lymph node transplantation. Ann Surg 2006;243:313–315
146. Lin CH, Ali R, Chen SC, et al. Vascularized groin lymph node transfer using the wrist as a recipient site for management of postmastectomy upper extremity lymphedema. Plast Reconstr Surg 2009;123:1265–1275
147. Masia J. TBAR: Total Breast Anatomy Restoration. Second European Conference on Supermicrosurgery, Barcelona, March 1–2, 2012
148. Masia J. TBAR: Total Breast Anatomy Restoration. Barcelona Breast meeting, Barcelona, March 13–15, 2013
149. Saaristo AM, Niemi TS, Viitanen TP, Tervala TV, Hartiala P, Suominen EA. Microvascular breast reconstruction and lymph node transfer for postmastectomy lymphedema patients. Ann Surg 2012;255:468–473

2 Starting a Perforator Flap Breast Program

Christina R. Vargas and Bernard T. Lee

Microsurgical options for breast reconstruction have gained popularity over the past 15 years as a result of better patient access to postmastectomy reconstruction, less abdominal morbidity, excellent long-term aesthetic results, and thus high patient satisfaction.[1–3] According to the American Society of Plastic Surgeons, deep inferior epigastric perforator (DIEP) flaps were the most commonly performed autologous reconstructive breast procedure in 2012, with over 6,500 cases in that year alone.[4] However, recent surveys of plastic and reconstructive surgeons indicate that fewer than one in five currently perform microsurgery as part of their breast reconstructive practice.

Several studies have suggested that disparities in decision making about reconstruction are heavily influenced by the availability of procedures, provider bias, and hospital factors rather than aesthetic, functional, or anatomic aspects of surgery.[5,6] Microsurgical reconstructive procedures are inherently more complicated than implant-based or pedicled methods, and they require more specialized training, extended operative time, and longer patient hospitalization. Thus, many breast cancer treatment centers have not yet developed perforator flap programs, and large geographic regions of the United States lack even low-volume institutions.[7] Not surprisingly, providers who do perform perforator breast flap reconstruction were more likely to be affiliated with a multidisciplinary cancer center, involved with resident training, and part of a larger group practice.[8]

The American College of Surgeons established the National Accreditation Program for Breast Centers, which has provided guidelines for comprehensive breast cancer care that emphasize access to plastic surgeons and perforator flap reconstruction.[9] Patients who are diagnosed and undergo oncological treatment at nonmicrosurgical centers are forced to travel to referral centers if they wish to seek perforator reconstruction, resulting in fragmentation of their overall cancer care.[10,11]

The development of a dedicated perforator flap program meets the demands of routinely performing these complicated procedures. Gaining microsurgical experience by performing a large number of procedures is important, because plastic surgeons who perform more microsurgical reconstructions have been shown to encounter fewer obstacles related to the logistic and financial aspects of the procedures as compared with surgeons who performed few or no perforator reconstructions.[8] Patient outcomes after reconstruction are known to correlate with institutional autologous and microsurgical operative volume.[7] Improvement in outcome measures after the implementation of designated subspecialty programs has also been reported in other surgical and oncological fields.[12,13] Establishment of a specialized program for perforator reconstruction can contribute significantly to existing breast cancer care centers and bring new referrals from other local and regional institutions.[10] Finally, creating comprehensive breast care programs in underrepresented areas increases patient access to these highly sought-after and highly successful reconstructive options. Key phases in the design and implementation of a perforator flap program include a preliminary assessment, faculty recruitment, program development, and expansion and growth **(Table 2.1)**.

Preprogram Assessment

Creation of a perforator flap program is a multifaceted process, and it requires both departmental and institutional commitment. Evaluation of current breast cancer care and postmastectomy reconstruction services is important in making the decision to proceed with subspecialty program development. Active communication among leaders in the departments of surgery, plastic and reconstructive surgery, breast surgery, and hospital administration is vital for program success. Assessment of current local and regional referral patterns for breast reconstruction should be performed to identify opportunities to offer advanced breast cancer care options and to increase reconstructive volume. Requirements for recognition by the National Accreditation Program for Breast Centers (NAPBC) should be reviewed, and any areas for improvement noted.[9] Current infrastructure should be evaluated for its ability to provide excellent, well-coordinated cancer care. Input should be sought from institutional specialists in breast

Table 2.1 Key Components of Perforator Flap Program Design and Development

Preprogram assessment	• Evaluation of current systems • Institutional support • Breast care infrastructure • Microsurgery infrastructure
Recruitment	• Surgeon recruitment • Adoption of team-based approach • Multidisciplinary collaboration
Program development	• Standardization of perforator flap management • Intraoperative standardization • Learning curve • Staff education • Negotiation of financial reimbursement
Expansion and growth	• Community and referring provider outreach • Addition of staff • Fellowship training program • Outcomes assessment • Quality improvement

surgery, medical oncology, radiation oncology, pathology, and breast radiology. It is also vitally important that physicians in these other disciplines understand the value of implementing a microsurgical breast surgeon.

As successful microsurgery requires a well-trained multidisciplinary team and education of operating room (OR) staff, anesthesia teams, residents, and recovery room and floor nurses. Clinic staff should be provided and routinely reinforced. Access to appropriate facilities and equipment must be secured, including OR block time, staffed recovery rooms with flap monitoring capabilities, microsurgical instruments, and operating microscopes. Surgeons must confirm that they will be able to allocate sufficient time to performing these long operative cases and to integrate microsurgery effectively into their clinical practice schedules.

Recruitment

Gathering a team of skilled microsurgeons is integral to perforator program success. In anticipation of a team-based approach to complex microsurgery, recruitment of surgeons interested in collaboration is important. Inclusion of multiple surgeons in the program results in shorter operating time with potential for breaks during long perforator flap cases, and provides for rotating, expert post-operative coverage should complications arise. Input from other members of the multidisciplinary breast care team, such as breast surgeons and oncologists, may also be helpful during the recruitment process.

Program Development

Standardization of Perforator Flap Management

Standardization of reconstructive microsurgical care results in efficient use of staffing and resources, provides opportunities for quality improvement, increases patient safety, and decreases costs of care.[10] Early in program development, consider designing or adapting perioperative clinical pathways and postoperative order sets for perforator reconstruction. Anticipating the clinical course of microsurgical patients can facilitate identification of specific areas for collaboration with other specialty units and services. The most appropriate level of care for postoperative monitoring and initial recovery may vary by institution, and could include either a prolonged recovery room or a brief intensive care unit stay. Incorporation of anesthesia or pain medicine consultation may be valuable, depending on the surgeon's preferred method of postoperative analgesia. On a larger scale, collaboration with breast oncology services within the institution enables streamlining the referral process and eliminates unnecessary delays in obtaining reconstructive consultation. Coordination of preanesthesia evaluation may also be considered.

Microsurgery staff may wish to standardize the approach to flap monitoring, as there is considerable variability in these techniques within the field. Other adjunctive measures, such as the use of surgical drains, anticoagulation or antiplatelet therapy, projected postoperative progression, management of complications, and expected time to discharge should be discussed with nursing administration. Coordination of standard instructions and follow-up procedures can help to eliminate confusion on the part of patients, nurses, house staff, and midlevel providers at the time of discharge.

A standard, well-organized approach to the reconstruction process can help patients and staff to anticipate the next steps in care. Surgeons may wish to develop their own methods for preoperative patient education, which can be tailored to each institution's needs. Consistent support staff education and training also translates directly to better pre- and postoperative clinical management and flap monitoring, and reduces costs.[14] A recent investigation of the use of simulation for nurse training in microsurgery patient care found high levels of staff satisfaction and good retention of knowledge and skills.[15] Reinforcement of key components of the pathway with OR staff, recovery room staff, and hospital floor nurses should be conducted at least every few months. Facilitation of ongoing feedback from these team members can help to identify areas for improvement in the perioperative process.

Intraoperative Strategies for Standardization

Creation of a standard intraoperative protocol permits plastic surgery and anesthesia team members, OR nurses, and support staff to work in synchrony, anticipate potential issues, and communicate more effectively during procedures.[16] It also decreases operative time and increases surgeon and OR staff satisfaction.[16] Several strategies for managing stress and fatigue in the OR during lengthy free tissue transfer procedures have been proposed. Training all team members in their role in the procedure more clearly delineates performance expectations, increases communication, and decreases stress.

Identifying and training a core team specifically for microsurgical breast reconstruction facilitates a task-specific focus and overall awareness of the responsibility of each team member. It also facilitates prompt orientation for rotating members, such as anesthesia providers who join the team on the day of surgery. A proactive discussion with anesthesia team leadership regarding specific aspects of the perforator flap protocol is advised to address patient and OR table positioning, the avoidance of vasoactive drugs, maintenance of normothermia, adequate systolic blood pressure, and any anticipated intraoperative issues.

Standardizing the equipment and supplies needed perioperatively allows the staff to prepare them in advance and can help to avoid costly last-minute delays. Carefully planned coordination of the OR team can help to eliminate ambiguity, support shared responsibility, and improve efficiency.[17] OR team training initiatives have been shown to effectively decrease surgical morbidity and mortality.[18,19] Encouraging discussion of variance from the planned protocol yields ongoing improvement and problem solving among all involved groups.[20]

A framework for creation of an intraoperative pathway includes standardized surgical techniques and equipment, distinct phases of the procedure, set time points that mark transitions during the case, structured opportunities to resolve anticipated issues, consideration of staff breaks and hand-offs for each discipline, and attention to medication and antibiotic dosing when necessary **(Fig. 2.1)**.[16] For each phase, detailed descriptions of the necessary personnel and their competencies, and the required instruments, supplies, and activities should be provided. The activities defining the start and end of each phase, as well as their expected duration, should be clearly noted. Real-time documentation of completion or variance from each step in the pathway is encouraged, and signatures from key staff should be required for team accountability.

	PREOPERATIVE HOLDING	INDUCTION	MASTECTOMY	PERFORATOR DISSECTION	RECIPIENT VESSEL HARVEST	DIVISION OF VESSELS/FLAP TRANSFER	MICROSURGERY	FLAP INSET + CLOSURE	END OF CASE
			SIMULTANEOUS PROCEDURE PHASES			SIMULTANEOUS PROCEDURE PHASES			
Phase	I	II	III	IV	V	VI	VII	VIII	IX
Surgeon ☐ Breast Surgeon ☐ Surgeon 2 ■ Surgeons 1 + 2	Patient identification Marking	Patient positioning	Surgical timeout Mastectomy Sentinal lymph node biopsy Dissect abdominal flap	Perforator dissection Division of all side branches	Prepare chest Isolate internal mammary vessels	Division of vessels and flap harvest Flap transfer	Microsurgical anastomosis of artery and vein Simultaneous abdominal closure	Flap inset Breast closure	Transfer patient in flexed position Doppler evaluation after transfer Resolution of variance
OR staff	Patient identification DVT prophylaxis Initial counts	Assist with positioning Place lower extremity stockings	Surgical timeout Page surgeon prior to end of mastectomy Document specimen Confirm counts	Open additional sutures Obtain additional RN for counts Drape microscope	Second scrub team	No hand-off period Record specimen weights Confirm counts Prepare heparin	No hand-off period Confirm counts	Give report Obtain additional RN for counts	Transfer patient to recovery Complete documentation Resolution of variance

Fig. 2.1 Intraoperative pathway design. DVT, deep venous thrombosis; OR, operating room; RN, registered nurse.

Perforator Flap Learning Curve

Several studies have described both the incidence of perforator flap complications and the typical microsurgery learning curve that leads to increased efficiency and fewer complications.[21–27] Detailed discussion of these studies is beyond the scope of this chapter, but acquisition of superior technical skill and excellent perioperative management certainly contributes to optimal patient outcomes. Gaining experience with patient selection, flap design, and intraoperative decision making are critical to long-term success for both reconstructive surgeons and perforator flap programs.

Financial Reimbursement

High-complexity microsurgical techniques are associated with higher short-term health care costs.[28] Financial viability is critical for a successful perforator flap program. Several studies have demonstrated the cost-effectiveness of microsurgical reconstruction relative to other autologous techniques.[29–31] As current reimbursement standards for microsurgical breast reconstruction are not well defined, negotiation with insurance providers may be necessary to ensure that fee schedules accurately reflect physician time, hospital resources, and case complexity. It has been found that high-volume institutions experience fewer surgical complications, resulting in reduced costs for managing complications associated with autologous reconstruction and reduced costs for the entire procedure.[28] Providing complex reconstructive options for patients who would otherwise seek specialist care outside of their provider network presents a strategy that is mutually beneficial to patients, surgeons, hospitals, and insurance carriers. Negotiation of fair reimbursement in light of these changes is advised when possible.

Expansion and Growth

Community and Referring Provider Outreach

Following the establishment of a perforator flap program for breast reconstruction, prospective patients and referring providers can be sought using a variety of strategies. Local and regional academic presentations and hospital grand rounds can raise awareness of the new program, as can direct-to-consumer marketing techniques. Development of web-based content to provide information about the comprehensive reconstructive options offered may also be useful. Creation of specialized patient educational resources can help guide patients who tend to self-refer for microsurgical reconstruction.[11] Increasing use of social media as a tool for practice exposure has also been recently highlighted in several journals.[32–35]

Addition of Staff and Fellowship Training

As the perforator program matures and operative volume increases, recruitment of additional faculty specialists in breast microsurgery may become necessary. Concomitant growth of clinic and midlevel support staff can assist in the management of increasing patient volume. Establishment of a microsurgery fellowship training program provides additional skilled assistance both in and out of the OR. The introduction of fellows has been associated with shorter operating times and shorter hospital stays for patients, as well as improved outcomes in other specialties.[36–39] Commitment to providing advanced, postgraduate surgical education for fellows is important for the sustainability and growth of the breast microsurgery field as a whole.

Outcomes Assessment and Quality Improvement

Program leaders should seek opportunities to continually evaluate both its successes and areas of weakness. The literature suggests that in addition to high-quality surgical care, establishment of perforator flap programs has been associated with increases in referral volume and patient satisfaction.[10] Careful attention to patient outcomes, consistent pathway variations, and staff feedback should allow further refinement of the program design as it expands. Evaluation of referral patterns can help to optimize outreach and distribution of program information.

Starting a perforator flap program presents a unique opportunity to improve access to comprehensive breast cancer care. Providing consistent, high-quality, specialized service is the foundation for increasing referral volume, mitigating cost, lowering complication rates, and improving patient satisfaction. Although components of the development process described here may not translate to every situation and institution, many key areas for establishing and growing a successful program were presented.

References

1. Damen TH, Timman R, Kunst EH, et al. High satisfaction rates in women after DIEP flap breast reconstruction. J Plast Reconstr Aesthet Surg 2010;63:93–100
2. Momoh AO, Colakoglu S, Westvik TS, et al. Analysis of complications and patient satisfaction in pedicled transverse rectus

abdominis myocutaneous and deep inferior epigastric perforator flap breast reconstruction. Ann Plast Surg 2012;69:19–23
3. Tønseth KA, Hokland BM, Tindholdt TT, Abyholm FE, Stavem K. Quality of life, patient satisfaction and cosmetic outcome after breast reconstruction using DIEP flap or expandable breast implant. J Plast Reconstr Aesthet Surg 2008;61:1188–1194
4. Plastic Surgery Procedural Statistics. 2012; http://www.plasticsurgery.org/news/plastic-surgery-statistics/2012-plastic-surgery-statistics.html. Accessed May 6, 2014
5. Kruper L, Holt A, Xu XX, et al. Disparities in reconstruction rates after mastectomy: patterns of care and factors associated with the use of breast reconstruction in Southern California. Ann Surg Oncol 2011;18:2158–2165
6. Albornoz CR, Bach PB, Pusic AL, et al. The influence of sociodemographic factors and hospital characteristics on the method of breast reconstruction, including microsurgery: a U.S. population-based study. Plast Reconstr Surg 2012;129:1071–1079
7. Albornoz CR, Cordeiro PG, Hishon L, et al. A nationwide analysis of the relationship between hospital volume and outcome for autologous breast reconstruction. Plast Reconstr Surg 2013;132:192e–200e
8. Kulkarni AR, Sears ED, Atisha DM, Alderman AK. Use of autologous and microsurgical breast reconstruction by U.S. plastic surgeons. Plast Reconstr Surg 2013;132:534–541
9. National Accreditation Program for Breast Centers. 2012. http://napbc-breast.org/standards/standards.html. Accessed May 6, 2014
10. Lee BT, Yueh JH, Chen C, Lin SJ, Tobias AM, Slavin SA. Establishment of perforator flap programs for breast reconstruction: the New England program experience. Plast Reconstr Surg 2009;124:1410–1418
11. Matros E, Yueh JH, Bar-Meir ED, Slavin SA, Tobias AM, Lee BT. Sociodemographics, referral patterns, and Internet use for decision-making in microsurgical breast reconstruction. Plast Reconstr Surg 2010;125:1087–1094
12. Dumon KR, Edelson PK, Raper SE, Foster-Kilgarriff K, Williams NN. Implementation of designated bariatric surgery program leads to improved clinical outcomes. Surg Obes Relat Dis 2011;7:271–276
13. Bible KC, Smallridge RC, Morris JC, et al. Development of a multidisciplinary, multicampus subspecialty practice in endocrine cancers. J Oncol Pract 2012;8(3, Suppl):e1s–e5s
14. Haddock NT, Gobble RM, Levine JP. More consistent postoperative care and monitoring can reduce costs following microvascular free flap reconstruction. J Reconstr Microsurg 2010;26:435–439
15. Flurry M, Brooke S, Micholetti B, et al. Nurse training with simulation: an innovative approach to teach complex microsurgery patient care. Ann Plast Surg 2012;69:459–461
16. Lee BT, Tobias AM, Yueh JH, et al. Design and impact of an intraoperative pathway: a new operating room model for team-based practice. J Am Coll Surg 2008;207:865–873
17. Wolf FA, Way LW, Stewart L. The efficacy of medical team training: improved team performance and decreased operating room delays: a detailed analysis of 4863 cases. Ann Surg 2010;252:477–483, discussion 483–485
18. Neily J, Mills PD, Young-Xu Y, et al. Association between implementation of a medical team training program and surgical mortality. JAMA 2010;304:1693–1700
19. Young-Xu Y, Neily J, Mills PD, et al. Association between implementation of a medical team training program and surgical morbidity. Arch Surg 2011;146:1368–1373
20. Awad SS, Fagan SP, Bellows C, et al. Bridging the communication gap in the operating room with medical team training. Am J Surg 2005;190:770–774
21. Cubitt J, Barber Z, Khan AA, Tyler M. Breast reconstruction with deep inferior epigastric perforator flaps. Ann R Coll Surg Engl 2012;94:552–558
22. Demir A, Kucuker I, Keles MK, Demirtas Y. The effect of learning curve on flap selection, re-exploration, and salvage rates in free flaps; A retrospective analysis of 155 cases. Microsurgery 2013;33:519–526
23. Hallock GG. Is there a "learning curve" for muscle perforator flaps? Ann Plast Surg 2008;60:146–149
24. Busic V, Das-Gupta R, Mesic H, Begic A. The deep inferior epigastric perforator flap for breast reconstruction, the learning curve explored. J Plast Reconstr Aesthet Surg 2006;59:580–584
25. Damen TH, Morritt AN, Zhong T, Ahmad J, Hofer SO. Improving outcomes in microsurgical breast reconstruction: lessons learnt from 406 consecutive DIEP/TRAM flaps performed by a single surgeon. J Plast Reconstr Aesthet Surg 2013;66:1032–1038
26. Gart MS, Smetona JT, Hanwright PJ, et al. Autologous options for postmastectomy breast reconstruction: a comparison of outcomes based on the American College of Surgeons National Surgical Quality Improvement Program. J Am Coll Surg 2013;216:229–238
27. Sullivan SR, Fletcher DR, Isom CD, Isik FF. True incidence of all complications following immediate and delayed breast reconstruction. Plast Reconstr Surg 2008;122:19–28
28. Albornoz CR, Cordeiro PG, Mehrara BJ, et al. Economic implications of recent trends in U.S. immediate autologous breast reconstruction. Plast Reconstr Surg 2014;133:463–470
29. Cheng MH, Lin JY, Ulusal BG, Wei FC. Comparisons of resource costs and success rates between immediate and delayed breast reconstruction using DIEP or SIEA flaps under a well-controlled clinical trial. Plast Reconstr Surg 2006;117:2139–2142, discussion 2143–2144
30. Thoma A, Veltri K, Khuthaila D, Rockwell G, Duku E. Comparison of the deep inferior epigastric perforator flap and free transverse rectus abdominis myocutaneous flap in postmastectomy reconstruction: a cost-effectiveness analysis. Plast Reconstr Surg 2004;113:1650–1661
31. Kaplan JL, Allen RJ. Cost-based comparison between perforator flaps and TRAM flaps for breast reconstruction. Plast Reconstr Surg 2000;105:943–948
32. Vardanian AJ, Kusnezov N, Im DD, Lee JC, Jarrahy R. Social media use and impact on plastic surgery practice. Plast Reconstr Surg 2013;131:1184–1193
33. Margolin DA. Social media and the surgeon. Clin Colon Rectal Surg 2013;26:36–38
34. Kuechel MC. Showcase your service: social media and marketing basics in a dynamic, over-populated, mixed-message, and highly

competitive world. Facial Plast Surg Clin North Am 2010;18:533–536
35. Martin A, Grundin E, Harrison D, Espinoza J. Marketing your practice in a social world. J Med Pract Manage 2012;27:227–229
36. Gonzalez R, Nelson LG, Murr MM. Does establishing a bariatric surgery fellowship training program influence operative outcomes? Surg Endosc 2007;21:109–114
37. Kohn GP, Galanko JA, Overby DW, Farrell TM. High case volumes and surgical fellowships are associated with improved outcomes for bariatric surgery patients: a justification of current credentialing initiatives for practice and training. J Am Coll Surg 2010;210:909–918
38. Goldfarb M, Gondek S, Hodin R, Parangi S. Resident/fellow assistance in the operating room for endocrine surgery in the era of fellowships. Surgery 2010;148:1065–1071, discussion 1071–1072
39. Arbabi S, Jurkovich GJ, Rivara FP, et al. Patient outcomes in academic medical centers: influence of fellowship programs and in-house on-call attending surgeon. Arch Surg 2003;138:47–51, discussion 51

3 Essential Equipment Needed for Perforator Flap Breast Reconstruction and Operating Room Setup

David Greenspun

Every microsurgeon has a preference for specific instruments and operating room (OR) configurations. This chapter describes an approach to instrumentation and OR setup that has proved useful and reliable for the successful performance of perforator flaps. There is no absolute right or wrong way to organize the OR, and the equipment will not in itself determine the outcome of the surgery. However, giving careful thought to these matters will doubtless increase the surgeon's comfort and efficiency.

Regardless of specific instrumentations used, familiarity with equipment and establishing consistency in the OR setup are important elements for achieving microsurgical success.[1] Maintaining consistency of instrumentation and setup is extremely helpful, not just for the surgeon, but for the entire OR team. Therefore, it is certainly worth surgeons' investing the time and energy in developing an approach that works well for them. The microsurgery equipment must always be well maintained, and owing to the delicate nature of certain microsurgical instruments, replaced with some frequency.

Evaluation and Selection of Instruments

For successful performance of perforator flap surgery, surgeons should evaluate microsurgical instrumentation and equipment and select the instruments with which they feel comfortable. This may require inspecting the myriad instruments that are already available in the OR. Surgeons' height, hand size, and experience will likely have significant influence over their personal preferences. For example, surgeons who have larger hands may prefer instruments with longer length. It is important to point out that the selection of instruments and OR setup is a somewhat iterative process, subject to continual reevaluation. Continually try to eliminate extraneous instruments from the setup. Simplification of the setup by reducing the number of instruments facilitates operative efficiency, makes procedures easier for the nursing staff, and has obvious economic advantages. Of course, even infrequently used instruments that can be vital in certain challenging situations remain as components of the regular setup. In addition, the introduction of new technology and equipment sometimes requires the addition of instrumentation. My selection of instruments for flap harvest and microsurgical anastomosis are shown in **Figs. 3.1** and **Fig. 3.2,** respectively.

It is important to note that regardless of the specific instruments that one chooses to use for perforator flap surgery, it is critical that a duplicate set of sterile, case-critical instruments be maintained and easily accessed, so that if a patient requires urgent reoperation and the primary set of instruments is unavailable (for example, the instruments are being cleaned and sterilized), another set is available. This principle applies to all microsurgical cases.

The use of a "case cart" specifically designated for perforator flap microsurgery enables all of the specialized equipment, instruments, and supplies used for these cases to be grouped and maintained together. This helps ensure that all of the necessary items will be available in the OR, and also allows for convenient transport of these items to the OR. This also means that key equipment will always be present in the OR, reducing the time spent searching for it and the burden put on the OR staff. It is also a good idea to maintain on hand a small stock of "extra" delicate microsurgical instruments, such as fine-tipped forceps, that are sometimes inadvertently damaged and rendered unusable, often at a most inopportune time. To this end, it is also preferable that instruments designated specifically for perforator flap surgery be used only for this purpose and not for general plastic surgery or hand surgery cases.

Given the complexity of perforator flap surgery, it is helpful to have one individual such as an OR nurse designated as a team leader to provide oversight of OR preparedness. Having an individual who understands the intricacies of this type of surgery, the importance of maintaining the equipment, and the value of consistency in the OR setup is extremely helpful to the whole team.

Key Concepts

- Familiarity
- Consistency
- Duplication set of key instruments for possible take back
- Maintenance and replacement

Surgical Setup

Three instrument stands are used for free flap procedures. Instruments and equipment for flap harvest **(Fig. 3.1)** are set up on one stand, instruments for performing microsurgical anastomoses are set up on another **(Fig. 3.2)**, and a third stand is used for additional instruments, retractors, sutures, lap pads, and the like that are shared by the two microsurgical teams. Placing a silicone mat (such as the type used to line the bottom of sterilization containers) on the stand used to set up microsurgical instruments helps to protect the tips of these delicate instruments and to preserve their longevity **(Fig. 3.2)**. The use of a mobile Mayo stand facilitates the movement of microvascular instruments to a position beside or opposite the surgeon performing the microsurgery or, if necessary, to opposite sides of the OR table. When an oncological or general surgeon is also involved, that surgeon's instruments are maintained on a fourth and separate instrument stand. Larger ORs clearly facilitate this type of setup and minimize the possibility of inadvertent contamination as the staff moves about the OR.

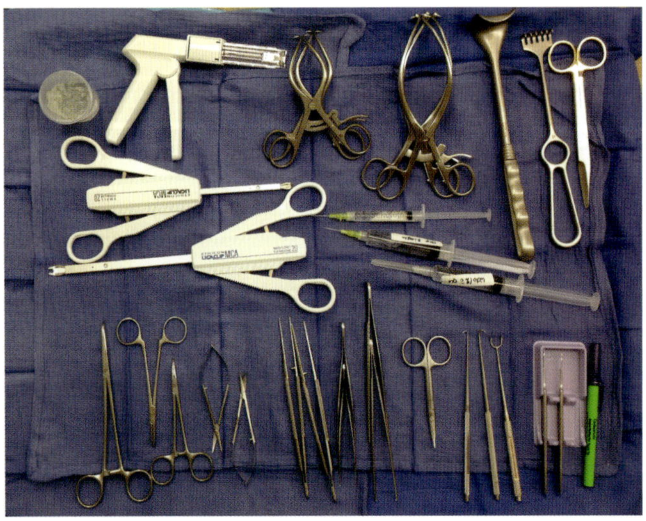

Fig. 3.1 Perforator flap harvest instrument setup. *Top row (left to right):* ultrasonic transmission gel for Doppler, skin stapler, small and large self-retaining Gelpi retractors, Richardson retractor, rake retractor, suture scissor. *Middle row (left to right):* automatic clip appliers, syringes. *Bottom row (left to right):* large right-angle clamp, small right-angle clamp, mosquito clamp, Westcott scissors, various forceps, tenotomy scissors, skin hooks, scalpels, marking pen.

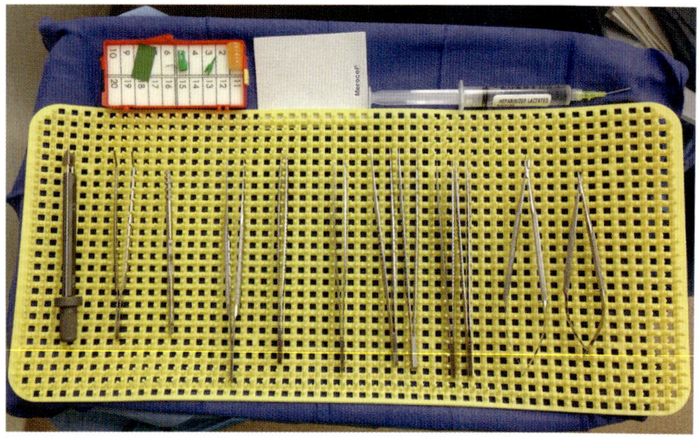

Fig. 3.2 Microsurgical Mayo stand setup. Microsurgical instruments are arranged atop a silicone mat to help protect their delicate tips. *Top row (left to right):* needle park housing containing microsurgical visibility background, microvascular occluding clamps, and cartridge of GEM MicroClips; Merocel gauze; syringe with heparin-containing irrigant. *Bottom row (left to right):* GEM microvascular anastomotic coupler, microvascular occluding clamp applier, vessel measuring gauge, coupler forceps, right-angle forceps, curved forceps, dilator forceps, fine-tipped forceps, needle holder, dissecting scissors.

When working with an oncological or extirpative surgeon, at our center maintain the instruments used for the resection separately from the instruments used for free flap reconstruction. These instruments are set up on their own stand during the case. When the oncological portion of the procedure is completed, the instruments used for the resection are counted and set aside in the OR. It is important that the instruments not be removed from the room until every portion of the surgery is complete: in case there is a discrepancy in the final count, all instruments will be present for enumeration.

At our center, our approach involves two microsurgeons in every procedure. One surgeon focuses on flap harvest and the other on the recipient site. Each surgeon is assisted by a separate scrub nurse or scrub technician. The use of two scrub nurses or technicians facilitates the efficiency of the two-team approach. The OR is set up with duplicate mono- and bipolar cauteries as well as suction tubing for each team. Ellman radiofrequency bipolar cautery for flap elevation is another bipolar option that seems to produce less tissue adherence to the bipolar forceps than traditional diathermy cautery. With this efficient system, it is helpful to label each cautery generator and its corresponding cautery handpieces and foot pedals so that the surgical teams can readily distinguish one setup from the other. Stickers or colored tape is used for this purpose. Round cautery foot pedals are preferred to the traditional flat spring-loaded hinge pedals that resemble pedals in a car, because the round foot pedal does not require any specific spatial orientation.

To help maintain normothermia, a combination of warm water-based and warm air-based systems are used. A warm-air blanket and an insulated head cap are placed on the patient in the preoperative area so that the patient does not arrive in the OR with a low body temperature. A water-based warming pad is placed on the operating table below the patient. Water-based systems are preferable to underbody warm-air systems, as they do not puff up and potentially obstruct the surgical field. Whenever possible, a warm air system blanket is additionally utilized to cover the patient to help maintain core body temperature.

Flap harvesting and recipient-site vessel preparation are performed with the aid of loupe magnification. Whenever possible, try to obtain exposure without the aid of an assistant; doing so minimizes the need for additional help and crowding around the OR table. Self-retaining retractors and elastic stays with sharp hooks (Lone Star Retractor System, Cooper Surgical, Trumbull, CT) enable the surgeon to gain excellent exposure without an assistant holding retractors (**Fig. 3.3**). A Doppler probe (Koven Technology Corp., St. Louis, MO) equipped with a sterile probe and a surgeon-controlled on/off switch is advantageous because the surgeon can utilize the ultrasound without delay and without distracting the circulating nurse from other tasks (**Fig. 3.4**). The surgeon may find a headlight helpful, because overhead surgical lights may not provide optimal illumination. Battery-powered LED headlight systems are generally more convenient than traditional fiber-optic cable headlight systems, but both work well. The latter requires a light source connected to a wall outlet as well as connection of the surgeon's headlight to the light source via a fiber-optic cable. This configuration requires equipment that is bulkier than the battery-powered light sources, creates obstacles in the OR, and requires the help of OR staff to reposition the system when the surgeon moves about the OR.

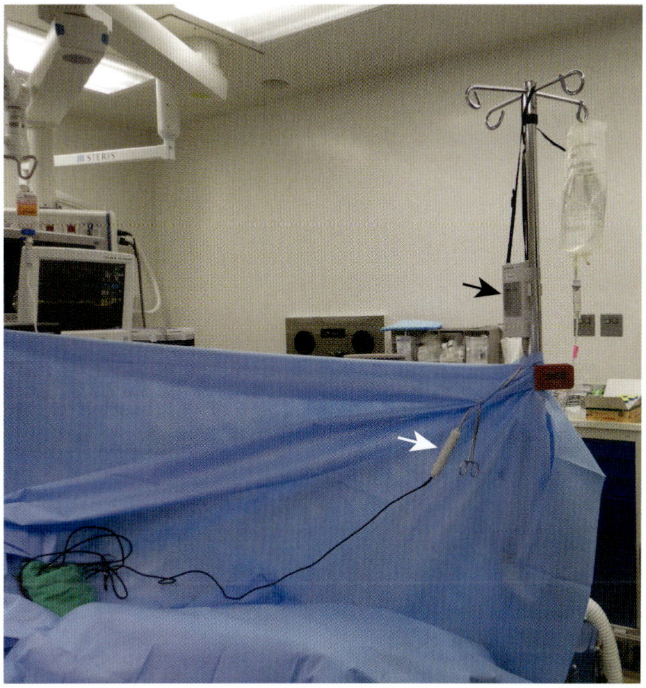

Fig. 3.4 A Doppler ultrasound *(black arrow)* with a surgeon activated on/off switch *(white arrow)* on a sterile probe is mounted to an IV pole at the head of the bed.

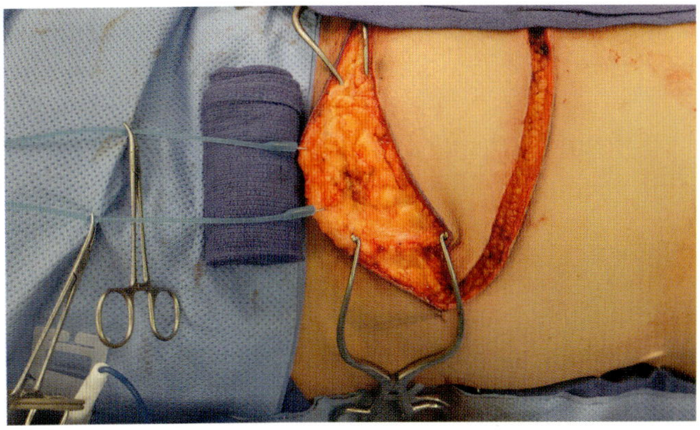

Fig. 3.3 Two self-retaining Gelpi retractors are used in combination with hooks (Lone Star Retractor System) to provide exposure during dissection of the superficial inferior epigastric vessels. The hooks are draped over a rolled-up towel and clamped to the drapes to help retract the soft tissue below the incision.

Although some surgeons perform microsurgical anastomoses under loupe magnification,[2] I find that a microscope with excellent optical resolution, oculars oriented opposite each other, and a foot pedal control for zoom, focus, and X-Y axis control is essential. An integrated video adapter on the microscope enables broadcast of the microsurgical field to video monitors in the OR theater. This is extremely helpful, because it enables the OR staff to visualize the performance of the microsurgery itself and thus best anticipate the needs of the surgeon.

Disposable microvascular clamps provide consistent closing pressure for vascular control during the anastomotic portion of the procedure. Single clamps with closing pressures of 20 or 30 g/mm^2 are used generally for proximal control of recipient veins, and double-opposing clamps with the same closing pressures are used for arterial anastomoses. Venous anastomoses are almost universally performed with the GEM microvascular anastomotic coupler (Synovis, Birmingham, AL), whereas arterial anastomoses are usually hand-sewn with nylon suture. The coupler system has advantages over hand-sewn venous anastomoses, in that anastomoses can be performed more expeditiously, vessel size mismatch can be managed with relative ease, and anastomotic patency has been shown to be higher than that for hand-sewn venous anastomoses.[3–5] In challenging situations, for example when insetting repeatedly compromises flow within the pedicle of a flap, in our practice, a Cook-Swartz implantable Doppler probe is employed to continuously evaluate flow in the pedicle. It is worth noting that some surgeons use a vascular coupler that contains a built in flow-monitoring probe (Flow Through Coupler, Synovis), but our experience is that the use of the Cook-Swartz on a case-by-case basis is more cost-effective, and both methods of direct vessel monitoring have been shown to be comparable.[6]

Although the ideal method of flap monitoring remains a topic of much debate, there is general consensus that prompt recognition of vascular compromise is a prerequisite for flap salvage. Any combination of various parameters, such as clinical judgment, surface temperature monitoring, pencil Doppler probe analysis, and mixed tissue oxygen saturation, can be used according to the surgeon's preference.[7,8] Some mixed tissue oxygen saturation monitors such as that from ViOptix (Fremont, CA) provide continuous uninterrupted monitoring and facilitate remote monitoring with an Internet-connected device such as a cell phone—two features I have come to find invaluable. Although I employ all of the above methods in combination, I have found, as has been described in the literature, that mixed tissue oxygen saturation monitoring is an extremely valuable tool for early detection of vascular compromise.[9]

Conclusion

There is no single best way to approach perforator flap surgery, but following these general principles will help achieve the best possible outcomes in a consistent and reliable manner. Give careful consideration and reconsideration to instrument selection and OR setup, being aware that each surgeon's approach will likely evolve over time. Surgeons should select instruments with which they are comfortable, and should maintain the instruments well and use them often.

References

1. Lee BT, Yueh JH, Chen C, Lin SJ, Tobias AM, Slavin SA. Establishment of perforator flap programs for breast reconstruction: the New England program experience. Plast Reconstr Surg 2009;124:1410–1418
2. Vega S, Smartt JM Jr, Jiang S, et al. 500 Consecutive patients with free TRAM flap breast reconstruction: a single surgeon's experience. Plast Reconstr Surg 2008;122:329–339
3. Ardehali B, Morritt AN, Jain A. Systematic review: anastomotic microvascular device. J Plast Reconstr Aesthet Surg 2014;67:752–755
4. Jandali S, Wu LC, Vega SJ, Kovach SJ, Serletti JM. 1000 consecutive venous anastomoses using the microvascular anastomotic coupler in breast reconstruction. Plast Reconstr Surg 2010;125:792–798
5. Sullivan SK, Dellacroce F, Allen R. Management of significant venous discrepancy with microvascular venous coupler. J Reconstr Microsurg 2003;19:377–380
6. Um GT, Chang J, Louie O, et al; Um GT1. Implantable Cook-Swartz Doppler probe versus Synovis Flow Coupler for the post-operative monitoring of free flap breast reconstruction. J Plast Reconstr Aesthet Surg 2014;67:960–966
7. Lohman RF, Langevin CJ, Bozkurt M, Kundu N, Djohan R. A prospective analysis of free flap monitoring techniques: physical examination, external Doppler, implantable Doppler, and tissue oximetry. J Reconstr Microsurg 2013;29:51–56
8. Smit JM, Zeebregts CJ, Acosta R, Werker PM. Advancements in free flap monitoring in the last decade: a critical review. Plast Reconstr Surg 2010;125:177–185
9. Lin SJ, Nguyen MD, Chen C, et al. Tissue oximetry monitoring in microsurgical breast reconstruction decreases flap loss and improves rate of flap salvage. Plast Reconstr Surg 2011;127:1080–1085

4 Deep Inferior Epigastric Perforator Flap for Breast Reconstruction

Robert J. Allen, Sr., Constance M. Chen, and Maria M. LoTempio

Carl Hartrampf's contribution of the transverse rectus abdominis musculocutaneous (TRAM) flap in the early 1980s was a great advance in autogenous breast reconstruction. He popularized a technique that could be performed by all plastic surgeons to reconstruct a breast without a prosthesis. However, as the procedure became more popular, the donor-site morbidity became more obvious. Agreeing that the ideal donor tissue in the parous female lies transversely across the lower abdomen, investigations began in the late 1980s to utilize this coveted donor area without sacrifice of the rectus abdominis muscles. An early free flap from the 1970s was the superficial inferior epigastric artery (SIEA) flap, usually oriented vertically. By injecting fresh abdominoplastic specimens with radiopaque dye and methylene blue, it was determined that a transverse abdominoplasty flap could be transferred. Seven breast reconstructions with the SIEA flap were performed at Louisiana State University Medical Center by the senior author in 1989 and 1990.[1] The chief problem with the SIEA flap was the variable vascular anatomy, with the artery being either absent or very small in a significant percentage of patients.

Given its limitations, the SIEA flap for breast reconstruction was temporarily abandoned, and investigations of the perforators of the deep inferior epigastric vessels began. Following vascular injection studies, the first deep inferior epigastric perforator (DIEP) flap for breast reconstruction was performed in 1992.[2] Plastic surgeons now had a technique that could be done in any patient who was a candidate for a TRAM flap but without muscle sacrifice.[3]

The DIEP flap steadily gained acceptance worldwide until it became the gold standard for autogenous breast reconstruction. The main drawbacks with the DIEP technique is the requirement of microsurgical expertise and the extended duration of the procedure. The success rate with free tissue transfer is higher than that with any other technique. In over 2,000 DIEP flap breast reconstructions, our success rate has been over 99%. The advent of preoperative imaging with computed tomography angiography (CTA) or magnetic resonance angiography (MRA) in the past decade has contributed to reduced operating room (OR) times. Unilateral DIEP flap breast reconstructions are now routinely completed in under 4 hours, and bilateral DIEP flap breast reconstructions are completed in about 4 hours.

In 2013, a total of 232,340 women in the United States received a breast cancer diagnosis, and an additional 64,640 women received a diagnosis of in-situ breast cancer. The overwhelming number of women who receive a breast cancer diagnosis will go on to live a long and cancer-free life. Of women who undergo surgical treatment, two thirds elect to undergo breast-conserving therapy (BCT) and one-third elect to undergo mastectomy. For most women, the crucial element that drives their choice is trying to balance their concern about cosmetic result with their fear of recurrence. Thus, the ideal solution for most women faced with a breast cancer diagnosis would be to reduce the risk of breast cancer while preserving breast appearance.

In 2013, a total of 95,589 women in the United States underwent breast reconstruction, a number that is almost quadruple that of 15 years earlier. Eighty percent of these breast reconstructions were done with tissue expanders and implants, and 20% were done with autologous tissue. Interestingly, a 2009 University of Michigan study demonstrated that although there is no difference in short-term (<5 years) patient satisfaction after implant-based or autologous tissue breast reconstruction, over the long term (>9 years) there is significantly less patient satisfaction after implant-based breast reconstruction, whereas patient satisfaction after autologous tissue breast reconstruction remains consistently high.

Of all the types of autologous tissue breast reconstruction, the current gold standard is perforator flap breast reconstruction. In particular, the DIEP flap breast reconstruction has achieved popularity as a consistent and reliable method of creating a long-lasting and natural-appearing breast with minimal patient morbidity.[4,5] By using the skin and fat of the abdominal tissue to re-create the breast mound, the DIEP flap achieves the plastic surgery principle of "replacing like with like."

Indications

The best candidates for DIEP flap breast reconstruction are women with adequate abdominal fat and no major medical comorbidities who have not previously undergone autologous tissue breast reconstruction. In particular, women who have undergone multiple pregnancies often have experienced a "tissue expander" effect on their abdominal skin and fat that renders their abdomen an ideal donor site for DIEP flap breast reconstruction. The abdominal fat must incorporate an adequate blood supply from the deep inferior epigastric vessels, however. Thus, women who have undergone abdominoplasty are not candidates for DIEP flap breast reconstruction, as the perforators from the deep inferior epigastric vessels will have been taken. Likewise, women who have undergone gynecologic exenterations or extensive intra-abdominal procedures should also obtain preoperative imaging prior to a DIEP flap breast reconstruction to ensure that the perforating vessels from the deep inferior epigastric vessel are still intact. Liposuction is not an absolute contraindication to DIEP flap breast reconstruction, but very thin women with no abdominal fat may not have enough subcutaneous tissue to enable the surgeon to re-create a satisfactory breast mound. If a woman does not have adequate abdominal fat for a DIEP flap breast reconstruction, she may still be able to undergo autologous tissue breast reconstruction using the thigh, back, or buttock as donor sites.

Another common indication for DIEP flap breast reconstruction is failed implant-based breast reconstruction.[6] About 20% of our breast reconstruction patients are women who have experienced problems such as infection, capsular contracture, implant displacement, or other such problems after implant-based breast reconstruction. Particularly in women who have had to undergo radiation therapy as an adjunct to their breast cancer treatment, autologous tissue breast reconstruction can create a new breast mound that looks and feels natural while using the woman's own tissues.

Besides abdominoplasty, the primary contraindications to DIEP flap breast reconstruction are severe medical comorbidities. For example, significant heart disease, pulmonary disease, or other systemic disease may preclude any reconstructive effort. Breast reconstruction is an elective operation and, despite its significant psychological benefits, it should not endanger the welfare of the patient. Other risk factors in the medical history that should influence decision making include coagulopathies, autoimmune disease, obesity, previous history of abdominal surgery, and prior radiation therapy. Additionally, smoking has been found to be significantly associated with overall complications. Active smokers should be counseled to abstain from tobacco and nicotine use for a minimum of 4 weeks prior to any reconstructive procedure. For potential postmastectomy radiotherapy patients, it may be prudent to place a tissue expander as a skin spacer or to delay reconstruction to avoid the complications that can result from irradiating a free flap.

Preoperative Planning

All patients require an extended preoperative consultation to delineate goals, explain alternatives, discuss expectations, and review potential complications. In doing so, the patient becomes actively involved in the decision-making process and participates in the selection of a reconstructive technique.

During the initial consultation, potential patients are informed that DIEP flap breast reconstruction entails three stages. The first stage involves the actual microsurgical breast reconstruction with the DIEP flap. (In a unilateral breast reconstruction, a symmetrizing procedure on the contralateral breast such as mastopexy, augmentation, or reduction may be performed either at the first or second stage.) The second stage involves nipple reconstruction, and if nipple-sparing mastectomy has been done, any revision to the donor site, breast flap, or the contralateral breast in a unilateral reconstruction. For example, any excess tissue at the donor site or fat necrosis in the breast flap may be excised in this stage. The third stage involves tattooing of the nipple-areolar complex if nipple reconstruction is needed. The first stage is an inpatient procedure that requires an average hospital stay of 3 to 4 days. The second stage is performed as an outpatient procedure in the hospital or in the office. The third stage is always performed in the office. Increasingly, most patients are candidates for nipple-sparing mastectomy and immediate DIEP flap breast reconstruction. In these patients, one stage is possible, but a second stage is often done to achieve the optimal results.

Suitable patients who elect DIEP flap breast reconstruction undergo routine presurgical testing, including appropriate laboratory and diagnostic studies and anesthesia consultation. Blood typing and screening is not necessary. Preoperative imaging, either CTA or MRA, is obtained to delineate the topography of the deep inferior epigastric perforators.[7] Preoperative imaging reduces our operative time significantly, and it also contributes greatly to patient safety the surgeon can be confident about exactly which perforating vessels will be the largest and most robust to use for the DIEP flap. The dissection can be planned preoperatively, and no time is wasted guessing which perforating vessels to use while the patient is under general

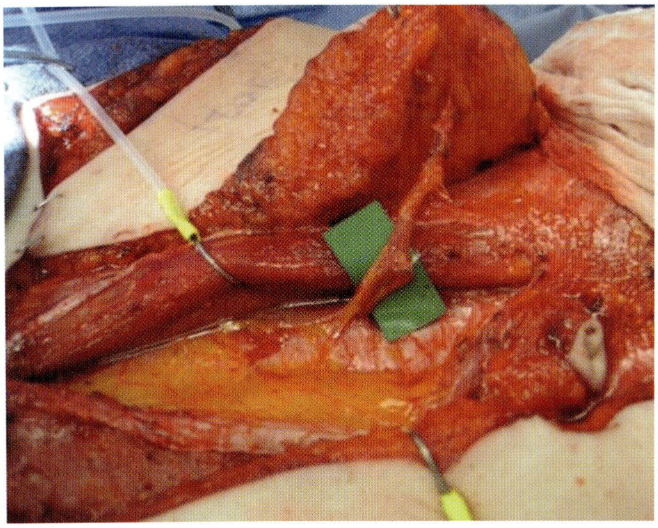

Fig. 4.1 In 8% of patients, a septocutaneous perforator may be found in which the dominant perforator vessel travels around the medial edge of the rectus abdominis muscle with no intramuscular course at all.

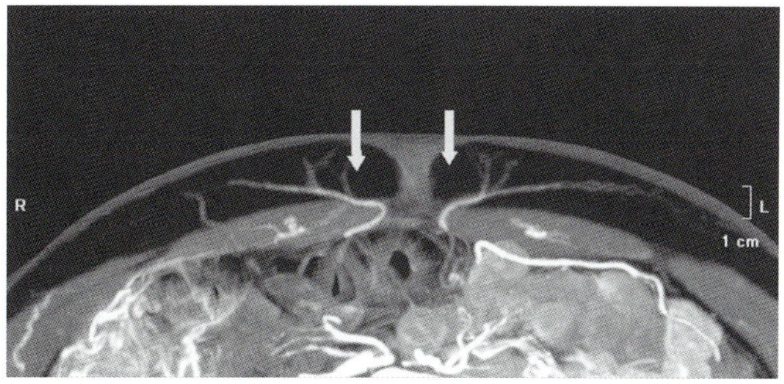

Fig. 4.2 The best way to identify a septocutaneous perforator is via preoperative imaging. *Arrows* are pointing to septocutaneous perforators.

anesthesia. In addition, imaging facilitates preoperative mapping of the recipient vessels and helps provide an estimate of the flap volume from the DIEP flap.

Anatomy

Detailed knowledge of the deep inferior epigastric vasculature and its perforator topography is required for successful execution of the DIEP flap. Accurate knowledge of the perforator topography may be obtained via preoperative imaging—either CTA or MRA. The largest perforator vessels may be chosen preoperatively and then mapped on an X-Y axis. A large perforator trumps the location. Prior to the era of preoperative imaging, the flap was based on one perforator 20% of the time and usually used the lateral row.[8] With preoperative imaging, one perforator flap is used 70% of the time, and the medial row is used in 75% of cases. In 8% of patients, a septocutaneous or paramuscular perforator may be found in which the dominant perforator vessel travels around the medial edge of the rectus abdominis muscle with no intramuscular course at all **(Fig. 4.1)**. This completely eliminates any intramuscular dissection and damage to the musculature, and the best way to identify a septocutaneous perforator is via preoperative imaging **(Fig. 4.2)**. Often, the best perforator vessels are around the umbilicus or slightly above the umbilicus. In these situations, The DIEP flap is designed to incorporate the largest and most robust perforator vessels as seen on preoperative imaging.

Interestingly, our 10-year review of DIEP flaps prior to the era of preoperative imaging has demonstrated that the incidence of any complication increases with the number of perforator vessels used **(Fig. 4.3)**.[8] For example, univariate analysis of partial flap loss indicated significance of any complication with the use of five perforators ($p < 0.05$). Both univariate and multivariate analysis demonstrated significantly fewer complications with the use of one perforator ($p < 0.05$). For fat necrosis, there was a steady trend of increased incidence of fat necrosis with increasing number of perforators ($p < 0.05$). Thus, it is generally best to harvest one perforator for a DIEP flap, as long as the single perforator chosen is large and the best perforator. Ideally, this is delineated on preoperative imaging and confirmed intraoperatively.

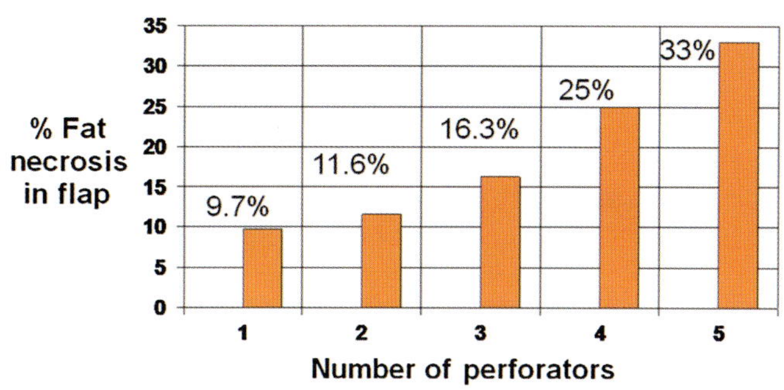

Fig. 4.3 The incidence of fat necrosis increases with the number of perforators used. (From Gill P, Hunt J, Guerra A, et al. A 10-year retrospective review of 758 DIEP flaps for breast reconstruction. Plast Reconstr Surg 2004;113:1153. Reprinted with permission.)

Surgical Technique

The DIEP flap is based on the perforating vessels that originate from the deep inferior epigastric system. These perforators travel through or around the rectus abdominis muscle, pierce the anterior rectus sheath, and supply the overlying skin and fat **(Fig. 4.4)**. During DIEP flap surgery, the lower abdominal soft tissue is mobilized on one or more perforators in preparation for free tissue transfer. Because the rectus abdominis muscle is not harvested, the pedicle length is substantially longer than in a TRAM flap. The longer pedicle length makes the DIEP flap easier to position in the chest wall and also simplifies the microsurgical anastomosis. In addition, less dissection is required inferiorly toward the external iliac vessels.

Patients are marked preoperatively in the standing position for anatomic landmarks on the breast and abdomen **(Figs. 4.5 and 4.6)**. On the anterior chest wall, this includes the boundaries of the existing breast mound. On the lower abdomen, marks are placed at the midline, at the perimeter of the umbilicus, and on the proposed outline of an elliptical flap in the hypogastrium. With the patient in the supine position, the key perforators are then marked according to the findings of the CTA or MRA. A handheld Doppler can also be used to confirm the position of key vessels. The upper mark of this proposed flap is placed above the umbilicus if needed to incorporate paraumbilical perforators. The lower mark is placed in a suprapubic crease, and may be shifted superiorly during surgery to ensure less tension in the abdominal closure. The abdominal scar can be lowered 7 cm at the second stage.

The patient is positioned supine on the operating table with the arms at 60 degrees or tucked by her side, depending on surgeon preference. Tuck the arms unless the breast surgeon needs to have the arms extended for a sentinel lymph node biopsy and possible axillary dissection. Simultaneous abdominal flap harvest and mastectomy, followed by preparation of the chest wall vasculature is performed via a two-team approach. The internal mammary system is used as a recipient site. The vessels are usually approached at the second interspace between the second and third costal cartilages. Some or all of the third costal cartilage can be removed if needed, but in patients with appropriate anatomy the anastomosis can be achieved without removing any rib

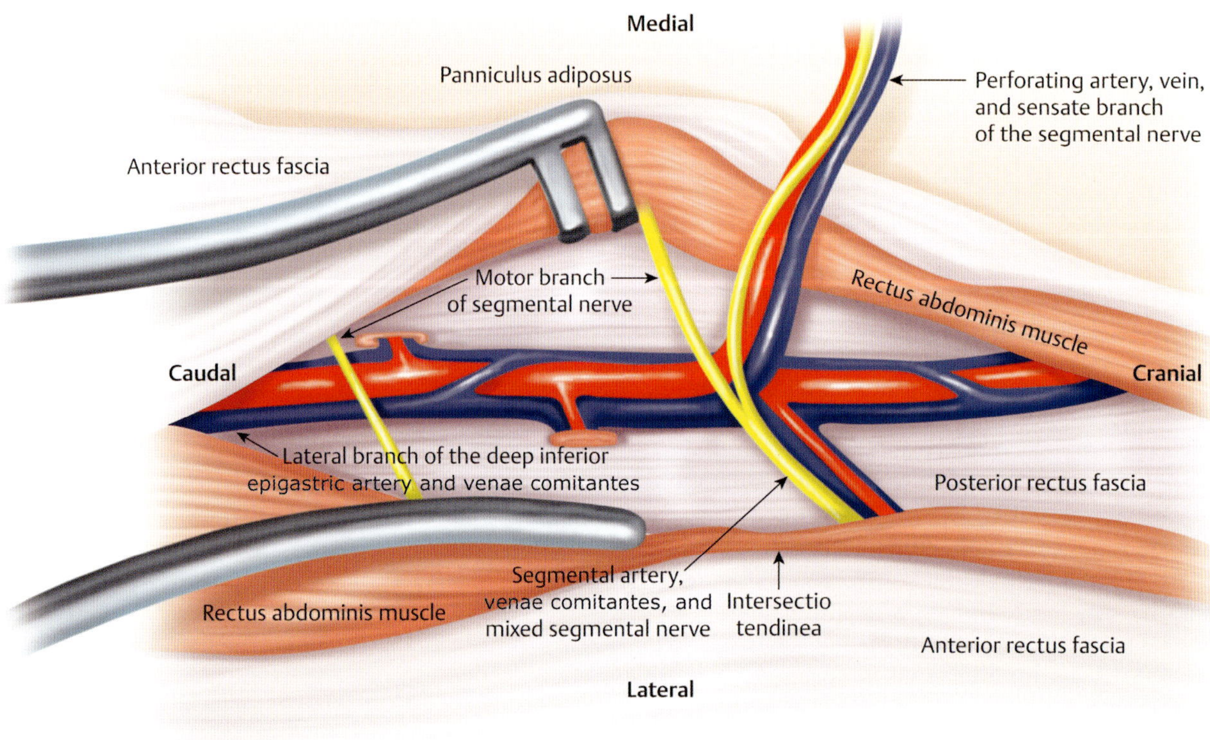

Fig. 4.4 The DIEP flap is based on perforating vessels that originate from the deep inferior epigastric system, travel through the rectus abdominis muscle, pierce the anterior rectus sheath, and supply the overlying abdominal skin and fat.

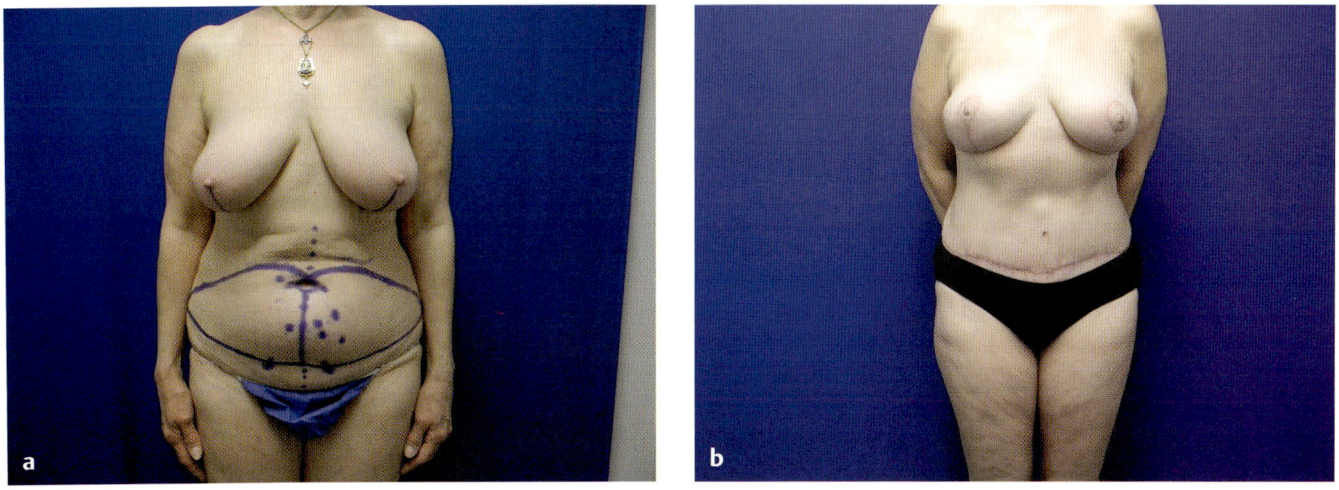

Fig. 4.5 **(a)** Patient is marked preoperatively in the standing position for anatomic landmarks on the breast and abdomen. **(b)** Postoperative photograph of the same patient following a nipple-sparing mastectomy on the right and a skin-sparing mastectomy on the left with DIEP breast reconstruction.

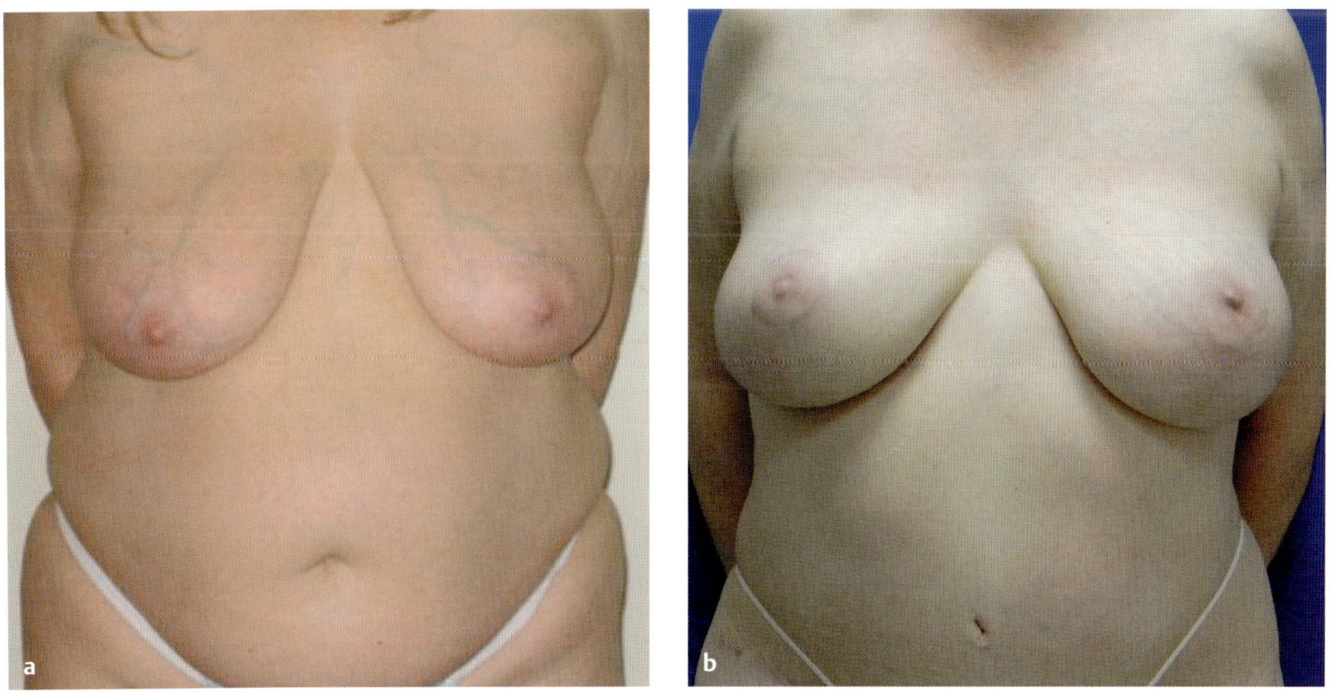

Fig. 4.6 **(a)** Preoperative photograph of a patient prior to bilateral nipple-sparing mastectomy. Even patients with an obese body habitus who are in good health can safely undergo DIEP flap breast reconstruction. **(b)** Postoperative photograph of the same patient following nipple-sparing mastectomy with immediate DIEP flap breast reconstruction and subsequent mastopexy.

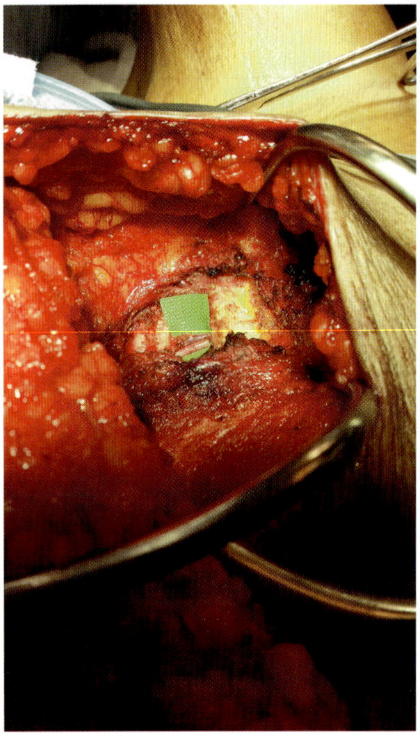

Fig. 4.7 The vessels are usually approached at the level of the third rib and in the interspace above or below it, depending on which interspace has the greatest width.

at all **(Fig. 4.7)**. The diameter of the internal mammary vessels is largest in the second intercostal space. When technically feasible, a rib-sparing technique is used to preserve the pectoralis muscle and prevent a chest wall deformity. Occasionally, the internal mammary system may have adequately sized perforators that can be used for microanastomosis, thus precluding the need to dissect through the rib space to the deeper internal mammary vessels. However, in nipple-sparing mastectomies these perforators should be preserved to provide needed blood supply and sensation to the nipple-areola complex.

Increasing numbers of microsurgeons who routinely perform perforator flap breast reconstruction identify the main perforators of the deep inferior epigastric vasculature preoperatively via CTA or MRA. This enables them to obtain precise information on perforator diameter and three-dimensional course. A handheld Doppler probe is used to confirm the vessels that they choose preoperatively, and then identify them with direct visualization during flap harvest and perforator isolation.

Harvesting of the DIEP flap begins with an incision at the upper marked line, dissection through the full thickness of the abdominal wall to the anterior fascia, and elevation of a superior abdominal wall flap. If the perforator has already been identified via preoperative imaging, then the dissection can continue directly to the chosen perforator. In a bilateral DIEP flap, the midline incision is made first. If the perforator is a medial row or a septocutaneous paramuscular perforator, then the chosen perforator is isolated prior to elevating the lateral edges of the abdominal flap. Once the largest perforator has been identified, the dissection proceeds efficiently with elevation of the skin-fat flap from the underlying rectus fascia. The remainder of the perforators are divided. Care is taken when making the inferior incision to look for superficial inferior epigastric vessels. In particular, it is helpful to preserve the superficial inferior epigastric vein in case the flap has a superficial-dominant drainage system.

Isolation of the DIEP flap proceeds under loupe magnification, and begins by opening the anterior rectus sheath around the selected perforator. Some surgeons incorporate a 1- to 2-mm cuff of the sheath around each perforator, but no fascia is needed. Using a Westcott microsurgical scissors or bipolar electrocautery, the perforator is followed through the rectus muscle, carefully clipping or coagulating all small side branches. If a second or third perforator has been selected, particular attention must be paid to maintaining its continuity in line with the first. Preoperative imaging is very helpful in determining the vascular course.

As dissection proceeds, the muscle is split along the direction of its fibers, preserving all intercostal nerves that do not lie between two perforators. A divided nerve between two perforators should be repaired. The dissection is continued inferiorly until the main trunk of the deep inferior epigastric vessels are reached. An optimal pedicle length is 8 to 10 cm.

The DIEP flap is then harvested by individually dividing the deep inferior epigastric artery and its one or two venae comitantes. It is helpful to mark the anterior surface of the vessels with methylene blue prior to vessel division. In addition, the smaller vena comitantes can be clipped, leaving the larger vena comitantes and artery open for anastomosis. The flap is weighed at this time to determine its comparability to the mastectomy specimen or implant. It is then transferred to the anterior chest wall and temporarily secured in position. This can be done by suturing the flap to the chest wall or by wrapping the flap in a moist lap sponge that is stapled to the chest wall.

The operating microscope is positioned at the recipient site and the pedicle prepared for microanastomosis, taking care to avoid twisting of the vessels. An end-to-end venous anastomosis is completed with a microvascular coupling device **(Fig. 4.8)**. The end-to-end arterial anastomosis is hand-sewn with 9-0 nylon sutures. Some microsurgeons use a Doppler flow-through venous coupler or implant a

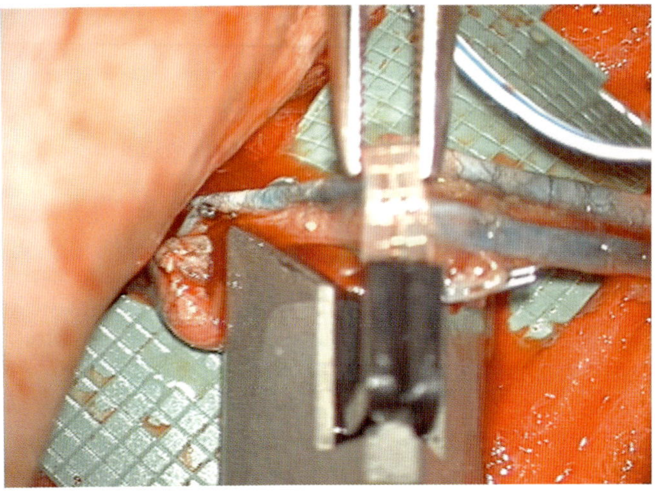

Fig. 4.8 An end-to-end venous anastomosis is completed with a microvascular coupling device.

venous or arterial Doppler cuff at the completion of microsurgery for postoperative monitoring. Preferably, leave a skin island for postoperative monitoring.

The DIEP flap is then debulked, contoured, and inset to achieve the desired breast size and shape (**Fig. 4.9**). Areas underlying the native mastectomy flaps are de-epithelialized in situ. The pedicle position is secured and protected with deep absorbable suture. Peripheral absorbable sutures inset the flap in the appropriate position. A closed suction drain is placed and brought out through the lateral edge of the skin closure or through a separate stab incision. After the flap has been shaped and inset, the skin is closed with subcutaneous absorbable sutures.

Ideally, closure of the abdomen begins as soon as the flap(s) are harvested and finished by the time the flaps are inset. The anterior rectus sheath is closed with two-layer running barbed suture. Because no fascia has been harvested, mesh is not used. Any diastasis is repaired with running suture as well. The remainder of the abdominal closure is in layered fashion, using interrupted 2-0 absorbable suture or running barbed suture in Scarpa's fascia, and running subcuticular skin closure. Two closed suction drains are placed in the abdomen and brought out through the lateral incision. The umbilicus is then brought through the abdominal wall at a predetermined site after de-epithelializing an elliptical patch of skin. It is secured in place using 4-0 half-buried mattress sutures.

Postoperative Management

The patient is monitored in the recovery room for 1 to 2 hours postoperatively. Flap checks are performed every 15 to 30 minutes during this time, and consist of assessments of skin paddle color, temperature, capillary refill, and Doppler signals. The patient is then moved to a regular room, where flap checks are performed every 2 to 4 hours overnight. Deep venous thrombosis prophylaxis with anticoagulation and sequential pressure hose are continued during hospitalization. In the morning, the Foley catheter and intravenous lines are removed. The patient is started on a regular diet, and is required to ambulate. Flap checks are continued every 4 hours while the patient is in the hospital. The patient is usually discharged on postoperative day 3 or 4. After 4 weeks, patients are encouraged to resume their preoperative levels of activity. The importance of postoperative flap monitoring is changing. One study reviewed take-backs in a series of 400 breast free flaps over 7 years at New York University Tisch Hospital. There were four take-backs. Two occurred early while the patient was still in the postoperative acute care unit (PACU) and were salvaged with venous drainage through the superficial system. The other two occurred after discharge, with one total flap failure and one near-total fat necrosis. Flap monitoring on the ward was not helpful in this series, and flap failure after discharge is usually not salvageable. At present, flap monitoring after the PACU is de-emphasized. Strategies to decrease the take-back rate are being emphasized and taught to residents and fellows.

Complications

The DIEP flap represents a significant advance in autologous tissue breast reconstruction. Unlike the pedicled and

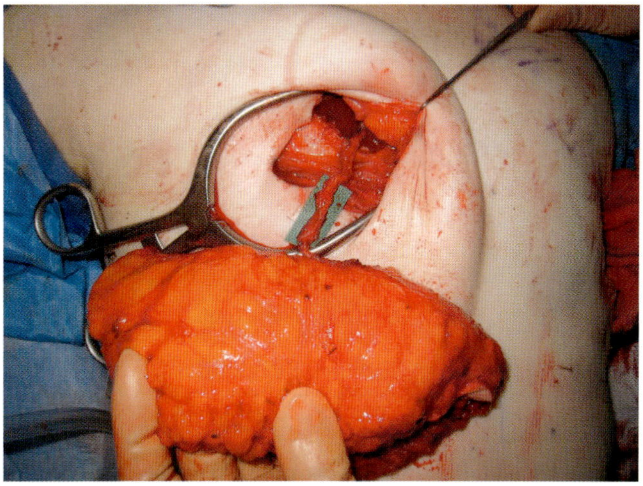

Fig. 4.9 The DIEP flap is then debulked, contoured, and inset to achieve the desired breast size and shape.

free TRAM, the DIEP flap preserves the rectus abdominis muscle to maintain abdominal wall strength and minimize the risk of abdominal bulge or hernia.[9,10] Preservation of the rectus abdominis muscle decreases abdominal wall morbidity, resulting in improved abdominal wall strength and contour. This translates into less postoperative pain, shorter hospital stays, and quicker recovery. In addition, the longer vascular pedicle enables greater freedom of design that optimizes the aesthetics of breast reconstruction. Because it minimizes the adverse impact on activities of daily living, preserves quality of life, and maximizes cosmesis, the DIEP flap is becoming the standard of care for breast reconstruction.

Patients reconstructed with the DIEP flap report less postoperative pain and experience a quicker recovery compared with those with pedicled and free TRAM flaps. These differences have been noted by patients, nurses, and surgeons. Studies confirm that patients with DIEP flap procedures have less postoperative pain, a lower perioperative narcotic requirement that is statistically significant, and earlier conversion to oral analgesics.[11] Recovery is also faster, and DIEP flap patients have shorter hospital stays. They are routinely discharged on postoperative day 3 or 4. Indeed, a 2001 study at M.D. Anderson Cancer Center comparing DIEP and TRAM flap breast reconstruction demonstrated that DIEP flap breast reconstruction halved postoperative morphine use with patient-controlled analgesia (PCA) and significantly shortened hospital stay.[11]

In our series of 1,536 DIEP flaps from 1992 to 2014, the total complication rate compares favorably with that in other forms of autologous tissue breast reconstructions **(Table 4.1)**.[8] Our complication rates include a 10.3% abdominal wound healing complication. In DIEP flap patients with a history of smoking, hypertension, and previous radiotherapy, a higher incidence of complications can be expected. There may also be an association of complications with higher body mass index (BMI). Early complications included the need to return to the operating room in 4% of patients: 2% for venous occlusion, 1% for arterial occlusion, and 1% for hematoma. Adoption of a coupling device for venous anastomosis has decreased the take-back rate even further. The rate of total flap loss was 0.5%, with a partial flap loss rate of 2.3%. The incidence of these complications is favorable compared with those reported for breast reconstruction with other free-flap techniques.

The most common complication following autologous breast reconstruction with abdominal tissue is fat necrosis. This is thought to arise in areas of deficient perfusion, often at the flap periphery farthest from the vascular supply. The rate of fat necrosis in DIEP flap breast reconstruction is comparable with that for free TRAM flaps, and less than that for pedicled TRAM flaps. Our retrospective review of 1,536 DIEP flaps found a 12% fat necrosis rate, which is significantly correlated with smoking and post-reconstruction radiotherapy. Similarly, the rate of fat necrosis in free TRAM reconstructions has been routinely reported as being between 10% and 13%. Studies of pedicled TRAM reconstruction have shown rates ranging from 11% to 25%.

Late complications of the DIEP flap included a postoperative bulge rate of only 0.5%. This is markedly lower than the rate for pedicled TRAM reconstruction, which was 9% in a similarly sized cohort. A higher hernia and abdominal bulge rate has also been reported for free TRAM reconstruction, typically between 1% and 15%, but as high as 82%. A considerable advantage of DIEP flap reconstruction is also the avoidance of prosthetic mesh placement, often seen during pedicled and free TRAM reconstruction.

Perforator flap opponents continue to argue against the routine use of the DIEP flap because of increased operative time. However, after an initial learning curve, microsurgeons committed to performing perforator flap breast reconstruction can perform a unilateral reconstruction in under 3 hours and a bilateral reconstruction in under 4 hours. This is comparable with the length of time needed for pedicled TRAM or implant-based reconstructions. Furthermore, it can be argued that a DIEP flap breast reconstruction is actually easier and safer to perform than a muscle-sparing TRAM, especially when preoperative imaging is used, because the selected perforator can be visualized throughout the dissection. Modern microsurgery has evolved to a point where the arguments of high failure rates and long operative times may be obsolete.

The DIEP flap technique has expanded the pool of potential reconstructive candidates by allowing for autologous breast reconstruction in previously unsuitable patients, such as obese individuals or those with prior abdominal surgery. With the increasing use of preoperative imaging, operative times are decreasing and the procedure itself has become safer and more predictable. DIEP flap breast reconstruction is particularly well suited for physically active women, irradiated women, women with bilateral reconstructions, and women in whom other modalities are contraindicated, failed, or deemed unsuitable. The DIEP flap represents the state-of-the-art technique in autologous breast reconstruction using the abdomen and provides the best long-term aesthetic outcome. The increased demand for microsurgical expertise is more than offset by the rewards of minimized donor-site morbidity and increased patient satisfaction.

Table 4.1 Comparisons of Complications Following Deep Inferior Epigastric Perforator (DIEP) and Free Transverse Rectus Abdominis Musculocutaneous (TRAM) Flaps

Source	No. of Flaps	Partial Loss	Total Loss	Fat Necrosis	Abdominal Wound Complication	Hernia/ Bulge	Return to Operating Room	Venous Occlusion	Arterial Occlusion
Allen, 1992–2014[12]									
DIEP	1536	2.3%	0.5%	12.0%	10.3%	0.5%	3%	2%	1%
Chen et al, 2007[13]									
DIEP	41	0%	0%	12.2%	n/a	n/a	n/a	n/a	n/a
TRAM	159	1.3%	0.6%	12.8%	n/a	n/a	n/a	n/a	n/a
Scheer et al, 2006[14]									
DIEP	84	1.1%	6%	42.9%	22.6%	9.5%		7.1%	0%
TRAM	46	6.5%	4.3%	8.7%	10.9%	19.6%		4.3%	0%
Bonde et al, 2006[15]									
DIEP	44	n/a	4.5%	0%	n/a	2.3%	n/a	n/a	n/a
TRAM	233	n/a	2.1%	3.9%	n/a	5.6%	n/a	n/a	n/a
Bajaj et al, 2006[16]									
DIEP	43	2.3%	4.7%	11.6%	n/a	9.3%	6.3%	n/a	n/a
TRAM	150	0.7%	0%	9.3%	n/a	10.0%	3.2%	n/a	n/a
Nahabedian et al, 2005[17]									
DIEP	110	0%	2.7%	6.4%	n/a	1.8%	n/a	4.5%	n/a
TRAM	113	0%	1.8%	7.1%	n/a	7.1%	n/a	2.7%	n/a
Kroll et al, 2000[18]									
DIEP	31	16.1%	0%	29%	n/a	n/a	n/a	n/a	n/a
TRAM	279	1.1%	1.4%	12.9%	n/a	n/a	n/a	n/a	n/a
Blondeel et al, 1997[4]									
DIEP	18	n/a	n/a	n/a	n/a	0%	n/a	n/a	n/a
TRAM	20	n/a	n/a	n/a	n/a	15%	n/a	n/a	n/a

Abbreviation: n/a, not available.

Conclusion

Beginning in the 1990s, it was apparent that one DIEP flap did not always provide enough volume for one breast reconstruction. To address this, stacked bilateral DIEP flaps for unilateral breast reconstruction were employed with excellent results. Over the past decade, the rate of bilateral mastectomies has increased tremendously. Much of this increase is thought to be due to genetic testing, improved breast reconstruction options, and the rise of nipple-sparing mastectomy. Bilateral reconstructions are now much more common than unilateral reconstructions. Extending the two flaps are often better than one for unilateral reconstruction, and in bilateral reconstruction this can mean using four flaps for bilateral reconstructions. Our first choice when using four flaps is combining the DIEP and profunda artery perforator (PAP) flaps for each breast. The entire procedure of bilateral mastectomy and bilateral combined DIEP/PAP flaps is done with the patient in the supine position and takes about 7½ hours.

References

1. Allen RJ, Glass CA, Dupin CL, et al. Breast reconstruction with the superficial inferior epigastric arterial system. Presented at the annual meeting of the Southeastern Society of Plastic and Reconstructive Surgeons, Kiawah, SC, June 1990
2. Allen RJ, Treece P. Deep inferior epigastric perforator flap for breast reconstruction. Ann Plast Surg 1994;32:32–38

3. Blondeel PN. One hundred free DIEP flap breast reconstructions: a personal experience. Br J Plast Surg 1999;52:104–111
4. Blondeel N, Vanderstraeten GG, Monstrey SJ, et al. The donor site morbidity of free DIEP flaps and free TRAM flaps for breast reconstruction. Br J Plast Surg 1997;50:322–330
5. Futter CM, Webster MH, Hagen S, Mitchell SL. A retrospective comparison of abdominal muscle strength following breast reconstruction with a free TRAM or DIEP flap. Br J Plast Surg 2000;53:578–583
6. Levine SM, Lester ME, Fontenot B, Allen RJ Sr. Perforator flap breast reconstruction after unsatisfactory implant reconstruction. Ann Plast Surg 2011;66:513–517
7. Agrawal MD, Thimmappa ND, Vasile JV, et al. Autologous breast reconstruction: preoperative magnetic resonance angiography for perforator flap vessel mapping. J Reconstr Microsurg 2014
8. Gill PS, Hunt JP, Guerra AB, et al. A 10-year retrospective review of 758 DIEP flaps for breast reconstruction. Plast Reconstr Surg 2004;113:1153–1160
9. Nahabedian MY, Dooley W, Singh N, Manson PN. Contour abnormalities of the abdomen after breast reconstruction with abdominal flaps: the role of muscle preservation. Plast Reconstr Surg 2002;109:91–101
10. Nahabedian MY, Momen B, Galdino G, Manson PN. Breast Reconstruction with the free TRAM or DIEP flap: patient selection, choice of flap, and outcome. Plast Reconstr Surg 2002;110:466–475, discussion 476–477
11. Kroll SS, Sharma S, Koutz C, et al; Evans GRD. Postoperative morphine requirements of free TRAM and DIEP flaps. Plast Reconstr Surg 2001;107:338–341
12. Healy C, Allen RJ Sr. The evolution of perforator flap breast reconstruction: twenty years after the first DIEP flap. J Reconstr Microsurg 2014;30:121–125
13. Chen CM, Halvorson EG, Disa JJ, et al. Immediate postoperative complications in DIEP versus free/muscle-sparing TRAM flaps. Plast Reconstr Surg 2007;120:1477–1482
14. Scheer AS, Novak CB, Neligan PC, Lipa JE, Zoller JE, Kubler AC. Complications associated with breast reconstruction using a perforator flap compared with a free TRAM flap. Ann Plast Surg 2006;56:355–358
15. Bonde CT, Christensen DE, Elberg JJ. Ten years' experience of free flaps for breast reconstruction in a Danish microsurgical centre: an audit. Scand J Plast Reconstr Surg Hand Surg 2006;40:8–12
16. Bajaj AK, Chevray PM, Chang DW. Comparison of donor-site complications and functional outcomes in free muscle-sparing TRAM flap and free DIEP flap breast reconstruction. Plast Reconstr Surg 2006;117:737–746, discussion 747–750
17. Nahabedian MY, Tsangaris T, Momen B. Breast reconstruction with the DIEP flap or the muscle-sparing (MS-2) free TRAM flap: is there a difference? Plast Reconstr Surg 2005;115:436–444, discussion 445–446
18. Kroll SS. Fat necrosis in free transverse rectus abdominis myocutaneous and deep inferior epigastric perforator flaps. Plast Reconstr Surg 2000;106:576–583

5 Superficial Inferior Epigastric Artery Flap for Breast Reconstruction

Aldona J. Spiegel

Abdominal adipose tissue is the closest match in texture to breast tissue that the body has to offer. Because of this texture characteristic, abdominal tissue transfer has become the preferred choice in autologous breast reconstruction. To provide optimal care to breast reconstruction patients, techniques to minimize dissection of the abdominal musculature have been developed, which include the deep inferior epigastric perforator (DIEP) flap and the superficial inferior epigastric artery (SIEA) flap as methods of breast reconstruction.[1] These flaps both involve the use of adipocutaneous tissue with the lower abdomen as a donor site **(Fig. 5.1)**.

In 1971, Antia and Buch[2] published the first article on the SIEA free flap, describing this flap for repair of a soft tissue deformity in the face. The first use of the SIEA flap for autologous breast reconstruction was done by Allen[3] in 1989.

Autologous flaps from the lower abdomen have evolved over the years, becoming less and less invasive. The free transverse rectus abdominis musculocutaneous (TRAM) flap, the first abdominally based free flap, requires partial- or full-thickness excision of the rectus abdominis muscle. Next came the DIEP flap, which requires only incision of the fascia, without excising any muscle. Next, in 1989, the SIEA flap for breast reconstruction was described, which requires neither excision nor incision of the abdominal wall. This is important, as violation of the rectus musculature or fascia can lead to a decrease in abdominal wall strength and integrity. Studies have shown that the SIEA causes significantly less donor-site morbidity than the DIEP or free TRAM flaps.[4,5] The DIEP described by Allen in 1994 has the advantage of a more reliable pedicle than the SIEA flap.

Indications and Contraindications

The SIEA flap is the least invasive option when using an abdominal donor site. However, it can be used only in selective cases when certain requirements are met. This is mostly an intraoperative decision, and if the criteria are not met, the DIEP flap is used instead. We have designed an algorithm for selection of the SIEA flap that has been previously published.[6] This algorithm will be discussed at length later in the chapter. Some patients may not be candidates for abdominally based autologous tissue reconstruction. These patients may be better suited for reconstruction with an autologous flap from another donor site, such as the superior gluteal artery perforator (SGAP) flap or the profunda artery perforator (PAP) flap from the posterior thigh, to name just two. If the patient has enough abdominal laxity but does not have sufficient tissue to reconstruct an adequately sized breast, it is possible to add an implant to provide additional volume, or to perform a double ("stacked") free flap.

Contraindications to the SIEA flap include, first and foremost, patients who smoke. In a previous study, we observed a higher rate of donor-site complication in patients who were current smokers at the time of reconstruction (odds ratio, 15.8; $p = 0.016$).[6] We require patients to refrain from smoking for at least 2 months prior to surgery and for 6 weeks after surgery. Patients with a history of prior abdominoplasty or abdominal surgery with excessive scaring in the flap region, and patients with other medical comorbidities that would hinder flap survival, such as coagulation disorders require careful preoperative medical and radiographical evaluation, and may be poorer candidates for microsurgical breast reconstruction. Lastly, certain intraoperative conditions must be met for the use of an SIEA flap. These will be discussed as part of the aforementioned algorithm.

Anatomy

The SIEA flap is sometimes incorrectly referred to as a perforator flap; however, this description is untrue as the superficial inferior epigastric vessels do not perforate a muscle or septum. The SIEA flap is more correctly termed a direct axial adipocutaneous flap as opposed to the DIEP and free TRAM flaps that are supplied by perforating vessels. The vascular supply for the SIEA flap comes from a subdermal vascular plexus that courses superficially and

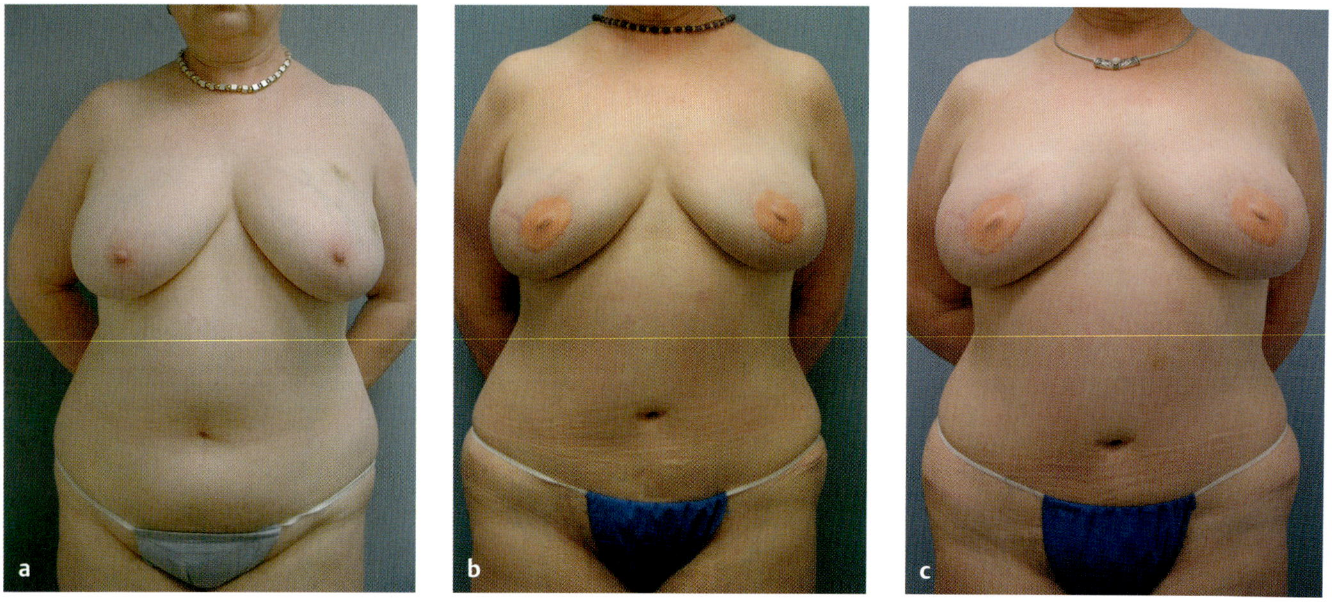

Fig. 5.1 (a) A 48-year-old woman with left invasive ductal carcinoma elected to undergo a bilateral skin-sparing mastectomy and superficial inferior epigastric artery (SIEA) flap reconstruction. **(b)** At 1-year follow-up. **(c)** At 4-year follow-up.

includes many smaller vessels that originate from the superficial inferior epigastric axial vessels.

In 1975, Taylor and Daniel[7] published the preeminent anatomic study of the SIEA. This study found the SIEA to be missing in 35% of the study participants. In the remaining participants, the SIEA origins were examined and found to be variable: 48% of the time the SIEA shares a common trunk with the superficial circumflex artery, whereas 52% of the pedicles had the SIEA originate as a direct branch off of the common femoral artery. In 2011, Piorkowski et al[8] conducted a study using computed tomography angiography (CTA) to evaluate the superficial inferior epigastric artery for potential use in an SIEA flap. They concluded that of their patients, 43% had at least one SIEA; however, only 21% had an SIEA of adequate caliber for use in an SIEA flap. Our own clinical experience with donor-site dissection of the lower abdomen for free flap breast reconstruction concurred with the results of these studies, as 42% of our 278 patients lacking an identifiable SIEA. Furthermore, of the 58% with an identifiable SIEA, only 54% of those had a suitable caliber (1.5 mm or greater). SIEA flap selection requires a minimum arterial external diameter of 1.5 mm when measured at the level of the lower abdominal incision. Thus, only 31% of the patients in our study had an SIEA adequate for use in a free flap, which is consistant with the findings of the previous studies.

The origin of the SIEA can be found 2 to 5 cm inferior to the inguinal ligament as it leaves the common femoral artery. As mentioned above, although it may branch off alone in some patients, it often shares a trunk with the superficial circumflex iliac artery. Of note, a variety of other origins have been noted in a small percentage of patients, from the deep femoral artery or even the pudendal artery. The SIEA and its adjacent venae comitantes are generally found running lateral to the lateral row of the deep inferior epigastric perforators. The origin of the SIEA is deep to Scarpa's fascia; however, as it courses superiorly the artery penetrates the fascia and continues cranially in the superficial subcutaneous tissue. There are two options for venous drainage of the SIEA flap, the two venae comitantes that course alongside the SIEA before terminating into the femoral vein and the superficial inferior epigastric vein (SIEV), which drains into the saphenous bulb. The SIEV usually has a sizable caliber, between 2 and 3 mm; however, it runs medial and away from the SIEA, which causes pedicle inset difficulties and can cause arterial kinking. For this reason the, venae comitantes are usually our vessels of choice and are used beyond the point when they merge together into one vein. The average pedicle length for the SIEA flap can range from 5 to 8 cm with arterial diameters anywhere from 1.1 to 1.9 mm.[9,10] The area of the SIEA flap is composed of the lower abdomen that is perfused by the SIEA; however, the lateral aspect of the flap may have some overlapping perfusion from the superficial circumflex iliac artery (SCIA).[11–14] The 10th to 12th intercostal nerves provide sensation to the region and can be used for reinnervation if a sensate flap is desired.[15]

The reliability of tissue perfusion and venous drainage across the midline in an unipedicled SIEA flap has been a topic of great debate in the literature. Some studies have concluded that drainage and perfusion across the midline is quite unpredictable, whereas others have shown that the use of tissue across the midline, in zone III and zone IV, is actually possible.[16,17] We will address evaluation of cross-flap perfusion and viability of this tissue later in the chapter.

Preoperative Preparations

Preoperative CTA may be ordered to determine if the SIEA is present and of sufficient caliber.[8] The imaging will also help to map the path of pertinent vessels within the flap.

Preoperative marking takes place on the morning of surgery. It begins with marking of the abdomen while the patient is supine, and we mark for the harvest of both an SIEA flap and a DIEP flap **(Fig. 5.2)**. The algorithm for deciding between the SIEA and the DIEP flap occurs intraoperatively.[6] All patients have both hemiabdomens marked for possible use of the ipsilateral or contralateral flap for reconstruction.

Marking begins with the use of a pencil Doppler to locate and mark the SIEA and venae comitantes, which are usually located approximately midway between the anterior superior iliac spine (ASIS) and the pubic symphysis, just superior to the inguinal crease. Next, the SIEV is marked, most often medial to the SIEA, followed by the arterial and venous periumbilical perforators bilaterally. At this point, the medial and lateral rows of the deep inferior epigastric perforators are marked.

When marking the inferior incision line, it is important to design this incision low enough to dissect out the SIEA with a suitable diameter. If the diameter fails to meet the 1.5-mm minimum diameter required by the algorithm, a DIEP is performed, which is why preoperative location and marking of the deep inferior epigastric perforators is crucial even when an SIEA flap is expected. The inferior incision mark begins in the midline, immediately superior to the pubic hairline, and extends laterally, with a slight superior curve, terminating at the ASIS. The superior abdominal incision mark begins approximately 1 cm superior to the umbilicus and extends laterally, with a gradual inferior curve, attaching to the inferior incision line at its terminus. The abdomen is then marked down the midline from umbilicus to the mons pubis. The average SIEA flap is 14 cm vertically by 17 cm horizontally from midline to ASIS.

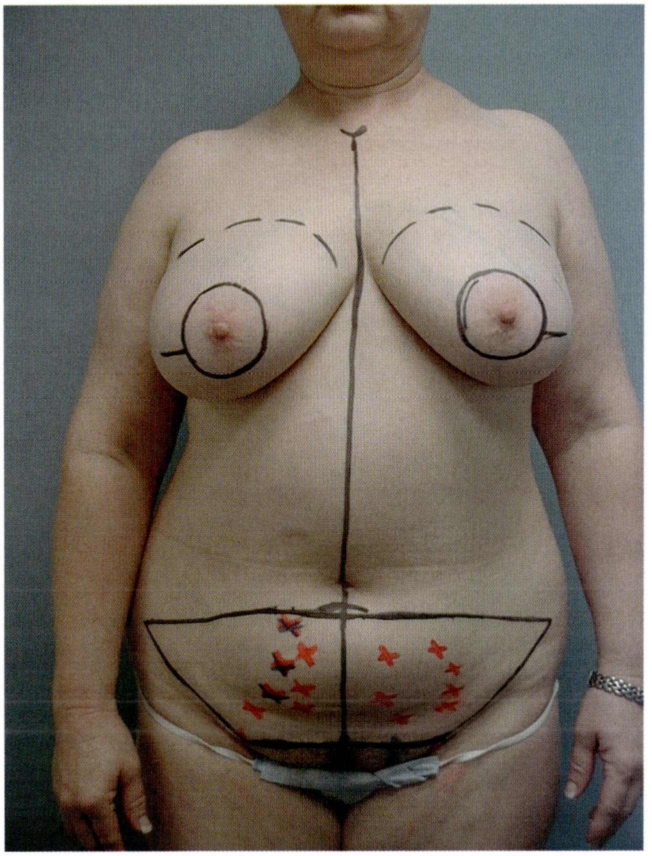

Fig. 5.2 Preoperative markings.

Further marking is continued with the patient standing and depends greatly on the procedure that is scheduled. In patients having immediate breast reconstruction, it is necessary to bilaterally mark the inframammary folds (IMFs) and superior breast poles. Patients undergoing skin-sparing mastectomies should also have the anticipated periareolar line marked as well. If the patient is scheduled for delayed unilateral reconstruction, the IMF and superior breast pole markings should match the current contralateral breast; however, in delayed bilateral reconstruction, the "proposed" IMF lines of both breasts should be marked. Previous mastectomy scars should be marked, with all of the aforementioned procedures. Lastly, the rest of the midline is marked from suprasternal notch to umbilicus and the second and third intercostal spaces are palpated and marked for easy identification of the recipient vessels and nerves.

Procedure

Flap Harvest

The patient is placed supine with both arms tucked to her side. This facilitates moving the microscope in and out of the surgical field as needed. While the flap is harvested under loupe magnification ×5.5, the microscope is necessary for vessel anastomosis and nerve coaptation in the recipient field. Local anesthetic or vasoconstrictors at the donor site as well as the recipient site are not used.

Harvesting the SIEA flap begins on the side ipsilateral to the breast being reconstructed with the inferior abdominal mark. Carefully create an incision along this line just deep to the dermis, and then perform a cautious subcutaneous dissection, making sure not to injure the SIEV, which has a fairly superficial course through this area **(Fig. 5.3)**. Next, locate the SIEA and SIEV and dissect away the adjacent tissue without skeletonizing the vessels. The SIEA should now be evaluated for appropriate caliber at the level of the skin incision.

Before proceeding with the SIEA flap, it is important to use the venous coupler's vessel sizer to measure the artery's external diameter. If the vessel meets the 1.5-mm criterion and has a palpable, visible, and audible Doppler pulse, then we will move on to the dissection of the artery and venae comitantes. It is important to continue dissection only as long as the vessel diameter is increasing. There is generally no need to dissect a vessel to its origin. Pedicle length is seldom an issue with the SIEA flap, unlike the DIEP, so there is no need to continue dissection once the vessel diameter becomes constant.* A small amount of subcutaneous tissue or fat deep to the vessels for protection of the pedicle is left around the vessels; however, it should be noted that leaving too much tissue in this area could lead to unnecessary seroma formation. Only the distal end of the vessel should be fully skeletonized, as this is necessary for anastomosis.

For unilateral breast reconstruction, the ipsilateral hemiabdomen is used for three reasons. First, the pedicle of the SIEA enters the abdominal tissue from the lateral border, so when an ipsilateral flap is rotated 180 degrees for inset on the chest, the pedicle will be closer to the recipient vessels on the medial aspect of the chest. Second, when attempting to shape the flap, by suturing an ipsilateral flap around the umbilical excision site, the flap will form a coned shape that sits in the more natural lateral position. Third, the inset position of an ipsilateral flap puts the area with the least reliable blood supply in the least prominent (lateral) position, as opposed to a contralateral flap, which places this at-risk tissue medially, where it is far more visible if it were to necrose. Regardless of the surgeon's preference of side, both SIEAs are evaluated before pedicle selection, which more often than not is determined by the caliber of the artery. If the caliber is less than 1.5 mm or it shows a weak pulse, the contralateral SIEA will be evaluated. If this contralateral SIEA proves satisfactory, the dissection is continued, and the reconstruction is done with the contralateral SIEA. If neither SIEA is sufficient for our needs, we assume deep perforator system dominance and revert to a DIEP flap. Evaluation for a DIEP flap begins, like with the SIEA flap, on the ipsilateral side for the same reasons mentioned above. The lateral row of perforators is explored first, and then the medial row. If neither is acceptable, the perforators of the contralateral hemiabdomen are evaluated. Bilateral reconstruction similarly favors ipsilateral SIEA flaps over contralateral for all of the aforementioned qualities.

In unilateral breast reconstruction patients who require more tissue than is available in one hemiabdomen to match the contralateral breast, some of the tissue across the midline must be incorporated. Although this is controversial in the literature, as mentioned above, we have seen in our own practice no evidence of increased fat necrosis or partial flap loss with our experience of well over 100 SIEA flaps, as long as the tissue is carefully evaluated for perfusion and nonviable tissue excised before final inset. We have observed reliable perfusion across the midline of an SIEA flap to approximately the lateral row of deep inferior epigastric perforators. Once the flap anastomosis is complete, zone IV and the poorly perfused area of zone III should be resected. Inspection and evaluation of this tissue will be discussed later in the chapter.

Once all the criteria of the algorithm have been met and the decision to proceed with the SIEA flap has been made, the relevant vessels should be identified and flap dissection continued. The superior incision begins at the lateral intersection of the abdominal incision lines marked preoperatively, near the ASIS, and continues medially along this superior marking to the midline. Continue this incision deeply, through the adipose tissue to the loose areolar tissue plane. This tissue lies immediately superficial to the muscular fascia of the abdominal wall. Next, elevate the flap off of the abdominal wall starting laterally and working medially, using Bovie cautery for complete hemostasis. Careful hemostasis is vital at this time to maintain a clear view of the correct surgical plane and prevent accidental incisions into the muscular fascia that can weaken the abdominal wall and increase donor-site morbidity.

Editor's note: Dissection of the SIEA all the way to its origin will provide a better size match with the internal mammary (IM) recipient vessel. This is especially true if there is a common trunk with the superficial circumflex iliac artery.

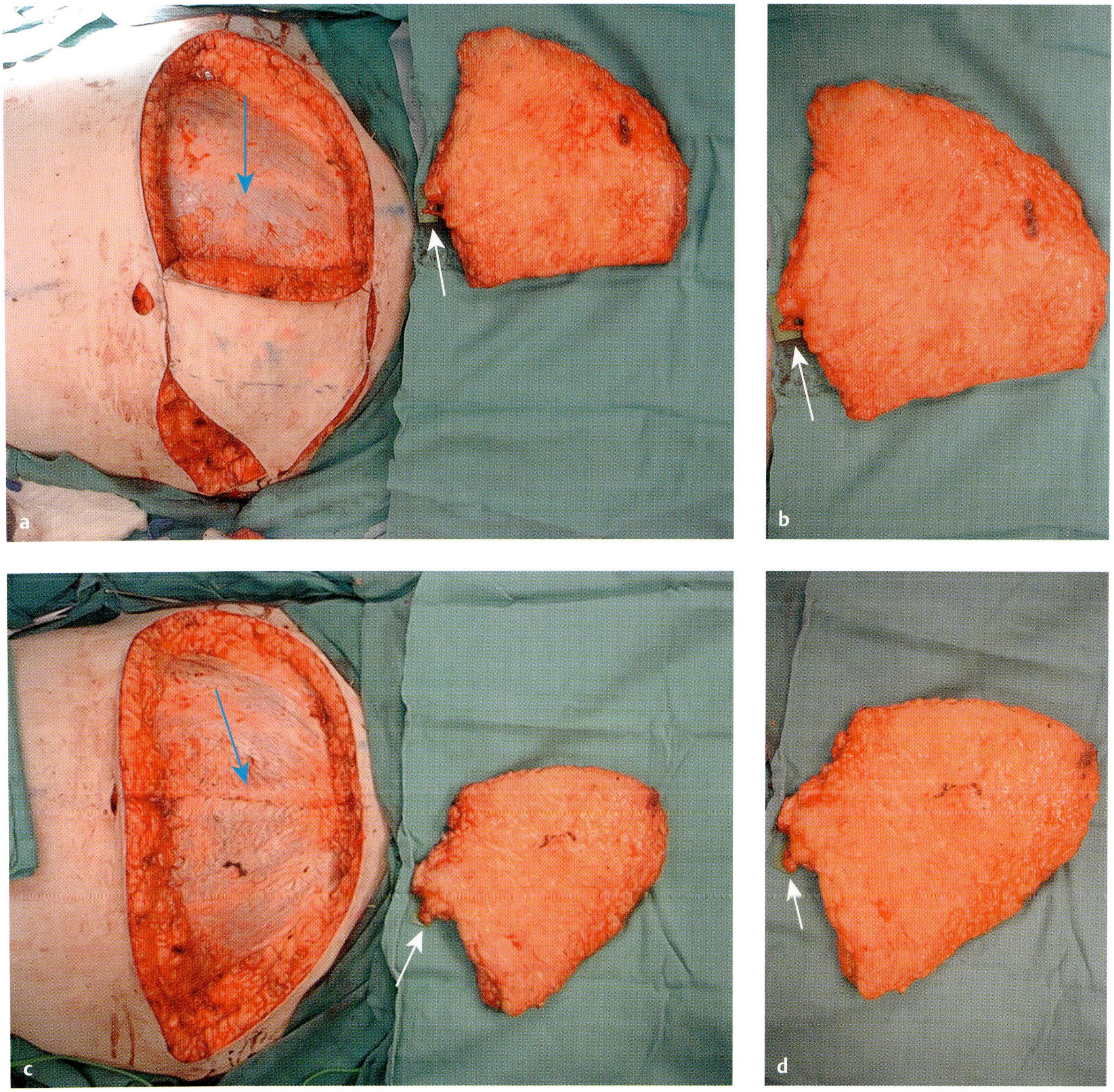

Fig. 5.3 **(a)** Left hemiabdominal flap is harvested and placed skin-side-down on the sheet to show the vascular pedicle *(white arrow)*. Note the preservation of the rectus fascia *(blue arrow)*. **(b)** Close-up of the left hemiabdomen with vascular pedicle *(arrow)*. **(c)** Both hemiabdomens have been harvested. The right hemiabdominal flap is turned over to show the vascular pedicle *(white arrow)*. note that the midline rectus diastasis has been plicated *(blue arrow)*. **(d)** The right hemiabdominal flap turned over to show the vascular pedicle *(arrow)*.

Next, use blunt dissection to free the umbilicus from the abdominal tissue. Then elevate the umbilicus with skin hooks and create a circumumbilical incision down to the rectus sheath to free the umbilical stalk, being careful not to skeletonize the stalk, as the surrounding blood supply is necessary for umbilical survival. While this region is exposed, the patient should be evaluated for periumbilical hernias, and any finding should be repaired with your closure and documented.

At this time it is important to test the superficial vascular system to see if it is able to support perfusion to the flap, before continuing. First, compare the recipient artery diameter to that of the SIEA and if there is a difference of more than 1 mm, strongly consider reverting to a DIEP flap. Next, to assess the vasculature, without removing the option of reverting to a DIEP flap, two or three deep perforators from the ipsilateral side should be preserved, and then use vascular clamps to occlude all the deep perforators on both sides as well as the contralateral SIEA and SIEV. At this point the flap is perfused only by the superficial system of the ipsilateral side and we can easily assess the flap for any areas being deprived of perfusion that would most likely not survive flap transfer. Now a decision is made as to whether or not the adequately perfused tissue will provide enough volume to reconstruct the breast, or if a DIEP flap, which generally provides more volume from better profusion across the midline, should be used.

Once flap elevation is completed, mark the superficial side of the pedicle with a marking pen, for future alignment, and then bring the flap edges back together on the abdomen and staple them in place while the recipient site is addressed. If a bilateral reconstruction is planned, the first flap should be anastomosed before evaluating the contralateral SIEA caliber and pulse to determine whether the superficial system is suitable for reconstruction or if a DIEP flap should be considered.

Recipient-Site Preparation

Patients who have either a skin-sparing mastectomy or nipple-sparing mastectomy with immediate breast reconstruction generally have the best aesthetic results. In these cases, the flap volume is used to simply refill the hollowed out skin envelope. With a skin-sparing mastectomy, a small circular skin paddle on the flap is left for perfusion monitoring after surgery and eventually nipple reconstruction and areolar tattooing. When reconstructing after a nipple-sparing mastectomy, a small, elliptical skin paddle is left in the inframammary fold for monitoring; however, this skin will be excised during a planned revision surgery at a later date. With either of these types of mastectomies, the IMF needs to be revised to the premarked height, and the lateral border of the breast pocket should be re-created if necessary. When re-creating an IMF, it is important to compensate for the abdominal closure. While closing the donor site, the skin of the superior abdomen and chest will be pulled down along with the re-created IMF, so it may be necessary to compensate by raising the IMF by 1 or 2 cm.

Some patients may require radiation therapy as part of their cancer treatment plan. In these cases, we delay reconstruction until 6 months after the completion of radiation therapy. The radiation changes and type of mastectomy directly affects how the mastectomy skin is treated. For instance, if the patient has a skin-sparing mastectomy and minimal to no skin changes after radiation, the patient is treated the same as a patient who did not require radiation, and we follow the same steps listed above, raising the hollowed-out skin envelope and replacing the volume with our flap. If, however, there are noticeable skin changes secondary to the radiation therapy that must be resected or if the patient had a simple mastectomy, there may not be enough skin left to re-create the breast skin envelope. In these situations, the skin inferior to the mastectomy scar is excised, while leaving the subcutaneous fat against the chest wall, and then bring a larger skin paddle with the flap to make up for this skin deficit.

Recipient Vessel Preparation

The internal mammary artery and vein are the recipient vessels of choice in the vast majority of our reconstructive cases. Other choices are available, if necessary, including the thoracoacromial vessels, internal mammary perforators, and serratus perforators. It is possible to use a contralateral "crossover" anastomosis from the contralateral IM if necessary, but this is rarely indicated. We prefer to save the thoracodorsal pedicle, which supplies the latissimus dorsi flap, as a backup plan in case of failure of the free tissue transfer.

Dissection to the internal mammary vessels is performed through the second or third intercostal space previously marked at the beginning of the case. The most important factor in choosing which space to use is the width, so that the vessels can fit through unimpeded. Next, an opening is made in the pectoralis major muscle, followed by resection of the intercostal muscles to expose the internal mammary vessels. If necessary, part of the costochondrium can be resected with a rongeur to widen this space, although we find this is usually not required. Then, using loupe magnification, prepare the recipient artery and vein for anastomosis.

Anastomosis

To prepare the field for microsurgical anastomosis, retract the mastectomy skin flaps very gently, taking care not to injure or strangulate this tissue. Next, prepare the recipient vessels for anastomosis using the microscope. Once these vessels are ready, move back to the donor site, ligate the SIEA, SIEV, and venae comitantes, and then transfer the flap to the prepared mastectomy field. It is important when ligating the venae comitantes to attempt ligation distal to their point of merging so that our venous anastomosis can be to a single combined vessel. Now rotate the flap 180 degrees from its original orientation on the abdomen so that the pedicle points medially, and then align the donor and recipient vessels for anastomosis. Next, staple the flap to the mastectomy skin and cover the flap with a moist laparotomy sponge while the microanastomosis takes place. Then trim back the distal end recipient vessels, making sure to leave enough for application of the vascular clamps.

If neurotization of the flap is planned, the third anterior intercostal is used as the donor nerve because it is more readily available in the current microvascular field.[18] The recipient nerve is usually a cutaneous branch of T11 or T12 and can be located during your abdominal dissection near the most inferior lateral perforator vessels. The donor nerve can generally be found at the junction of the inferior portion of the third rib and the sternum. The nerve travels across the superior portion of the intercostal vessels. Dissect the nerve away from the vessels and transect it medially. Now mobilize the nerve to give it the greatest length possible in preparation for neurotization. A conduit is used for nervous coaptation, as studies have shown that in this specific type of neurotization, the use of a conduit has provided a better return of sensibility than direct coaptation.[19] Now, anchor the donor and recipient nerves to opposite ends of the conduit with 8-0 nylon suture. When using a nerve conduit, it is important to complete the nervous coaptation before the microvascular anastomosis to prevent the conduit from compressing the vessels.

To begin the anastomosis, the venous system is addressed first by connecting the internal mammary vein (IMV) to the venae comitantes using a venous coupler. Most often the medial internal mammary vein is a better size match with the venae comitantes, but if the lateral internal mammary vein is of sufficient caliber as well, the lateral IMV is used for venous anastomosis as it can usually provide more length. Historically, the IMV would be anastomosed to the SIEV, but due to the proximity and size match, the venae comitantes are used in the majority of cases, as opposed to the SIEV, which has shown an increased risk of vessel kinking and flap complication. The SIEV may be used if the venae comitantes are inadequate or if an additional venous anastomosis is required for increased flap drainage.

Now the donor and recipient arteries are lined up for arterial anastomosis with double opposing clamps. The arteries are anastomosed by using a 9-0 nylon suture with either running or interrupted stitches. Next, an internal Doppler cuff is placed around the venous anastomosis for continuous monitoring of anastomotic patency.

Flap Inset and Closure

When insetting the flap, it is important to orient the pedicle correctly on the chest wall by using the previous marking of the superficial aspect of the SIEA. This will prevent twisting of the pedicle as it enters the flap, which could be devastating for flap perfusion. It is also important to note that once inset, the pedicle of the SIEA flap will take a sharp turn as it exits the intercostal space and travels into the flap. It is at this turn that problems may arise, so be careful not to compress or twist the pedicle beneath the flap. If the patient has had previous radiation to this breast, be leery of pedicle compression from the increased skin tension pressing against the flap and in turn against the pedicle. It is crucial to monitor the internal Doppler closely, and investigate any abnormality fully before the final inset. It may be necessary to reposition or reorient the pedicle or flap slightly to prevent vascular occlusion. Once set, the flap is sutured to the chest wall with interrupted 2-0 Monocryl stitches at the superolateral and inferior flap edges. The patient is then flexed to a nearly seated position to evaluate breast symmetry and to assist with abdominal donor-site closure by bringing the skin edges closer together.

In patients who had a simple mastectomy or who have a skin deficit due to resection from radiation changes, the skin paddle serves a dual purpose: to replace skin necessary for the new skin envelope, and to serve to monitor flap perfusion. Any flap skin not included in the skin paddle will be de-epithelialized and covered with the new skin envelope.

Two 15-French (F) drains are placed before final closure, one laterally and one inferiorly. The ends of the drains should be trimmed to avoid damaging or obstructing the pedicle and anastomosis. For breast skin closure, we prefer to close in layers, with 3-0 Monocryl used for the deep dermis, 4-0 Monocryl used for a running subcuticular stitch with buried knots, and finally liquid adhesive used to seal the skin edges together. Steri-Strips or tape over the wound immediately following a procedure are not used because edematous swelling after surgery will cause bruising in taped areas that are restricted from expanding with the swelling.

At the donor site, diastasis of the rectus is corrected, if necessary, by plicating the rectus fascia. A new opening is created for the umbilicus in the skin of the lower abdomen and then the umbilicus is delivered through that opening and attached with 3-0 and 4-0 Monocryl sutures. As with the breast, two 15F Blake drains are placed (this time both at the lateral edge) before closing in layers. Scarpa's fascia is closed with 2-0 Monocryl, the deep subcutaneous tissue with 3-0 Monocryl, and a running 4-0 Monocryl subcuticular stitch before sealing the skin edges with liquid adhesive and covering with a dry dressing.

Cautions to Take

Perfusion Assessment

When utilizing tissue across the midline in an SIEA flap, it is important to resect all potentially nonviable tissue including all of zone IV and any underperfused areas of zone III. The volume of tissue across the midline available for use in the reconstruction will differ in each patient based on her unique perfusion pattern. There are many ways to evaluate perfusion. A line of demarcation is identified between the sufficiently and insufficiently perfused tissue while the flap is still in situ, with the deep perforators and contralateral SIEA clamped shut. This line is marked before flap transfer and anastomosis, because it takes quite a bit of time for the reperfused flap to develop a clear delineation between viable and nonviable tissue. The SPY Elite® system (Novadaq, Bonita Springs, FL) may be used to aid in visualization of perfusion in real time, providing a more confident assessment of which tissue to resect after anastomosis, which may require adjustment of the previous marking for tissue resection.

Flap Orientation

Final inset of the flap requires careful orientation of the flap to prevent pedicle obstruction and perfusion compromise. The pedicle of the SIEA enters the flap superficially at the inferior edge, as opposed to perforator flaps where the pedicle enters from the deep aspect. Because the recipient inframammary vessels are within the chest wall, the pedicle must travel from superficial to deep for the anastomosis. Although the perforator flap pedicles are optimally oriented for this step, the SIEA pedicle enters the flap from the side, so it must turn 90 degrees to course deep toward the recipient vessels, which leads to an increased risk of pedicle kinking, and obstruction of blood flow. Another area where pedicle obstruction can be a problem with the SIEA flap is in the window resected out of the pectoralis. When creating this window, it is important to take the pedicle position into consideration. It is important not only to excise a window large enough to prevent the pedicle from being compressed against the muscle, but also to elevate the skin over the anastomosis off of the pectoralis muscle to prevent excess tension from compressing the pedicle. This is especially important in patients with previous radiotherapy, as radiation changes cause the skin to become less pliable and contract even more. A wider dissection over the area of anastomosis in radiated patients is recommended to compensate for these skin changes.

Abdominal Drains

In SIEA patients, donor-site drains generally stay in place for a longer period of time than in DIEP patients, possibly due a disturbance of lymphatics during the groin dissection that is more extensive for an SIEA flap. Drains should stay place in until drainage is less than 25 cc per day, which usually takes approximately 1 to 2 weeks.

Postoperative Monitoring

For the first 24 hours after surgery, Flaps are checked hourly. A sitting trial is performed a sitting trial on postoperative day 1 by advancing them to a reclining chair for 1 hour while the nurse keeps a watchful eye on the flap's capillary refill, color, and Doppler signals, as the change in the angle of the gravitational pull on the flap can cause a change in perfusion. If there are no complications during the sitting trial, the patient can be transferred to a regular room, as long as her vitals are stable and pain control is adequate. Patients are encouraged to progressively ambulate as tolerated and are usually discharged on postoperative day 3 or 4. A daily low-dose 81-mg aspirin regimen starts on postoperative day 1, which the patient continues for 2 weeks.

A second-stage revision procedure is performed 3 to 4 months after completion of the SIEA flap. This involves minor tweaks to the breast and abdomen contour as well as nipple reconstruction. In the case of a nipple-sparing mastectomy, it is at this stage that the elliptical skin paddle that was left for monitoring is removed. The final stage of the reconstruction is tattooing of the new nipple and areola, if necessary, to provide complete breast restoration.

References

1. Allen RJ, Treece P. The DIEP flap for breast reconstruction. Ann Plast Surg 1994;32:32–38
2. Antia NH, Buch VI. Transfer of an abdominal dermo-fat graft by direct anastomosis of blood vessels. Br J Plast Surg 1971;24:15–19
3. Allen RJ, Heitland AS. Superficial inferior epigastric artery flap for breast reconstruction. Semin Plast Surg 2002;16:35–44
4. Wu LC, Bajaj A, Chang DW, Chevray PM. Comparison of donor-site morbidity of SIEA, DIEP, and muscle-sparing TRAM flaps for breast reconstruction. Plast Reconstr Surg 2008;122:702–709
5. Chevray PM. Breast reconstruction with superficial inferior epigastric artery flaps: a prospective comparison with TRAM and DIEP flaps. Plast Reconstr Surg 2004;114:1077–1083, discussion 1084–1085
6. Spiegel AJ, Khan FN. An intraoperative algorithm for use of the SIEA flap for breast reconstruction. Plast Reconstr Surg 2007;120:1450–1459
7. Taylor GI, Daniel RK. The anatomy of several free flap donor sites. Plast Reconstr Surg 1975;56:243–253
8. Piorkowski JR, DeRosier LC, Nickerson P, Fix RJ. Preoperative computed tomography angiogram to predict patients with favorable anatomy for superficial inferior epigastric artery flap breast reconstruction. Ann Plast Surg 2011;66:534–536
9. Arnez ZM, Khan U, Pogorelec D, Planinsek F. Breast reconstruction using the free superficial inferior epigastric artery (SIEA) flap. Br J Plast Surg 1999;52:276–279
10. Stern HS, Nahai F. The versatile superficial inferior epigastric artery free flap. Br J Plast Surg 1992;45:270–274
11. Reardon CM, O'Ceallaigh S, O'Sullivan ST. An anatomical study of the superficial inferior epigastric vessels in humans. Br J Plast Surg 2004;57:515–519
12. Schaverien M, Saint-Cyr M, Arbique G, Brown SA. Arterial and venous anatomies of the deep inferior epigastric perforator and superficial inferior epigastric artery flaps. Plast Reconstr Surg 2008;121:1909–1919
13. Hester TR Jr, Nahai F, Beegle PE, Bostwick J III. Blood supply of the abdomen revisited, with emphasis on the superficial inferior epigastric artery. Plast Reconstr Surg 1984;74:657–670
14. Holm C, Mayr M, Höfter E, Ninkovic M. The versatility of the SIEA flap: a clinical assessment of the vascular territory of the superficial epigastric inferior artery. J Plast Reconstr Aesthet Surg 2007;60:946–951
15. Schlenz I, Kuzbari R, Gruber H, Holle J. The sensitivity of the nipple-areola complex: an anatomic study. Plast Reconstr Surg 2000;105:905–909
16. Granzow JW, Levine JL, Chiu ES, Allen RJ. Breast reconstruction using perforator flaps. J Surg Oncol 2006;94:441–454
17. Ulusal BG, Cheng MH, Wei FC, Ho-Asjoe M, Song D. Breast reconstruction using the entire transverse abdominal adipocutaneous flap based on unilateral superficial or deep inferior epigastric vessels. Plast Reconstr Surg 2006;117:1395–1403, discussion 1404–1406
18. Spiegel AJ, Salazar-Reyes H, Izaddoost S, Khan FN. A novel method for neurotization of deep inferior epigastric perforator and superficial inferior epigastric artery flaps. Plast Reconstr Surg 2009;123:29e–30e
19. Spiegel AJ, Menn ZK, Eldor L, Kaufman Y, Dellon AL. Breast reinnervation: DIEP neurotization using the third anterior intercostal nerve. Plast Reconstr Surg Glob Open 2013;1:e72

6 Gluteal Artery Perforator Flap for Breast Reconstruction

Richard Mahlon Kline, Jr., and James Ernest Craigie

In 1994, Robert J. Allen presented the gluteal artery perforator (GAP) flap for breast reconstruction at a meeting of the American Association of Plastic Surgeons in St. Louis, Missouri. Since that time, GAP flaps have become a reliable option for muscle-sparing autogenous tissue breast reconstruction. Advancements in the field of perforator flaps have increased the donor sites available to microsurgeons for breast reconstruction. Breast reconstruction scenarios are as varied as the human body in regard to shape, form, and volume requirements. When the perforator concept is employed, skin and fat are harvested without requiring removal of the underlying muscle. Also, emphasis is directed away from larger named blood vessels, donor sites confined to a template over certain muscles, and familiar anatomic landmarks. This enables a patient's donor site to be designed based on their distribution of fat and body shape. GAP flaps have been used when the lower abdominal tissues are inadequate to meet the desired result or when previous surgery compromised the lower abdominal perforators. When both the abdomen and the buttock are available and both meet the volume requirement, the flap of choice can be based on the patients' preference about donor-scar location. This is particularly the case in patients who are thinner and who would not benefit from a tummy tuck.

Indications

Gluteal artery perforator flaps are used for unilateral and bilateral cases. Breast reconstruction indications include developmental aplasia and postmastectomy cases. GAP flaps are utilized following mastectomies for both cancer and prophylactic indications. Immediate reconstruction cases include nipple-sparing and skin-sparing mastectomies **(Fig. 6.1)**. When radiation is indicated, a delayed reconstruction may be required following recovery from the radiation. Delayed reconstructions include failed implant cases and failed previous free flap procedures. A superior gluteal artery perforator (SGAP) flap can provide reasonable symmetry with a contralateral breast previously reconstructed with a deep inferior epigastric perforator (DIEP) flap. The gluteal fat and skin can be a very close match for a contralateral DIEP.

Preoperative Planning

Two microsurgeons who are experienced with perforator techniques and principles work together on each case. The primary surgeon meets with the patient the day before surgery at the presurgery planning appointment. At this time surgical markings are placed based on a review of the magnetic resonance angiogram (MRA) and the use of the handheld Doppler. Preoperative imaging with an MRA or a computed tomography angiogram (CTA) greatly enhances the application of the gluteal donor site and the perforator flap concept. Imaging combined with a handheld Doppler exam enables more detailed tailoring of the flap and is particularly helpful for bilateral simultaneous GAP (BSG) flap harvesting.

During the presurgery marking, the MRA is reviewed in detail.[1] The location of the largest GAPs are described by the radiologist using a coordinate system. Each large perforator is measured from a midline reference point on the patient's skin. The reference point is the top of the gluteal crease or tip of the coccyx. The radiologist records the horizontal distance and the vertical distance from the reference point. The perforator location is measured at the point it leaves the muscle, and the location is extrapolated to the position on the skin where the Doppler signal will be heard. It is important to note that the both the MRA and markings are performed with the patient in the prone position.

The images are reviewed, and the best perforators are chosen with regard to size, location, distribution of fat around the perforator, and the intramuscular/submuscular course of each vessel. For a bilateral case, note is made of the most symmetrical pair of perforators on the right and left side **(Fig. 6.2)**. There are two important points to note: (1) whether a perforator is located in the medial or lateral third of the flap, and (2) whether there is a septocutaneous (sc) GAP between the gluteus maximus and medius muscles.[2] The more lateral perforators and sc-GAP will

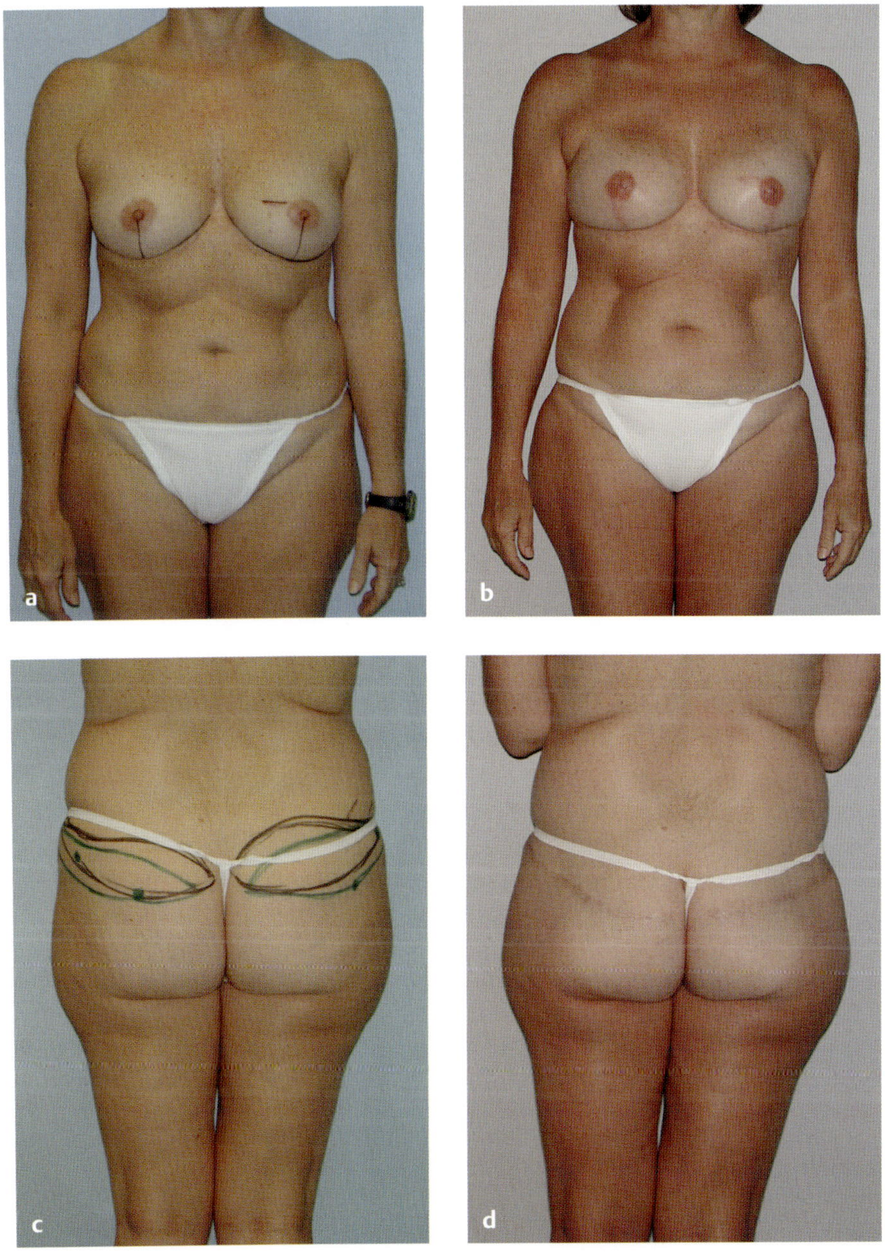

Fig. 6.1 **(a)** Preoperative photograph of a patient requiring bilateral nipple-sparing mastectomy and s bilateral simultaneous gluteal artery perforator (BSG) flap. **(b)** Postoperative photograph at 3 years. **(c)** Preoperative photograph of buttocks with markings. **(d)** Postoperative photograph of buttocks.

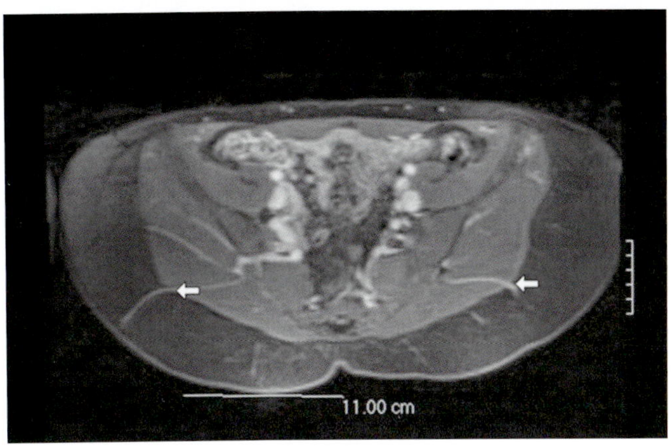

Fig. 6.2 Magnetic resonance angiogram: axial image. *White arrows* point to two superior gluteal artery perforators of large size and similar position on each buttock.

have a more tangential course around the gluteus maximus muscle and result in a longer pedicle, which is preferred. The medial perforators will have a more direct intramuscular course and shorter pedicle. Perforator selection is important for symmetry and for exposure during the microsurgical anastomosis.

If the MRA reveals large laterally positioned perforators, then the flap can be designed more laterally away from the gluteal crease and centered over the thicker fat and large perforator. Also, this places the resulting scar in a more aesthetic position, as it can be covered by underwear or a bathing suit.

The mastectomy defect is measured first or anticipated for immediate reconstruction so that the flap dimensions can be adequate. Caution is needed in patients with large skin requirements, particularly radiation defects. GAP flaps have a lower skin-to-fat thickness ratio and lower skin coverage compared with abdominal skin flaps. Typical skin paddle dimensions are 8 to 9 cm vertically, but occasionally 10 to 11 cm may be needed for significant skin deficits. If it is more than 12 cm, it may be difficult to close, and skin laxity of the donor site should be considered. The width of the skin paddle design varies more with the patient's shape but is typically 20 to 24 cm. Beveling is used to maximize the volume of harvested fat, so that upon reaching the muscle, the flap is longer and wider than the skin measurements. The base measurements are typically 12 to 14 cm, compared with an 8- to 9-cm skin pattern.

To aesthetically design the flap, the patient is marked first in the standing position so that the first flap design is over the most favorable contour of the buttock region. These marks are made without specific reference to the MRA measurements. Care must be taken to make sure the flap is not positioned too high. To avoid missing the dominate perforator, the patient is next marked in the prone position. A second pattern is designed at this time with specific note of the MRA measurements.

The markings are photographed with the patient in the standing position. The photo is taken to the operating room along with the MRA report measurements and the actual MRA disk for use during the surgery. The final markings include skin pattern and fat beveling outlines (**Fig. 6.3**). This becomes very important during bilateral simultaneous flap cases. The primary surgeon performs the markings, but both microsurgeons elevate a flap simultaneously, and the end result must be symmetric. It may be helpful to estimate flap weight at the beginning of the procedure and to attempt to shape the flap accordingly. Results improve with experience and with the surgeons working together.

Surgical Technique

Unilateral reconstruction cases can be done with the patient in the lateral decubitus position. The advantage of the lateral position is that the entire procedure can be done without a position change. The disadvantages of the lateral position are that the donor site is harder to close, and breast surgeons find it more difficult to perform the mastectomy. An alternative is to reposition the unilateral reconstruction patient similarly to a bilateral reconstruction patient.

If the patient is having immediate bilateral reconstruction, the mastectomies must be completed with the patient in the supine position before flap elevation can begin. After the mastectomies, the patient is maintained in the supine position, and the recipient vessels are dissected and prepared. After the recipient vessels are prepared, the patient is repositioned prone for simultaneous flap elevation. Both reconstructive surgeons review the perforator locations and the MRA for their respective flaps. Adjustments may be made in the skin paddle and fat beveling markings. After flap dissection and closure, the patient is returned to the supine position for microsurgical anastomosis and flap insetting.

Preparation of Recipient Site

The internal mammary vessels and perforators are the preferred recipients. The thoracodorsal vessels are used when the internal mammary vessels are not usable due to previous surgery. The gluteal perforator flaps have shorter pedicles than most perforator flaps. However, it is possible to reach the thoracodorsal vessels.

The gluteal vein can have a large diameter. It may be helpful to locate a branching point in the internal mammary vein to result in a larger caliber for better size match when anastomosing to the gluteal vein.

Gluteal Flap Harvest

When beveling of the fat is completed, the flap is elevated from the surface of the gluteus maximus muscle. If a septocutaneous perforator is present, it will be located between the gluteus maximus and medius muscles in the lateral portion of the flap.

Most of the base of the flap should be over the gluteus maximus muscle. When the flap is elevated from lateral to medial, dissection starts above the muscle fascia. When the gluteus maximus muscle is encountered, the dissection should be shifted below the muscle fascia and should progress row by row. This careful approach facilitates visualization of the perforator.

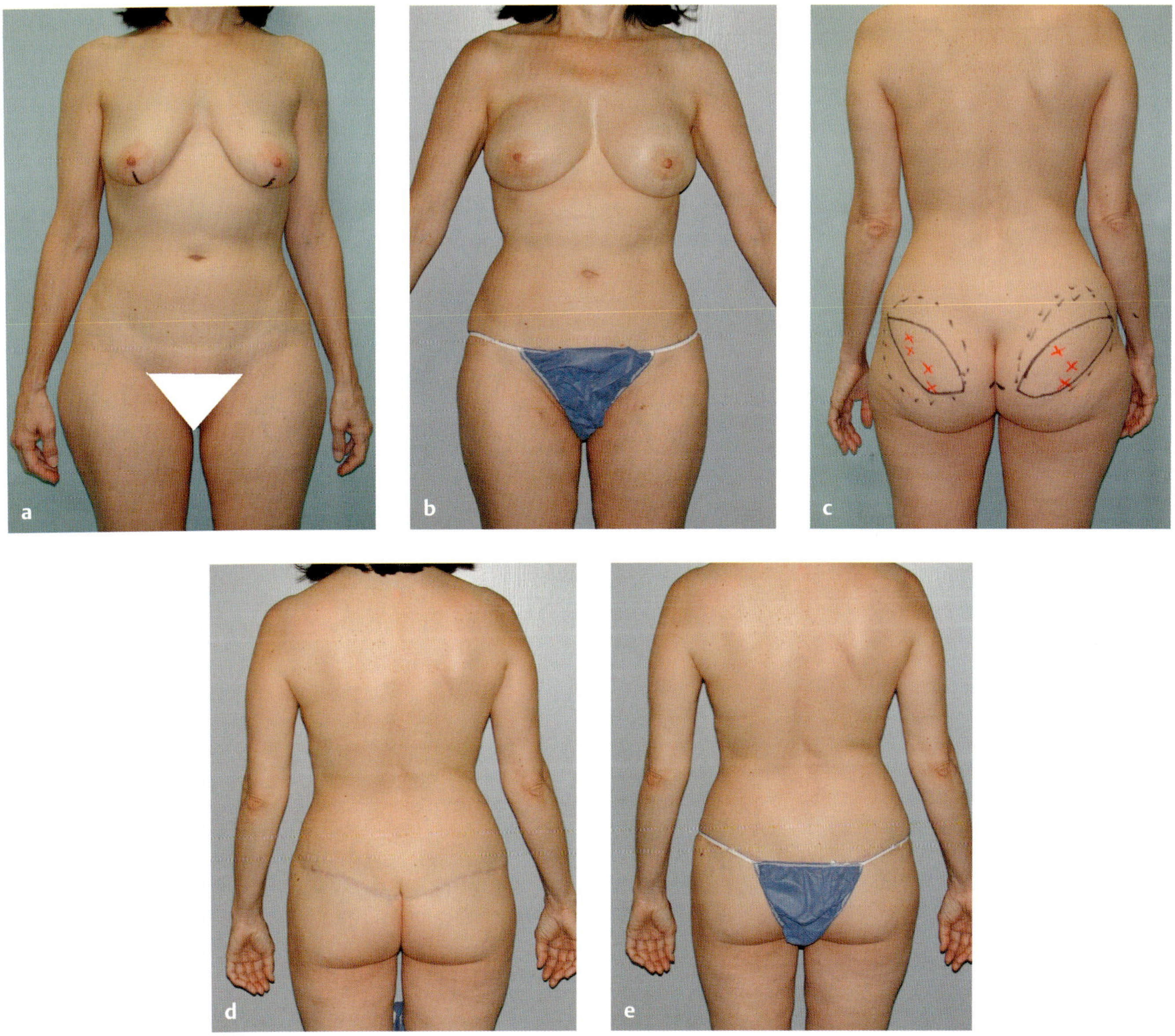

Fig. 6.3 (a) Preoperative photograph in a patient requiring bilateral nipple-sparing mastectomies and a BSG flap. **(b)** Postoperative photograph at 1 year. **(c)** Preoperative photograph of buttocks with markings. Note the skin flap designs, and markings for fat beveling. **(d)** Postoperative photograph of buttocks 1 year after revision surgery. **(e)** Postoperative photograph of buttocks with scar hidden.

The dominate perforator should be encountered and verified prior to dividing any substantial perforators in the central portion of the flap. If there is a question about the location of the target perforator, flap dissection can proceed from the opposite direction.

The flap pedicle dissection begins with the intramuscular course of the perforator. The flap is retracted with Lone Star surgical hooks (Cooper Surgical, Trumbull, CT) and wide exposure is obtained along the muscle fibers. Pedicle dissection continues until the pedicle has adequate length, and the artery and vein size adequately match with the prepared recipients. In our experience this usually requires dissection deep to the muscle. In the submuscular plane, the progress is slower and many side branches are divided carefully **(Fig. 6.4)**. At this point the goal is to identify an artery large enough and a vein not too large for the recipient vessels.

Editor's note: At this point in the procedure a thick layer of fascia is encountered prior to entering a submuscular fat pad. This fascia is divided widely to reveal

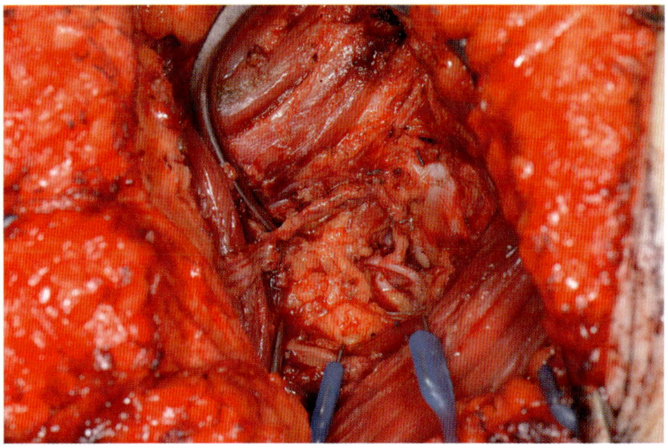

Fig. 6.4 Intraoperative photograph of a superior gluteal artery perforator (SGAP) pedicle deep to muscle, entering "Medusa's head." Note the right-angle branch point.

the gluteal vessels with many branches and tributaries. This part of the vascular anatomy is referred to as Medusa's head, and is potentially hazardous because bleeding here is very difficult to manage. However, it is very important to continue until the donor artery is wide enough to obtain a comfortable match with the internal mammary artery.

The flap is islanded on the chosen perforator and then the flap is harvested. The donor site is closed in layers over a drain and a dressing is placed.

Microsurgical Anastomosis and Insetting

The GAP flaps commonly have shorter pedicles than other perforator flaps used for breast reconstruction, and the fat is usually less flexible. These two factors combined have the potential to make positioning for anastomosis difficult. To secure the flap in place, it can be wrapped in a moistened laparotomy sponge and stapled to the inferior chest skin border of the wound, or stapled or sutured directly to the chest skin. Often, a single temporary 2-0 Vicryl suture is used to tether the inferior skin border of the wound to the perichondrium immediately below the prepared recipient vessels, thus enabling the flap to be placed in slightly better proximity by eliminating a step-off at the wound border. Occasionally, even these maneuvers will not allow the flap to be satisfactorily positioned for anastomosis. In these situations, the flap may be placed within the wound prior to anastomosis and secured to the chest wall (see below), and then its medial aspect may be retracted to provide exposure of the recipient vessels. In addition, or alternatively, the recipient vessels may be dissected further to provide sufficient length. Discretion should be used when considering removal of multiple levels of cartilage and intercostal muscle, however, as this can result in palpable and visible deformities.

The GAP flap pedicle at its most distal aspect has a few unusual properties. First, the vein is often significantly larger in diameter than either the artery or the recipient veins. Second, the length of vessel segments, both arterial and venous, between branch points is often quite short, and as the pedicle joins with larger branches it often does so at nearly right angles. This can have significant implications for clamp positioning during anastomosis, as well as for final pedicle positioning during insetting. There is usually a segment of artery that is very small in diameter, yet essential for pedicle continuity, situated proximal to the larger arterial segment that will be anastomosed to the recipient artery. It is important to avoid damaging this very narrow arterial segment with the microvascular clamp used to facilitate the anastomosis. Additionally, even attempting to flush the artery of the pedicle with heparinized saline can occasionally produce undesired consequences, as the many branch points and sudden caliber changes make the vessel unusually susceptible to iatrogenic damage from the catheter tip.

A mechanical coupler for venous anastomosis is recommend for its expediency and good patency. Rarely, is more than one venous anastomosis per flap indicated, as the vein is always large, and venous communications within the pedicle are extensive. A 9-0 nylon suture is typically used for end-to-end arterial anastomosis, as most arteries lack sufficient compliance to be joined with the mechanical coupler. The right-angle branching pattern often seen in the artery can sometimes make it difficult to position the arterial and venous portions of the pedicle in favorable orientations simultaneously. In this situation, conversion of the largest distal arterial segment to a Carrel patch allows 90-degree reorientation of the artery. In addition to simplifying orientation of the pedicle, conversion to a Carrel patch may reduce the risk of potentially thrombogenic nonlaminar blood flow by removing a sharp turn and a blind segment within the proximal pedicle.

Typically the largest (or only) vein on either side of the sternum will be medial, and therefore this is most commonly used for the single venous anastomosis. When the arterial anastomosis is completed lateral to the vein, it will form a shorter arc than the vein does as it moves away from the sternum toward the flap. Theoretically, the total artery length (internal mammary artery [IMA] + flap artery) should then be a little less than the total venous length to minimize the potential for arterial kinking. This is potentially a less important issue with the GAP flap than it is with some others (such as the DIEP flap) due to the unusual segmented nature of the GAP pedicle, but it nonetheless may be helpful to consider this in certain situations.

Perforator Pedicle Thrombosis

Postoperative vascular compromise is rarely caused by anastomotic problems, but more commonly the result of conformational changes in the pedicle. This assertion is supported by the following observations: First, the relatively consistently high quality and caliber of the internal mammary artery, combined with improved venous patency due to use of the intraoperative coupler device, has served to significantly reduce the incidence of anastomotic problems. Second, the perforator flap pedicle, with its decreased diameter (and often considerable length in non-GAP perforator flaps), typically deforms more easily when met with external forces than do non-perforator pedicles due to its higher compliance. Third, flaps for breast reconstruction tend to be bulky, and are subjected to significant changes in vectors of forces acting upon them as patients mobilize from the supine to the upright position in the postoperative period. Looking at these factors, one can conclude that the shifts in the flap position that occur with postoperative mobilization, combined with a pedicle that is susceptible to deformation from external forces, result in the conformational changes of the pedicle observed when reexploring for vascular compromise.

To secure the flap into position and reduce the risk of movement that could compromise blood flow in the pedicle, the flap is anchored at its deep surface only, placing sutures 2 to 3 cm inferior to the pedicle throughout its course. The sutures pass through the fascia at the deep surface of the flap, through the entire thickness of the pectoralis major muscle inferior to the muscle trough, and through periosteum or perichondrium. Skeletal fixation is important, as the pectoralis muscle is often fairly mobile, and fixation to it alone may not adequately stabilize the flap. With these sutures in place, the flap/pectoralis/chest wall becomes a fixed unit, and the pedicle is reliably protected from torsion and pressure within the muscle trough. There are some scenarios, most notably when prior attempts at prosthetic reconstruction in the submuscular plane have taken place, when the remaining pectoralis muscle may not be adequate to fabricate a trough. In this situation, the periprosthetic capsule, usually abundantly available in this setting, may be harvested and sutured to the chest wall in multiple layers to fabricate a trough, thereby mimicking the lower border of the transected muscle **(Fig. 6.5)**.

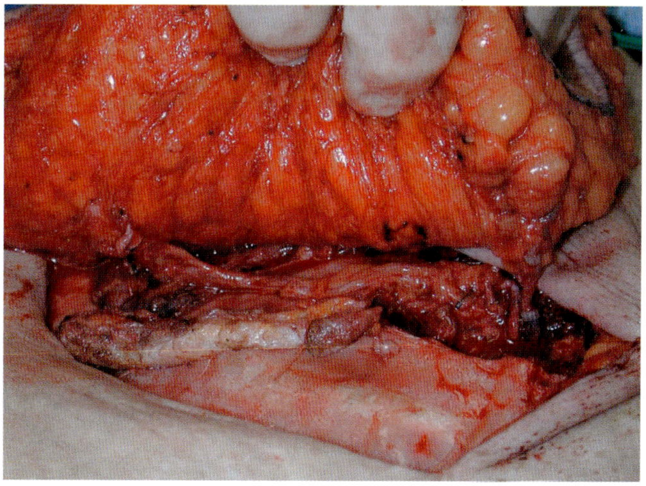

Fig. 6.5 Intraoperative photograph of a double layer of capsule sutured to the chest wall to fabricate a trough for the pedicle to lie in.

Second-Stage Surgery

Most patients require a second-stage revision of the reconstructed breasts or the donor-site incisions or both. Approximately 3 months following the first-stage reconstruction, second-stage procedures are performed. The buttock donor site is prone to contour deformities if healing problems develop. Contour deformities may be significant when seromas develop in combination with wound separation. In the rare event of a complicated wound healing problem and a persistent seroma, the following wound management can be helpful. The treatment includes combining a wound vacuum-assisted closure (VAC) device and a 19-French fluted Blake drain. The drain is first passed through the custom-shaped sponge and the grooves left in contact with the sponge. The tubing that normally connects to the bulb is excised. The functioning end of the drain is then positioned in the seroma cavity itself, which is usually located in the undermined area of the donor site. This approach allows the negative pressure generated in the wound VAC sponge to be directed to loculated pockets that would not be addressed with the sponge alone. As the wound heals, the drain is progressively pulled out and shortened with each wound VAC dressing change. Patients who do not have a healing complication may still develop a contour deformity of the buttock and may desire repair. An overlapping "pants over vest" fasciocutaneous flaps is useful **(Fig. 6.6)**. This approach makes it possible to precisely reposition the buttock scar in a more aesthetic position. The overlapping layers correct the contour depression resulting from flap harvesting and seroma development. Fat grafting may also be helpful for contour deformities that are less significant.

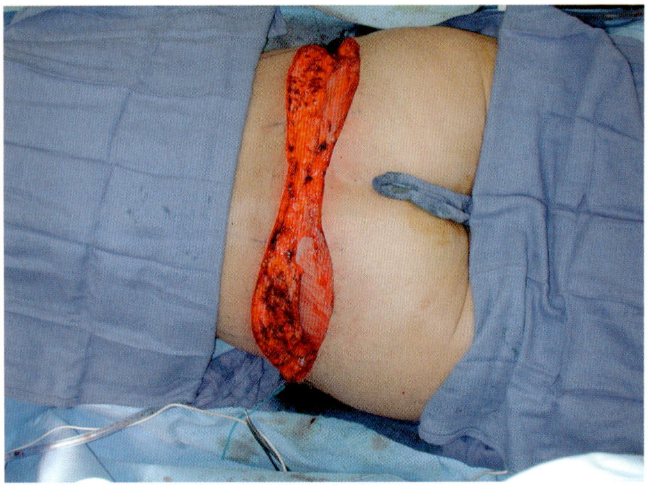

Fig. 6.6 Photograph of a second-stage revision donor site showing the "pants over vest" fasciocutaneous flaps.

Conclusion

Gluteal artery perforator flaps are a useful option for microsurgical breast reconstruction. The learning curve can be steep, but the techniques described in this chapter can improve results and minimize failure. The buttock donor site is amenable to the freestyle[3] concept of flap design, in which the flap encompasses the most beneficial tissue, given each patient's shape and reconstruction requirements. The limitations of the buttock donor site include intraoperative patient repositioning and, for bilateral cases, the need for two microsurgeons working simultaneously to create a symmetrical result. These hurdles can be managed effectively by a well-trained operative team and cooperation between two microsurgeons with expertise in perforator flaps. Preoperative planning and the use of preoperative imaging have also helped improve results and shorten operative times.

References

1. Vasile JV, Newman TM, Prince MR, et al. Contrast-enhanced magnetic resonance angiography. Clin Plast Surg 2011;38:263–275
2. Tuinder S, Chen CM, Massey MF, Allen RJ Sr, Van der Huist R. Introducing the septocutaneous gluteal artery perforator flap: a simplified approach to microsurgical breast reconstruction. Plast Reconstr Surg 2011;127:489–495
3. Wei FC, Celik N. Perforator flap entity. Clin Plast Surg 2003;30:325–329

7 Profunda Artery Perforator Flap for Breast Reconstruction

Robert J. Allen, Maria M. LoTiempo, and Constance M. Chen

Since its introduction by Allen[1] in 1992, the deep inferior epigastric artery perforator flap has become the gold standard for breast reconstruction. However, the lower abdomen is not an option in 25% of women. Absolute contraindications include previous abdominoplasty, and relative contraindications include previous liposuction, certain abdominal operations, and a paucity of subcutaneous fat. The profunda artery perforator (PAP) flap described by Allen[2,3] in 2010 is our first consideration if the abdomen is not a viable option. Other choices include the superior or inferior gluteal artery flaps[3,4] the thigh gluteal artery perforator (GAP) flap, and the lateral thigh flap.

The blood supply to the muscles surrounding the profunda artery perforators, specifically the adductor, has been described by Angrigiani et al.[5] The dominant blood supply to the posterior thigh is from the profunda artery perforators. The PAP flap has been used for breast reconstruction in over 200 cases over the past 4 years.

Indications

The ideal candidates for the PAP flap have breasts of small to moderate size, with excess body fat below the waist. A woman with a pear-shaped figure is a better candidate than one with an apple-shaped figure. Many of our patients have had previous abdominal surgery such as abdominoplasty, but a significant percentage of PAP patients have a paucity of abdominal fat, with more fat in the posterior thigh. Preoperative imaging with magnetic resonance angiography (MRA) or computed tomography angiography (CTA) is recommended on all patients to facilitate perforator mapping and dissection, and to reduce the operative time **(Fig. 7.1)**.

Vascular Anatomy

The profunda femoris artery arises from the common femoral artery ~3.5 cm distal to the inguinal ligament. Initially lateral to the femoral artery, it spirals posterior to the ligament to reach the medial side of the femur. The profunda femoris artery enters the posterior compartment of the thigh and gives off three main perforators. The first perforator is preferred as the pedicle to the PAP flap due to its more medial location and more ideal perfusion pattern.

Preoperative Planning

Preoperative markings are applied in the office the day prior to surgery. The patient starts in the standing position, and the inferior gluteal fold is marked for the superior extent of the incision. The second marking is 6 to 7 cm below this line, which is the lower extent of the skin flap. The lateral marking extends to the end of the infragluteal crease or slightly lateral to it. The patient is then moved to the supine position with the thigh in abduction, and the medial marking begins just posterior to the lymphatic-rich inguinal area posterior to the adductor longus muscle. The transverse crescent pattern is typically 26 cm × 7 cm. Then with the patient in the prone position, the key perforator[6] is marked based on the preoperative imaging. The key perforator is usually 3 to 6 cm below the infragluteal crease and within 4 cm of the posterior border of the gracilis muscle. The handheld Doppler confirms the location of the perforator(s). Most patients have adequate perforators through the adductor magnus muscle for the PAP flap, but sometimes the best perforator may be inferior to the skin island. In this case a perforator off the descending branch of the inferior gluteal artery (thigh gluteal artery flap) or more lateral profunda femoris perforator may be used. Another option with an inferiorly located perforator is to lower the skin pattern in a "boomerang" fashion to capture the key perforator.

Surgical Technique

The patient is placed in the supine position, and the lower extremities are prepped and draped into the sterile field. A two-team approach is used throughout much of the procedure. The skin incision is made with the thigh abducted

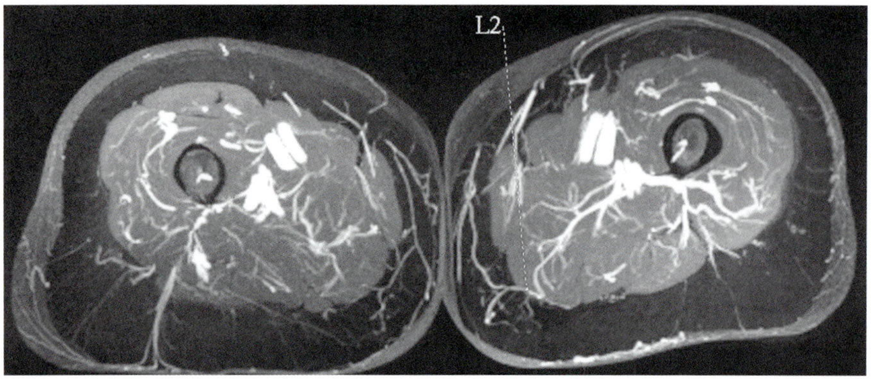

Fig. 7.1 Preoperative imaging with magnetic resonance angiography (MRA) or computed tomography angiography (CTA) is recommended on all patients to facilitate perforator mapping and dissection, and to reduce the operative time. Magnetic resonance angiography demonstrates a large perforator through the adductor magnus muscle. The perforator is located 2 cm posterior to the gracilis and 4 cm below the infragluteal fold.

for most of the incision and adducted for the most lateral incision. Superiorly beveling is avoided, particularly near the weight-bearing ischial fat pad, thus preserving it. Inferiorly the amount of beveling depends on the volume needed and the location of the key perforator. The flap is elevated from anterior to posterior. The gracilis fascia is opened vertically near the posterior border of the gracilis, retracting the muscle anteriorly. An incision is then made through the posterior gracilis fascia and on through the adductor magnus fascia. After elevating the adductor magnus fascia, the key perforator is located and followed through the muscle to its origin from the profunda femoris artery. It is important to reach the yellow fat space beyond the adductor magnus muscle before dividing the pedicle. This gives a pedicle length of 8 to 12 cm, with an average diameter of 2.2 mm of the artery and 2.7 mm of the vein. Once the flap harvest is completed, the donor site is closed in multiple layers over a suction drain, which is left in place for at least a week. The internal mammary vessels are most commonly used as recipient vessels, but the thoracodorsal vessels can be used as well. For insetting, the PAP flap is usually coned. A skin island is left for postoperative monitoring; it is removed at the second stage in nipple-sparing mastectomies. The total time for the PAP flap harvest ranges from 40 to 90 minutes **(Fig. 7.2)**.

Postoperative Care

After 1 to 2 hours in the recovery room, the patient is transferred to a regular room. The flap is checked every 4 hours, with a focus on evaluating the skin island. Photographic evaluation of the skin island is an extremely accurate method of monitoring. Nonsteroidal anti-inflammatory drugs are the mainstay of analgesia management. The intravenous (IV) and Foley catheters are removed the morning after surgery; then a regular diet is started and the patient begins ambulating. The patient is discharged 2 to 4 days after surgery.

Case Studies

Example 1: A patient with ductal carcinoma of the left breast. A PAP flap and bilateral mastopexy were performed **(Figs. 7.3** and **7.4)**.

Example 2: A patient with *BRCA1* gene mutation. A bilateral nipple-sparing mastectomy with PAP flaps was performed **(Fig. 7.5)**.

Example 3: A patient with carcinoma of the left breast. A thigh gluteal artery perforator (TGAP) flap was performed **(Figs. 7.6** and **7.7)**.

Discussion

In our experience with over 200 PAP flap breast reconstructions, all have been successful. Small areas of fat necrosis have been addressed at the second stage in fewer than 10% of flaps. Donor-site seromas occur in 10% of cases and resolved with aspiration or drain placement.

The posterior thigh is a potential donor site in most women. It is not uncommon that one flap is not quite enough to reconstruct one breast. Two flaps are often used for breast reconstruction. For bilateral reconstruction, our preference is to reconstruct each breast with a combined PAP and deep inferior epigastric perforator (DIEP) flap. Stacked PAP flaps for unilateral reconstruction can yield

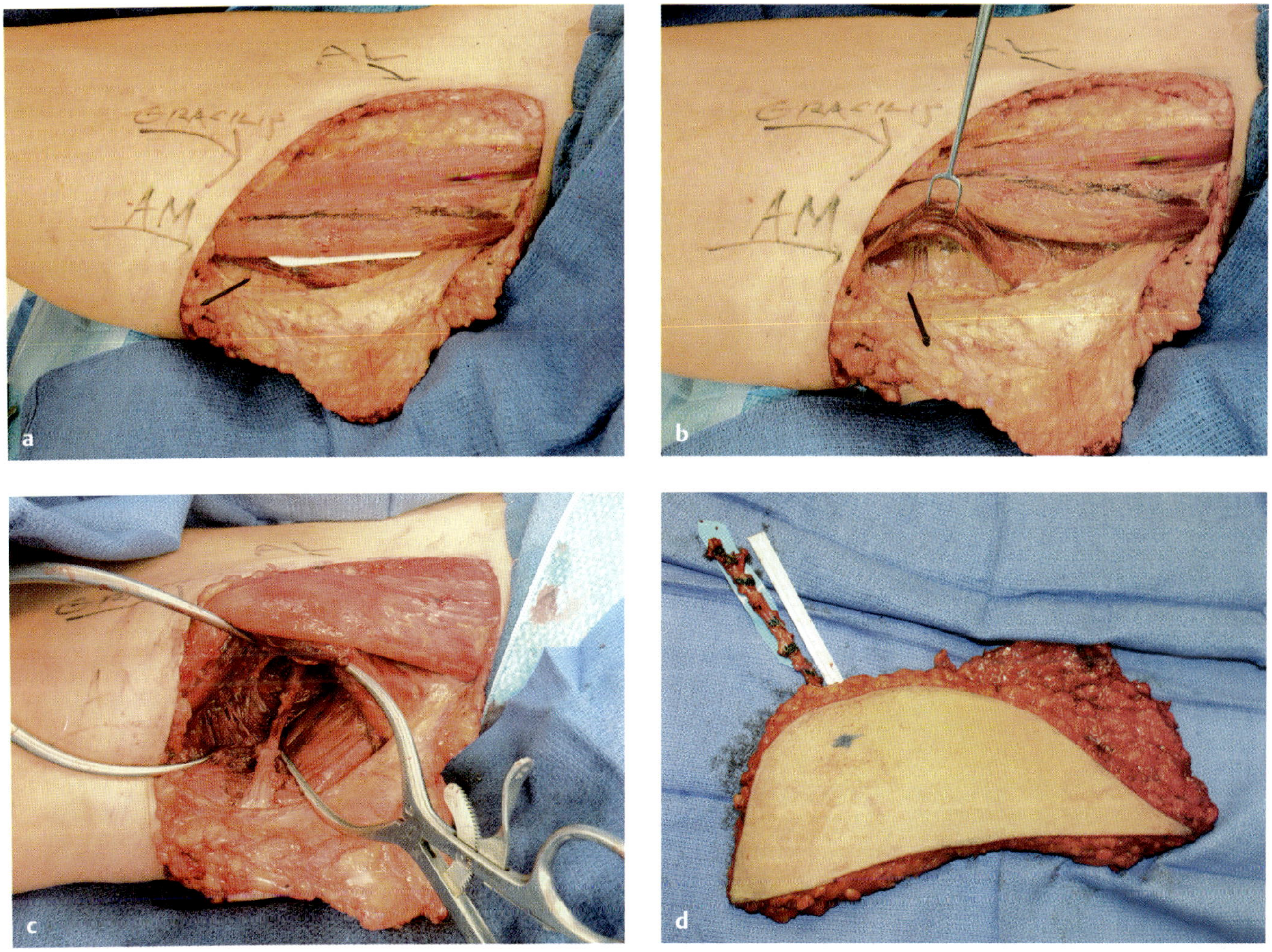

Fig. 7.2 (a) The gracilis fascia is opened vertically near the posterior border of the gracilis, retracting the muscle anteriorly. An incision is then made through the posterior gracilis fascia and on through the adductor magnus fascia. **(b)** By elevating the adductor magnus fascia, the key perforator is confirmed and followed through the muscle to its origin from the profunda femoris artery. **(c)** It is important to reach the yellow fat space beyond the adductor magnus muscle before dividing the pedicle, which gives **(d)** a pedicle length of 8 to 12 cm with an average diameter of 2.2 mm of the artery and 2.7 mm of the vein.

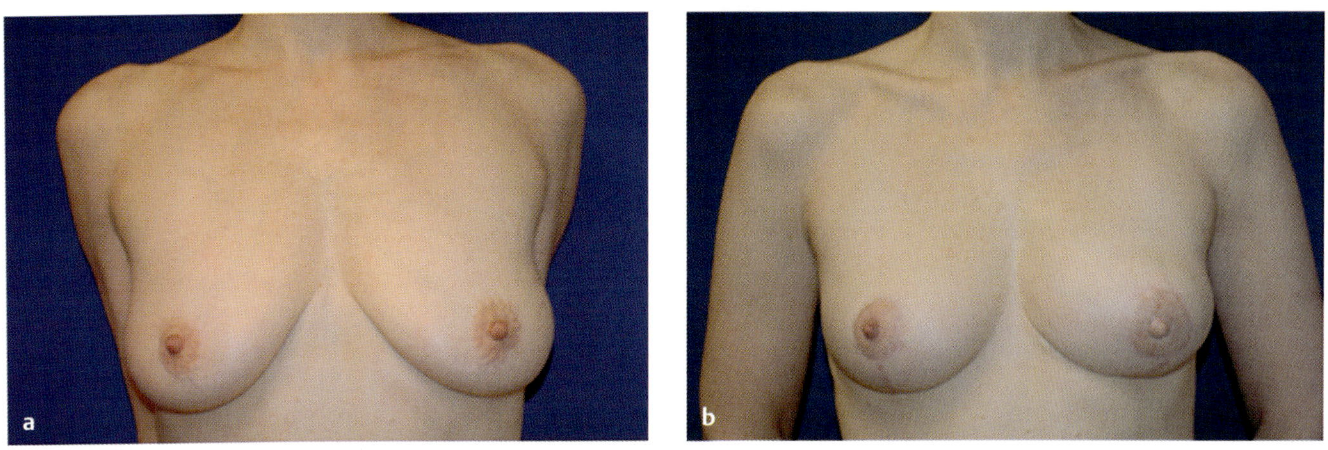

Fig. 7.3 A patient with ductal carcinoma of the left breast was treated with a left profunda artery perforator (PAP) flap with a bilateral mastopexy. **(a)** Preoperative. **(b)** Postoperative.

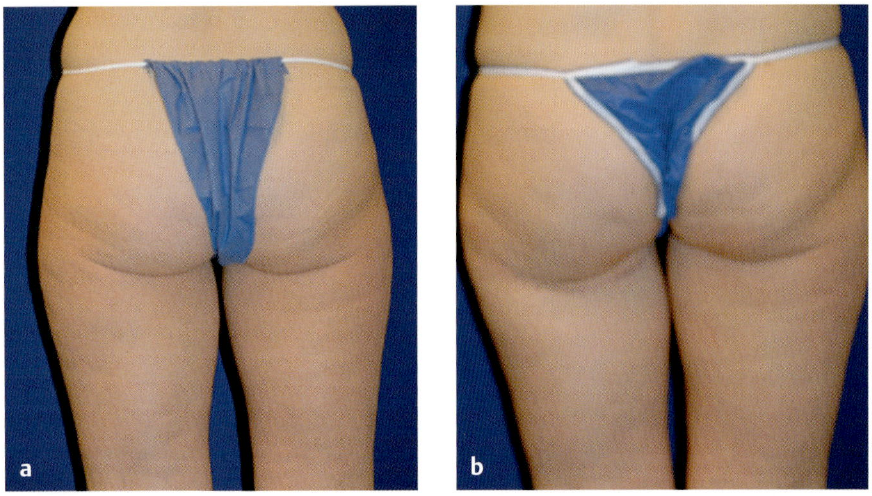

Fig. 7.4 Views of the donor site for the procedure in **Fig. 7.3. (a)** Preoperative. **(b)** Postoperative.

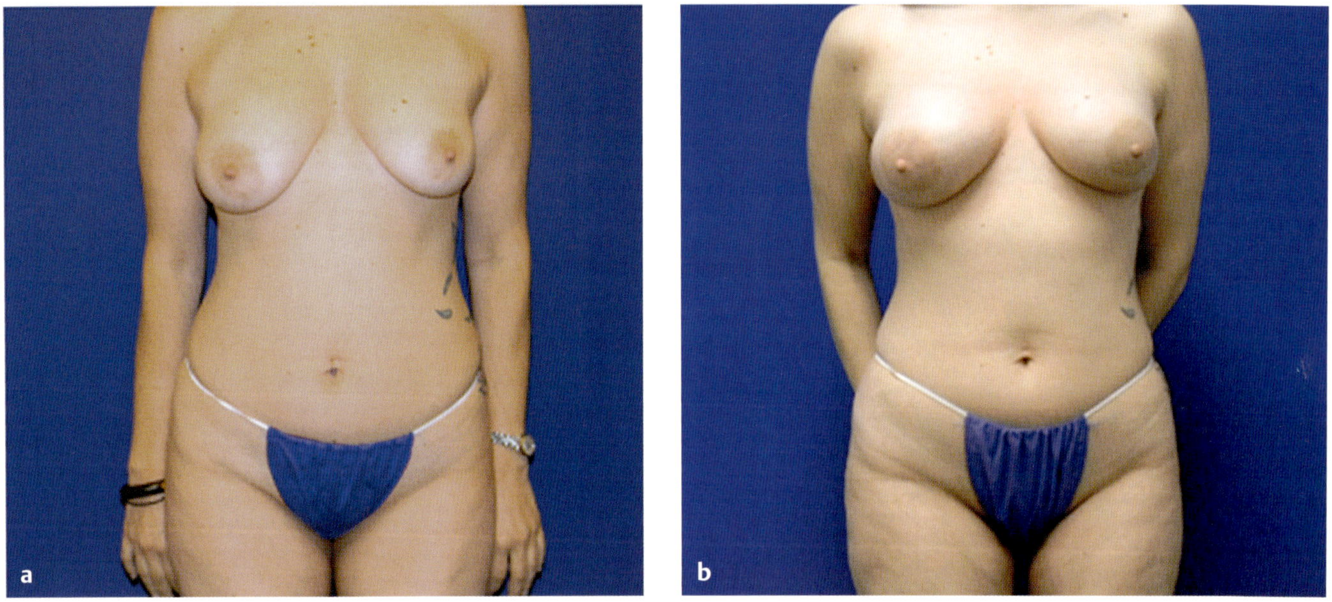

Fig. 7.5 A patient with a *BRCA1* gene mutation was treated with a bilateral nipple-sparing mastectomy with PAP flaps. **(a)** Preoperative. **(b)** Postoperative.

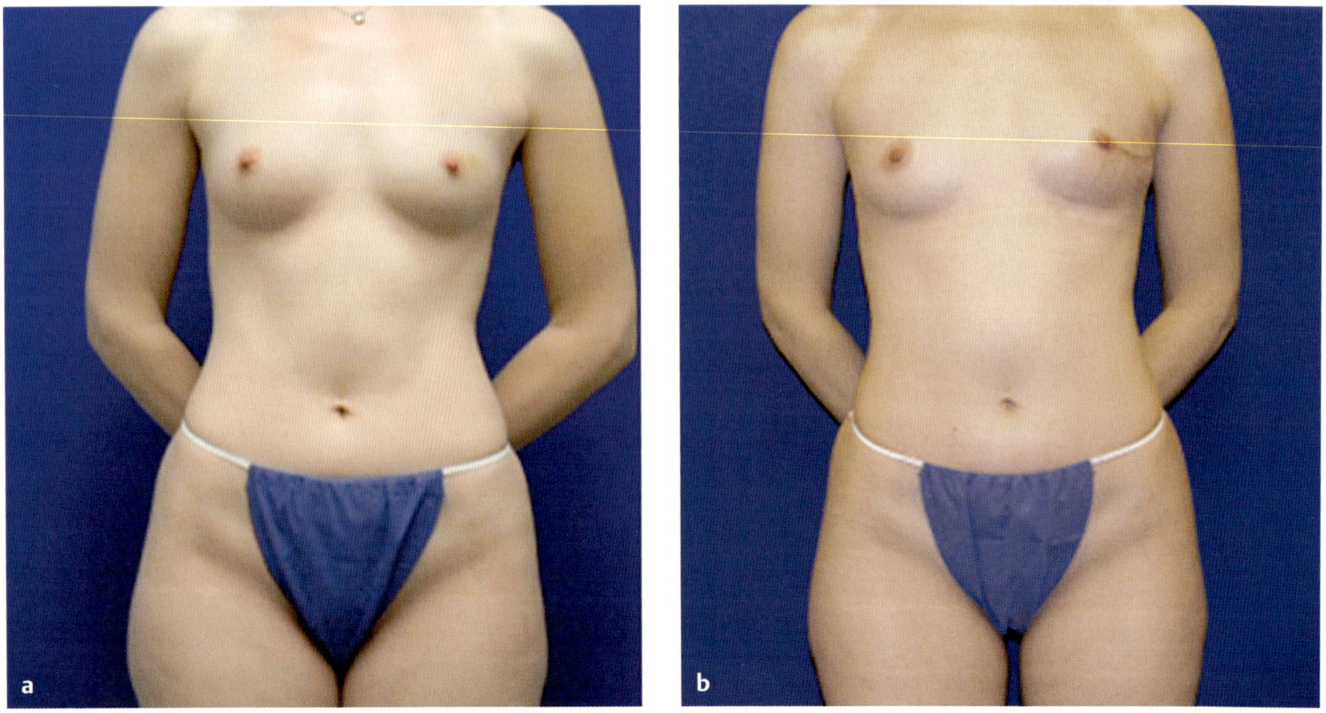

Fig. 7.6 A patient with carcinoma of the left breast was treated with a thigh gluteal artery perforator (TGAP) flap. **(a)** Preoperative. **(b)** Postoperative.

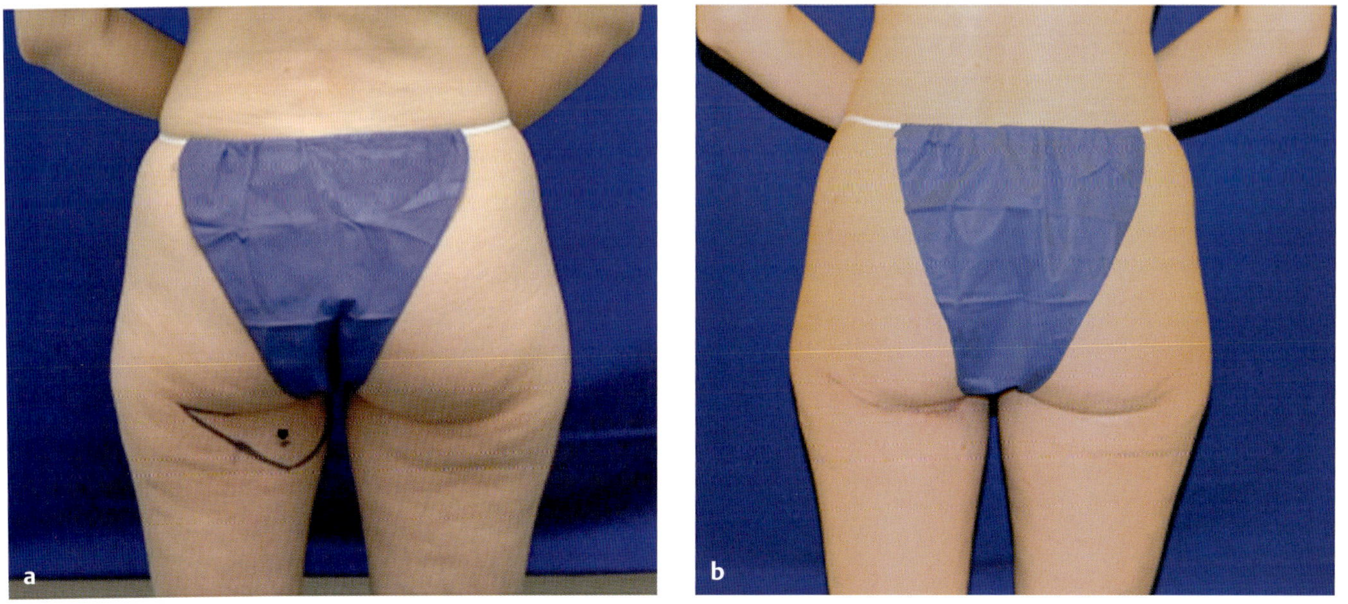

Fig. 7.7 Views of the donor site for the procedure in **Fig. 7.6. (a)** Preoperative. **(b)** Postoperative.

outstanding results. The PAP flap can also be combined with an intercostal artery perforator (ICAP) flap, using the PAP flap for the medial two thirds of the reconstruction and the ICAP flap for the lateral third.

Another advantage of the PAP flap is an artery and vein that matches the internal mammary recipient vessels well. The average 10-cm pedicle length makes the anastomoses and insetting quite easy. The crescent design provides a nice three-dimensional breast shape. Unlike GAP flaps, PAP flaps do not affect buttock contour. Adequate flap volume is routinely obtained to match the mastectomy weight despite a wide range of height and weight. PAP flap harvest avoids dissection near the inguinal lymphatics and has not resulted in any cases of lymphedema. This has been used as sensate flaps based on branches from the posterior cutaneous nerve of the thigh entering the deep surface of the flap.

Conclusion

Since its introduction in 2010, the PAP flap has rapidly become the choice for autogenous breast reconstruction when the DIEP is not a good option. The PAP flap provides a long pedicle with excellent vessel diameter, preserves muscle and function, can be optimally coned, and results in a well-hidden scar with good donor-site contour. The PAP flap is to the transverse upper gracilis (TUG) flap what the DIEP is to the transverse rectus abdominis musculocutaneous (TRAM) flap.

References

1. Allen RJ, Treece P. Deep inferior epigastric perforator flap for breast reconstruction. Ann Plast Surg 1994;32:32–38
2. Allen RJ, Haddock NT, Ahn CY, Sadeghi A. Breast reconstruction with the profunda artery perforator flap. Plast Reconstr Surg 2012; 129:16e–23e
3. Chen CM, LoTempio M, Allen RJ. Profunda artery perforator (PAP) flap for breast reconstruction. In: Spiegel AJ, ed. Breast Reconstruction: Current Perspectives and State of the Art Techniques. Rijeka, Croatia: InTech; 2013:161–171
4. Allen RJ, Tucker C Jr. Superior gluteal artery perforator free flap for breast reconstruction. Plast Reconstr Surg 1995;95:1207–1212
5. Angrigiani C, Grilli D, Thorne CH. The adductor flap: a new method for transferring posterior and medial thigh skin. Plast Reconstr Surg 2001;107:1725–1731
6. LoTempio MM, Allen RJ. Breast reconstruction with SGAP and IGAP flaps. Plast Reconstr Surg 2010;126:393–401

8 Free Lumbar Artery Perforator Flap for Autologous Breast Reconstruction

Koenraad Van Landuyt and Steven F. Morris

The development of the deep inferior epigastric perforator (DIEP) flap provided a major boost to the popularity of autologous breast reconstructions.[1,2] Unfortunately, with this increased demand there is a growing number of patients who may not be candidates for a DIEP flap because of scarring of the abdomen or, more frequently, because of a previous contralateral DIEP flap reconstruction, previous abdominoplasty, or insufficient abdominal volume. Although several methods have been developed to try to overcome a lack of volume, including harvesting additional venous outflow, bipedicled flaps, stacking of flaps, secondary lipofilling, or even adding a prosthesis, sometimes the abdomen is just not a good option as a donor site. In addition, some patients are not willing to accept the abdominal scar.

This led to the development of alternative donor sites, mostly around the gluteal area. The first of these was the traditional superior gluteal artery perforator (SGAP) flap.[3,4] However, at the dawn of perforator flap surgery, the drawbacks of a shorter pedicle, a more difficult dissection, cosmetic issues with a buttock scar, and the need of patient repositioning made the SGAP flap less desirable as an option.

New alternatives needed to be developed, and surgeons turned their attention downward to the inferior gluteal artery perforator (IGAP) flap[5–7]; the transverse gracilis muscle (TMG) flap,[8,9] either in its traditional myocutaneous form or perforator based; and lately the profunda artery perforator (PAP) flap.[10,11] Others looked for alternatives superiorly by slanting the SGAP flap superiorly, or by taking it higher on the upper part of the buttock on the septal superior gluteal artery perforators,[12] to try to minimize the donor-site contour deformity, which can be another disadvantage of the SGAP flap. Now that more surgeons are acquainted with, and feel comfortable performing, perforator flap dissection, the lumbar artery perforator (LAP) flap can be a valuable alternative in selected patients.

The LAP flaps were mainly introduced as local pedicled flaps to close defects in the lower back area. In 1988, Kroll and Rosenfield[13] described a local flap based on lumbar artery perforators, although the perforators were unnamed at that time. Other authors clarified the use of local LAP flaps for reconstruction of the lumbosacral region.[14–17]

The free LAP flap was first published as a case report in 2003 by de Weerd et al,[18] as an alternative free flap for autologous breast reconstruction. Though the LAP flap has gained greater acceptance, until now no major series have been published.

Anatomy

Four pairs of lumbar arteries arise from the posterior lumbar aorta. These are large 4-mm vessels that pass posteriorly to supply the posterior lumbar angiosomes including muscle, skin, and bone. The lumbar arteries then pass along the vertebrae and between the transverse processes before splitting into dorsal and abdominal branches. The dorsal branches have a variable course through the psoas major, quadratus lumborum, and erector spinae muscles or through the intermuscular septa (**Fig. 8.1**). The lumbar arteries anastomose freely with each other and the other main source vessels in the region, including the intercostal, subcostal, iliolumbar, and deep circumflex femoral arteries. The dorsal branch also gives off a spinal branch, which enter the vertebral canal. There have been several previous reports of the vascular anatomy of the region.[19–22]

In a study of seven fresh cadavers injected with lead oxide, we performed three-dimensional (3D) angiography to capture the distribution, size, and course of the lumbar artery perforators, which arise from the paired lumbar arteries (L1, L2, L3, and L4)[23] (**Fig. 8.2**). Most pairs pass posterior to the quadratus lumborum, but some take a route through the muscle. The L1 to L3 arteries course between quadratus lumborum and the erector spinae muscles, whereas the L4 vessels generally pass anterior to quadratus lumborum. Once the lumbar arteries pass the lumbosacral fascia, they branch into smaller vessels

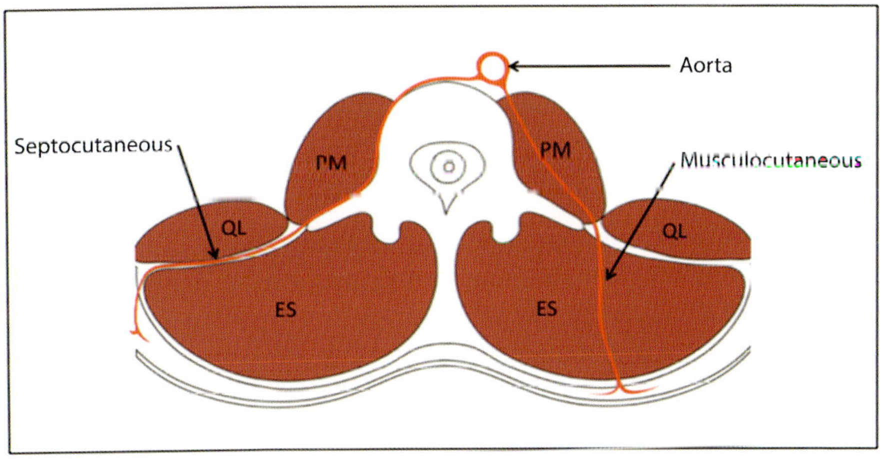

Fig. 8.1 Anatomy of the lumbar perforators as related to musculature: ES, erector spinae; PM, psoas major; QL, quadratus lumborum.

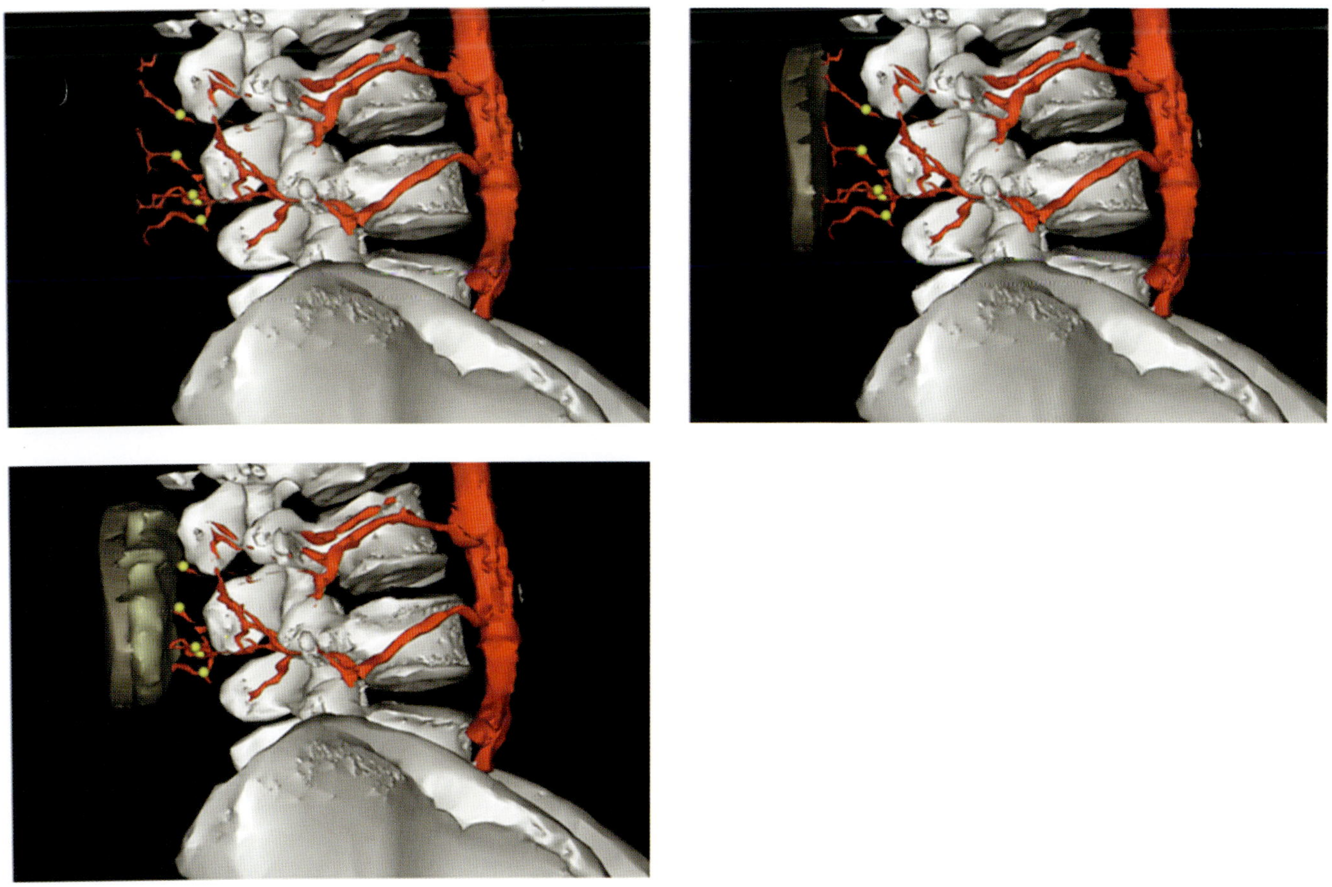

Fig. 8.2 3D reconstruction of the course of the different lumbar perforators.

supplying the lumbar integument. We observed that the individual perforator anatomy was quite variable, but in general the L4 perforators were often septocutaneous, whereas the L1 perforators were mostly musculocutaneous. Individual perforator anatomy was highly variable but septocutaneous perforators usually passed between the quadratus lumborum and erector spinae. Computed tomography angiography (CTA) shows the 3D course of lumbar artery perforators. More perforators arise from the L1 and L4 than from L2 and L3. Perforators measure ~1 mm in diameter where they penetrate the lumbosacral fascia (**Fig. 8.3**).

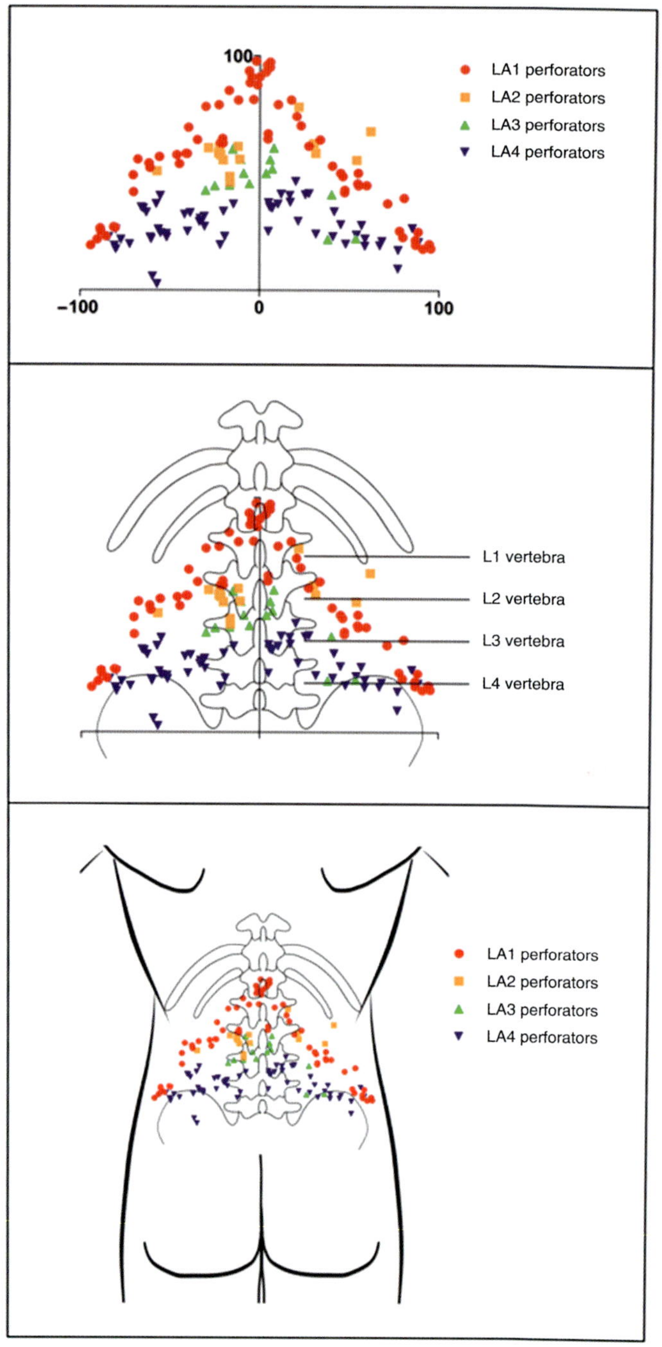

Fig. 8.3 Topographical distribution of the different lumbar perforators as they pierce the skin.

Indications

The DIEP flap reconstruction remains the workhorse of autologous breast reconstruction, as it does in our hands. However, as mentioned above, some patients seeking autologous reconstruction are not especially good candidates for DIEP flap reconstruction. Patients who underwent a failed DIEP flap procedure or who developed a secondary tumor in the contralateral breast after a previous DIEP flap reconstruction cannot have another DIEP flap. Also, some patients are seeking preventive bilateral subcutaneous mastectomy and immediate reconstruction because of genetic or familial breast cancer predisposition.

Surgical Procedure

Before surgery, the size, position, and course of the lumbar perforators is checked on a preoperative computed tomography (CT) or MRA scan. The patient should be positioned face down for the scan, so that the gluteal/lumbar perforators are not compresses. The X-axis is provided either by a horizontal radiopaque marker or by the height of the iliac crest (**Fig. 8.4**). The lowermost lumbar perforator (L4), crossing the posterior iliac crest, is usually preferred to enable positioning of the scar as low as possible.

With the patient in standing position, the skin island is marked as needed on top of the posterior iliac crest, pinching the posterior "love handles." The skin island is marked as low as possible above the gluteal prominence, slightly slanting upward from medial to lateral, mimicking the skin excision of a posterior buttock lift; however, care should be taken not to cross the posterior midline. In a primary breast reconstruction, the skin island should be kept as small as possible to avoid problems with donor-site closure; skin islands of 8 to 10 cm can be fairly easily closed. Vertical marks enable perfect closure of the donor site (**Fig. 8.5**). If a bilateral procedure is planned, the opposite side is marked symmetrically and covered with an

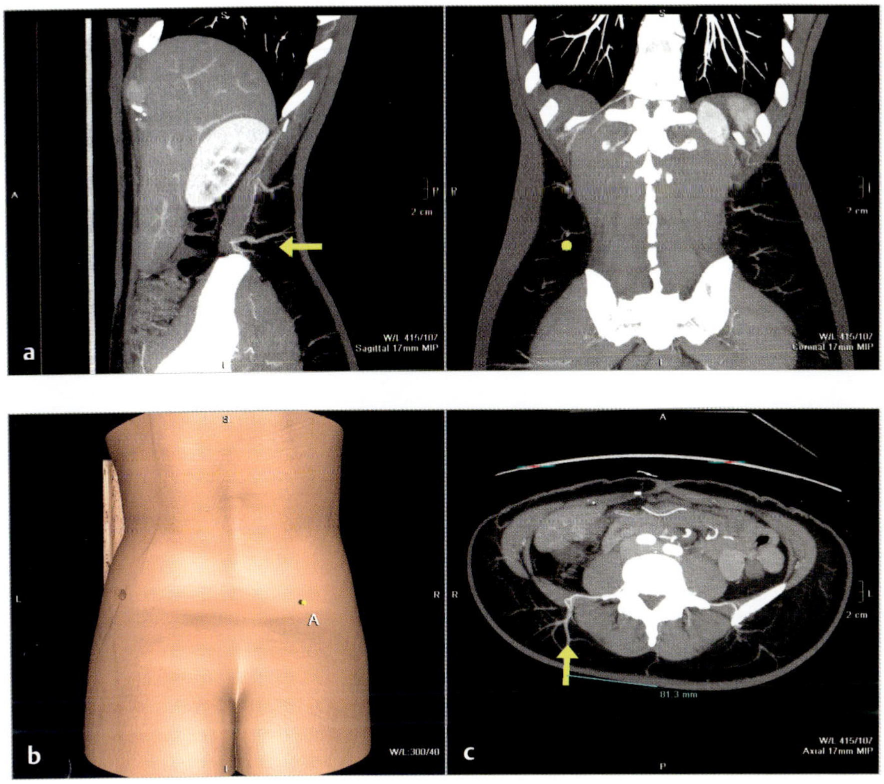

Fig. 8.4 **(a)** Computed tomography (CT) scan of a lumbar perforator, sagittal and coronal views. **(b)** Three-dimensional (3D) reconstruction of the perforators of the lumbar region. **(c)** Note the close proximity to the iliac bone and with the bone, the origin of the pedicle, crossing the foramen intervertebrale In front of the processus transversus.

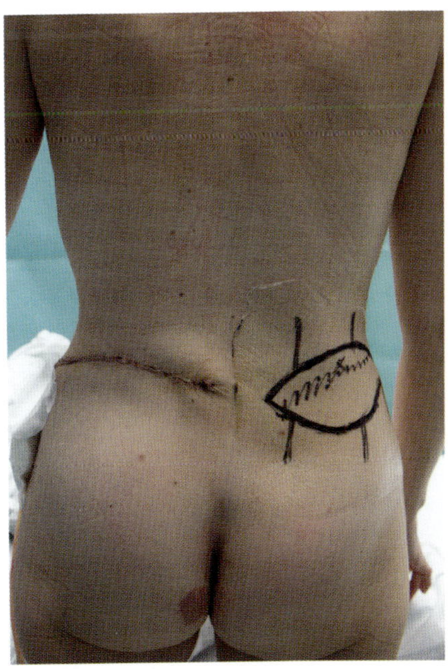

Fig. 8.5 Preoperative marking of the patient in standing position, dorsal view, for the second intervention 4 days after a previous left-sided lumbar artery perforator (LAP) reconstruction. Both markings are done simultaneously and are protected on the right side by a transparent dressing.

Opsite^{R} (Smith & Nephew, Andover, MA) dressing to save the drawings until the second intervention **(Fig. 8.6)**.

Markings on the chest are also performed with the patient in the standing position, including a small incision line in the groin area for the eventual harvest of an inferior epigastric pedicle graft.

The patient is repositioned on the operation table, face down, for transfer of the CT markings of the perforator in the same position as the patient was positioned in the scanner **(Fig. 8.7)**. Markings can be adjusted slightly to include the emergence of the perforator in the design of the flap, but should be kept as low as possible to prevent a high-rising scar.

After intubation and preparation of the patient (two peripheral IV lines, bladder catheter), she is placed in the lateral decubitus position, with the torso slightly twisted and the shoulder back to enable simultaneous surgery of the donor (LAP flap) and recipient (breast, vascular graft) sites; the ipsilateral arm is fixed in 90 degrees of flexion and 90 degrees of abduction, enabling eventual positioning of the microscope over the chest **(Fig. 8.8)**. Positioning of the patient should accommodate flexing the bed at the lumbar level, facilitating the dissection; breaking is released at the time of closure.

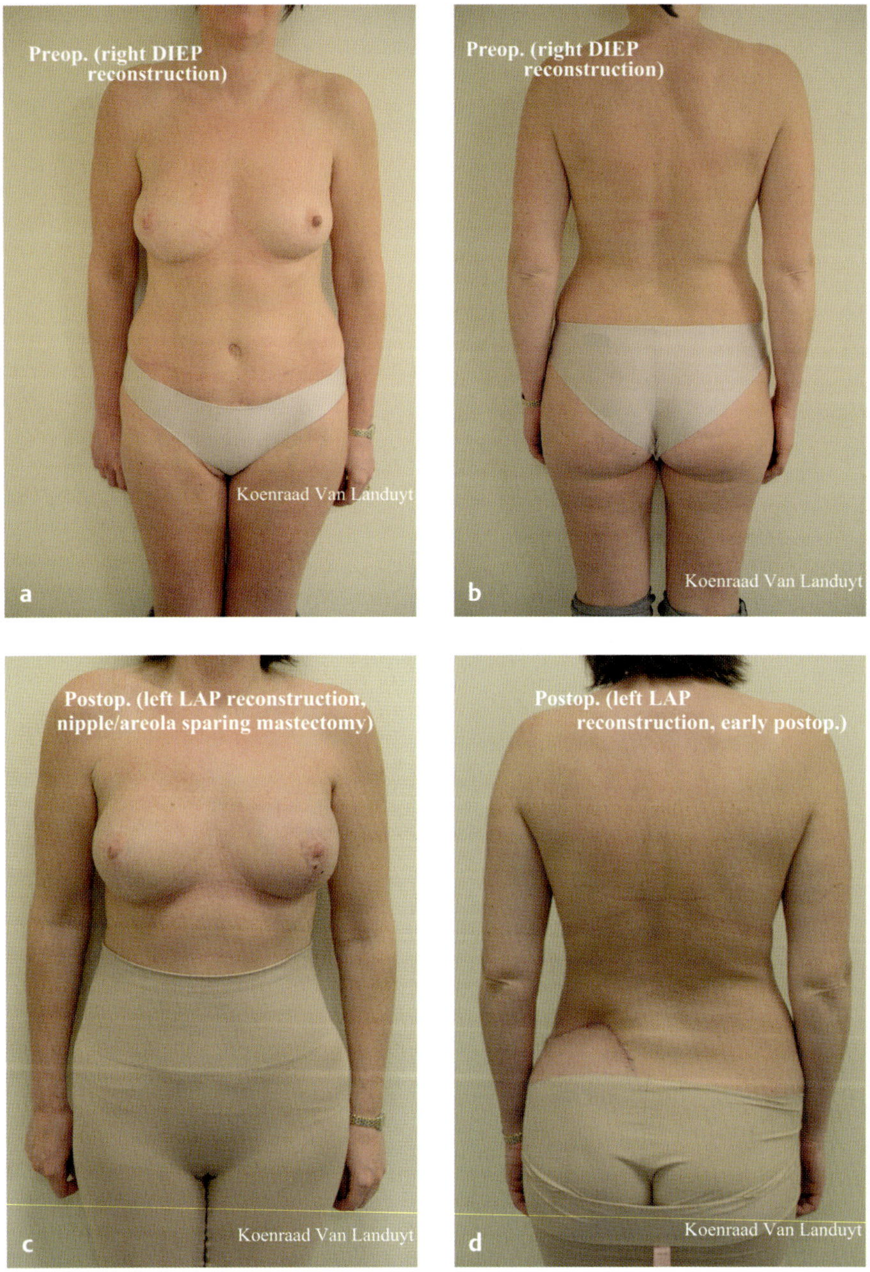

Fig. 8.6 (a) This patient is status post–right deep inferior epigastric perforator (DIEP) breast reconstruction, and is now scheduled for a left nipple-sparing mastectomy with left LAP flap reconstruction. **(b)** The left LAP flap will be harvested from the fatty hip area above the left buttocks. **(c)** Postoperative picture showing right DIEP and left LAP flap reconstructions. **(d)** Postoperative donor site after left LAP harvest.

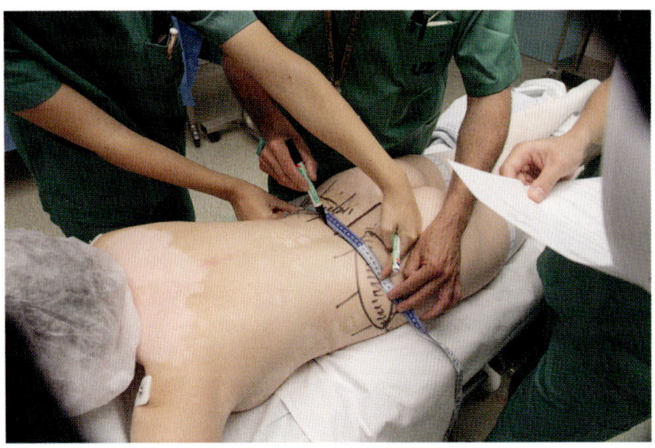

Fig. 8.7 Preoperative topographic transfer of CT markings on the patient, prior to anesthesia.

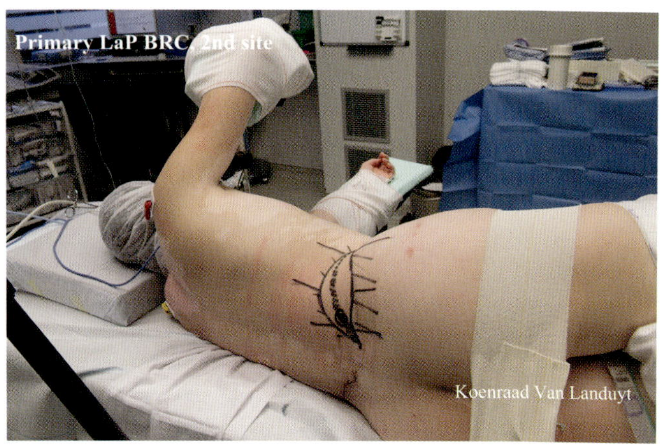

Fig. 8.8 Final positioning of the patient in the lateral decubitus position.

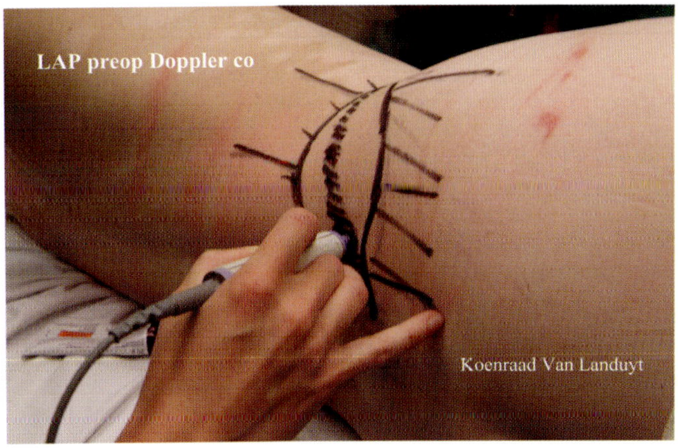

Fig. 8.9 Doppler control of the location of the perforator.

The exact position of the perforator is identified by Doppler evaluation at this time **(Fig. 8.9)**.

Surgery starts simultaneously on both the recipient site and the donor site. At the recipient site, a subcutaneous mastectomy is performed in the usual way, taking care to identify and spare for some length the medial and lateral branches of the fourth intercostal nerve supplying the breast. If a sentinel node dissection or lymphadenectomy has to be performed, a separate incision is preferred. The mammary vessels are dissected free after partial removal of the medial fourth costal cartilage, again leaving the vessels as long as possible. The vessels are not divided yet, to avoid twisting of the pedicle.

If a vascular graft is deemed necessary, the inferior epigastric vessels are approached through a small inguinal incision. The distal part of the epigastric pedicle is dissected over a length of 5 to 6 cm, from the exit point out of the rectus abdominis muscle, up to the collateral venous confluence; it is harvested and flushed with heparinized physiological solution **(Fig. 8.10)**.

The donor-site dissection of the LAP flap starts with an incision of the skin island on its superior, anterior, and inferior border, temporarily leaving the area over the perforator. The upper incision is slightly beveled and carried on to the underlying muscle fascia.

The upper beveling serves to provide upper pole fullness and avoids shelving, a problem typically encountered with the traditional SGAP flap. The lower beveling provides volume and projection to the breast. The main bulk of the flap is harvested on the inferior side, which is beveled as necessity, scooping the fat underneath the iliac crest, leaving the layer above the superficial fascia to avoid donor-site depression after closure. A large volume of tissue can be harvested in this way; care should be taken not to overdo the volume, as this can lead to a problem of depression at the donor site, necessitating secondary corrections **(Fig. 8.11a)**.

The flap is harvested from anterosuperior to posteroinferior on top of the obliquus externus muscle fascia, at first identifying the iliac crest. To limit donor-site morbidity, and especially seroma formation, one should avoid skeletonizing the iliac crest. Dissection below the iliac crest is superficial to the gluteus medius muscle, until one reaches the lateral edge of gluteus maximus. Perforators from the superior gluteal pedicle (septal perforators) can be identified here and temporarily spared as backup. The flap is allowed to fall backward in the process, which facilitates exposure.

Once the iliac crest is identified over a certain length, the upper skin and subcutaneous incision can be carried on, to enable approaching the lumbar perforators. Dissection is carried posteriorly on top of the muscle fascia. Based on the CT scan, the perforator can be anticipated close to the posterior iliac spine, or slightly higher in the space between the quadratus lumborum and spine musculature. Identifying the perforator here is the difficult part of the dissection, as the perforators tend to be compressed by the thoracolumbar fascia rendering them smaller and difficult to visualize. A hint can be the spot on top of the iliac crest where the muscle fascia of latissimus dorsi merges with the thoracolumbar fascia **(Fig. 8.11b)**. Sharp incision of the thoracolumbar fascia at this point facilitates subfascial dissection.

Once the perforator is identified, it is carefully freed from the surrounding tissue, ligating connections with the superior gluteal artery perforators and the deep circumflex iliac vessels. This dissection can frequently be performed by bluntly with the aid of a cotton tip. Cluneal

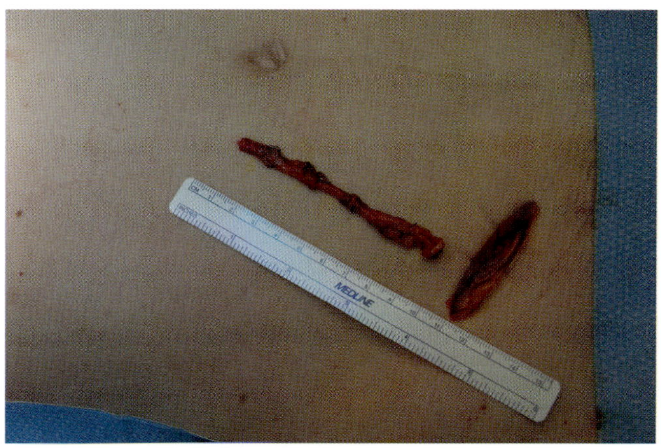

Fig. 8.10 Harvested epigastric pedicle.

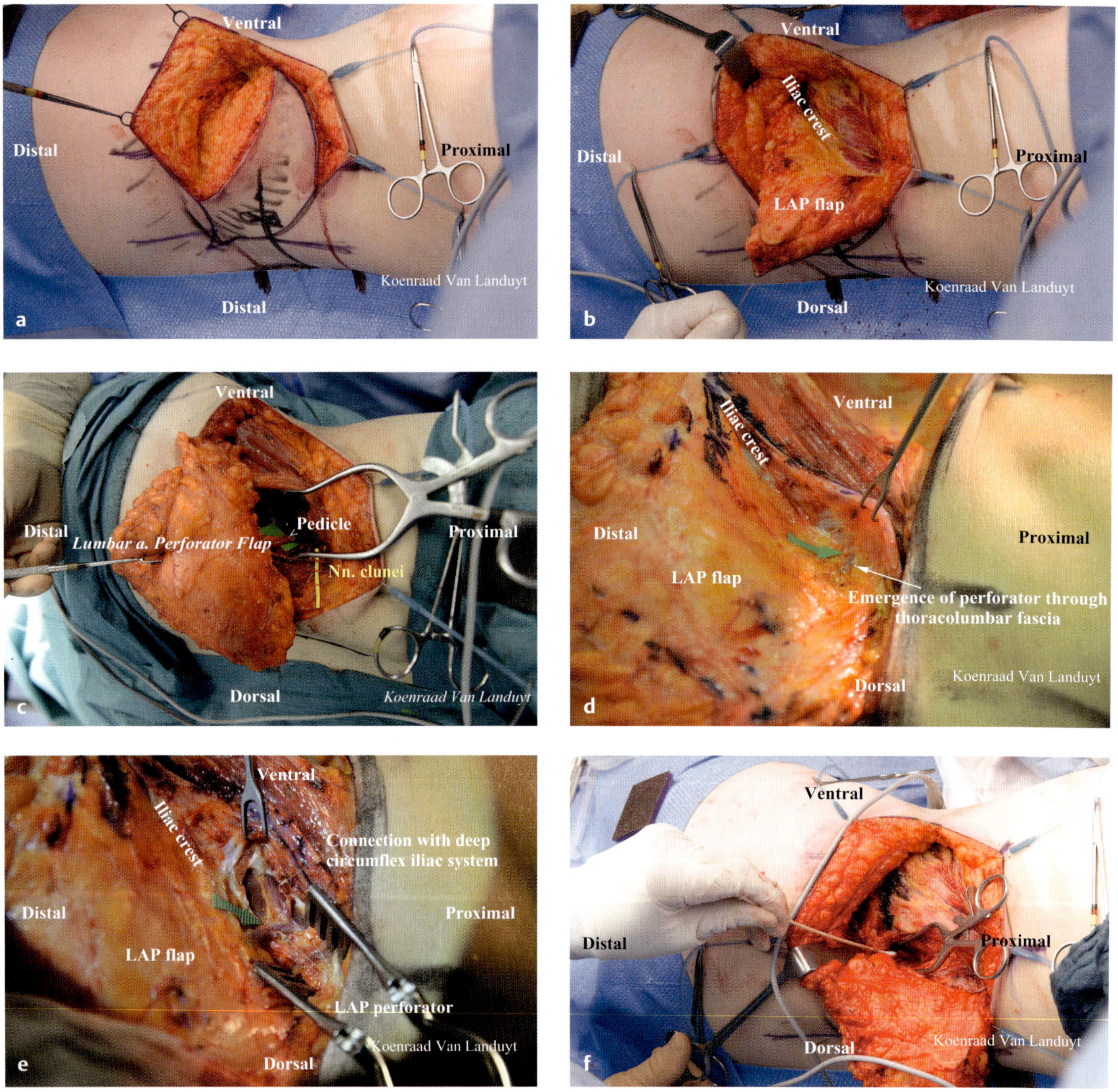

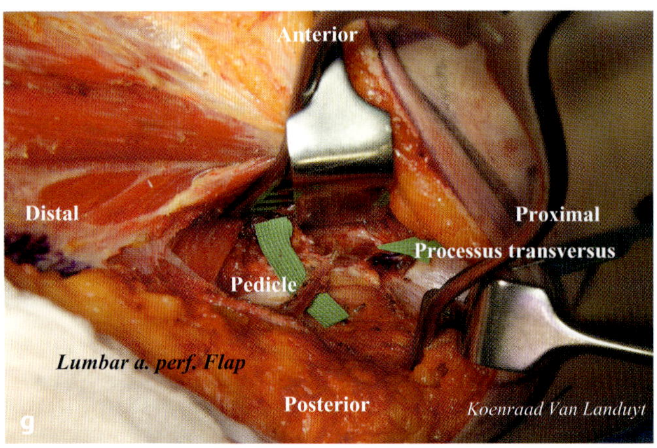

Fig. 8.11 (a,b) Initial dissection of the LAP flap, from lateral superior to medial inferior, toward the surgeon. **(c)** The course of the cluneal nerves. **(d)** The emergence of the lumbar perforator through the thoracolumbar fascia. **(e)** Dissection underneath the thoracolumbar fascia showing the connection with the deep circumflex iliac system. **(f)** Blunt freeing of the pedicle aided by the use of a cotton tip. **(g)** The length of the pedicle up to the processus transversus.

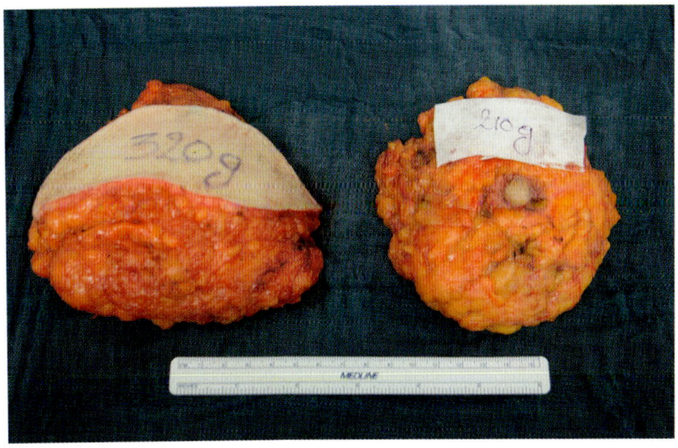

Fig. 8.12 The harvested free LAP flap. Note the slight beveling at the upper skin incision, and the bulk of the volume harvested from the lower part by liberal beveling at the lower skin incision. The epigastric pedicle is ready to be anastomosed to lengthen the pedicle. The harvested free lumbar flap accentuates the amount of upper and lower pole harvesting, and it resembles resected breast tissue.

nerves can be identified that cross the iliac crest almost together with the perforator, but they follow a different course, running up in between the fibers of the spinal musculature **(Fig. 8.11c)**. One or two of these nerves can be dissected out bluntly for a substantial length of 8 cm or more. Sensory denervation by harvesting them is limited to the flap itself and the upper part of the buttock, which seemingly does not pose a problem to the patients **(Fig. 8.11d,e)**.

Blunt dissection of the perforator with a cotton tip is carried on upward and into the depth of the intermuscular septum between the quadratus lumborum and the erector spinae musculature, carefully ligating or bipolar coagulating muscular side branches **(Fig. 8.11f)**. Dissection is stopped at the level of the processus transversus, regardless of the length or size of the pedicle **(Fig. 8.11g)**, to avoid injuring the spinal nerves emerging from the foramen intervertebrale in front of the processus transversus. Pedicle lengths of 5 to 7 cm can be obtained with the size of the vessels equaling those of the superficial epigastric artery perforator flaps (1- to 2-mm diameter). After harvesting of the pedicle and control of hemostasis, a small resorbable hemostatic wick is left in place at the site of pedicle harvesting. The pedicle itself is flushed with heparinized solution.

Fig. 8.12 demonstrates the LAP's resemblance to a mastectomy specimen.

As the LAP flap donor site is prone to seroma formation, careful closure of the donor site is mandatory. To obtain a buttock lift effect, undermining is continued but only inferiorly on top of the buttock musculature. If feasible, the gap in the thoracolumbar fascia is closed with interrupted resorbable sutures. The region around the iliac crest is injected subfascially with a long-acting local anesthetic to reduce postoperative pain. Two drains are left in place, tacking sutures are applied, and the wound edges are carefully approximated, following the preoperative vertical markings. Prior to closure, the wound is rinsed with an antibiotic solution.

If the pedicle is deemed of sufficient length and size, direct anastomosis with the mammary vessels can be performed with the patient in the lateral decubitus position **(Fig. 8.13)**, in the meantime closing the donor-site defect. Vessel length is frequently less of an issue than vessel size incongruence. The distal end of the inferior epigastric pedicle matches the mammary vessels quite nicely most of the time. In addition, the epigastric vessels taper down rather fast in their proximal part at the edge of the rectus abdominis, matching the lumbar vessels if taken shorter, which make the epigastric pedicle a good interposition graft of ~5 to 6 cm. Nowadays, we tend to more frequently use this interposition graft as compared with our initial experience with the LAP flap, a trick we tend to use also in the occasional SGAP reconstruction to

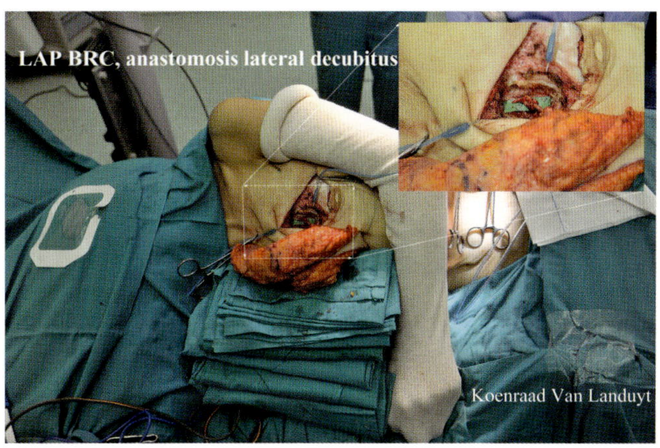

Fig. 8.13 Direct anastomosis of the LAP flap with the patient in lateral decubitus position.

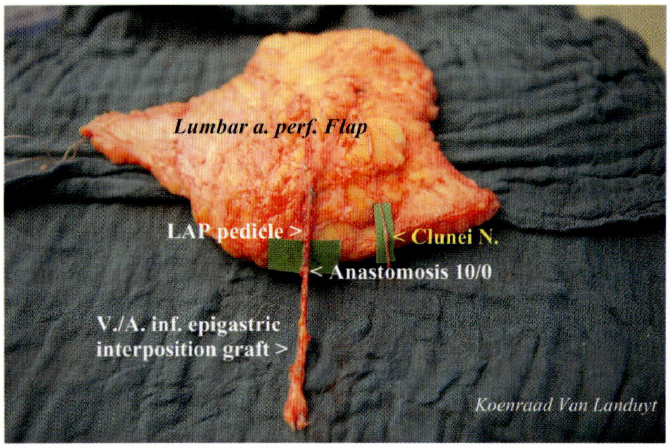

Fig. 8.14 Anastomosis of the interposition epigastric pedicle graft.

avoid vessel anastomotic incongruence. The interposition graft is anastomosed end to end, artery to artery, and vein to vein, with 10-0 sutures, on a side table in about the time it takes to close the donor site **(Fig. 8.14)**. Then the patient is placed in the supine position and an end-to-end anastomosis to the mammary vessels with 9-0 sutures is performed **(Fig. 8.15)**, and the nerve coaptation of the cluneal nerves is performed with the lateral or medial intercostal nerves **(Fig. 8.16)**. After control and careful positioning of the pedicle, the flap is shaped and inset; in cases of primary areola-sparing mastectomy, a small skin island is left in place for monitoring and for the nipple reconstruction. The flap is positioned as it is harvested, the thinner beveled upper side in the superomedial part of the breast, the thicker major inferior part of the flap in the lower part of the breast, eventually slightly folded underneath to provide for extra projection. Care should be taken to slightly overdo the medial upper filling to anticipate some secondary sagging of the flap. One drain is left in the breast.

Operative time is about 4 hours skin to skin. Including patient marking and positioning, this amounts to a total operative time of about 5 hours. If bilateral reconstruction is planned, surgery is scheduled 2 to 3 days apart. This limits hospitalization. Convalescence is one period of about 6 to 8 weeks.

Postoperatively, the patient is monitored for 1 day in the recovery unit, and kept in a semiupright position to alleviate the weight of the flap on the anastomosis, which sometimes is protected by pulling it through a short piece of silicon drain that is left in place. A Bair Hugger™ device (3M, St. Paul, MN) is applied until the patient regains normal body temperature; no specific anticoagulation is given apart from the usual postoperative low molecular weight heparin.

Drains in the gluteal area are left in place for ~ 10 days, even if the patient is usually discharged at the fifth postoperative day. Mobilization of the patient starts on the second postoperative day; at this time the bladder catheter and breast drain are usually removed. The patient should

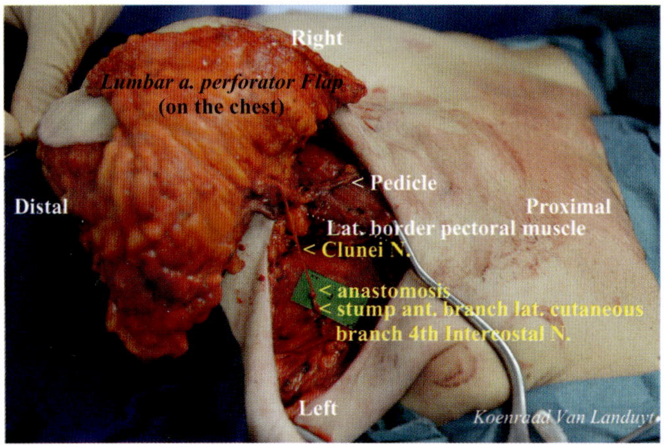

Fig. 8.15 Anastomosis of the harvested cluneal nerve with the lateral fourth intercostal nerve.

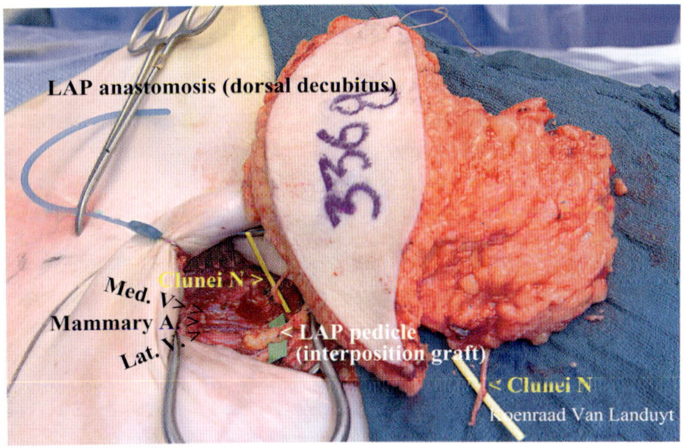

Fig. 8.16 Final anastomosis of the pedicle with the interposition graft, with the patient lying on her back.

wear a lumbar/gluteal compressive garment (contour correcting underwear or lipo-panty) with additional pressure pads at the donor site for at least 6 weeks and should be scheduled for weekly ambulatory control for the first 6 weeks to solve issues of eventual seroma formation. A paper tape (Micropore[R], 3M) is applied on the incision for ~3 months to control scar formation.

Secondary corrections are performed 3 to 6 months after the initial surgery including the usual nipple reconstruction, symmetrization of the breasts, and scar corrections. As to the donor site, symmetrization is also performed at this time by liposuction/lipofilling if necessary (**Fig. 8.17**).

Discussion

The LAP flap procedure should be performed by surgeons with experience in perforator dissection techniques and microsurgery. Its main difficulty lies in the preoperative identification of the perforator, which is why we stress preoperative imaging evaluation and Doppler in the correct patient position. The additional use of an interposition graft can be an issue in inexperienced hands, which offers better congruence of vessel size with the mammary vessels.

Although it is known that flaps regain some sensation through spontaneous neurotization of the skin, improving

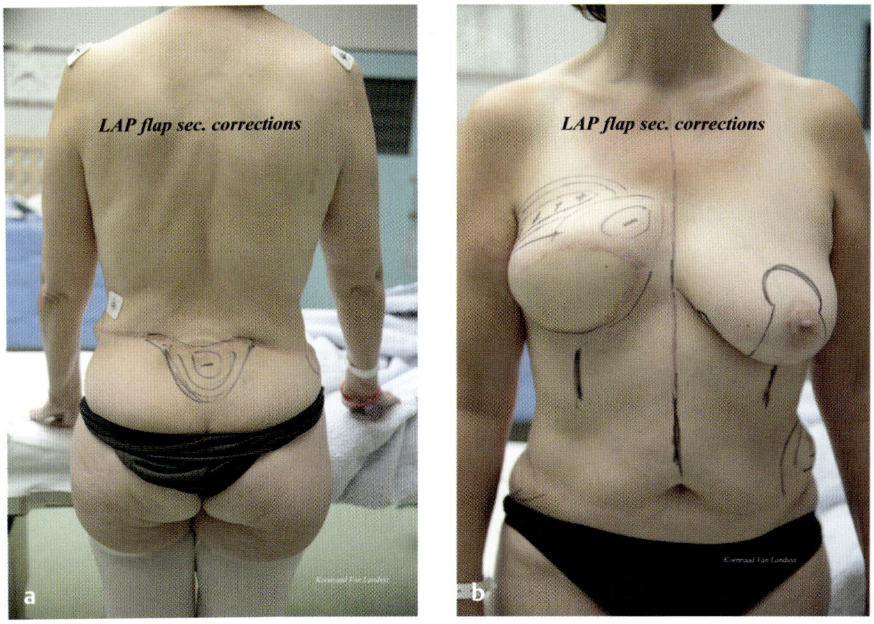

Fig. 8.17 **(a,b)** Secondary corrections.

sensation and especially erogenous sensation is the next step in breast reconstruction, especially as we start to treat younger patients who are genetically predisposed to breast cancer.[24–27] The LAP flap provides us with long vascularized sensate nerves, which makes coupling them directly, even to a stump of the lateral fourth intercostal nerve, rather easy; even double coupling of two cluneal nerves, both to the medial and lateral intercostal, is a possibility to explore.

The LAP flap provides us with ample volume to perform even a bilateral reconstruction in lean patients, without the need for secondary volume correction, and provide a good projection without the shelving of the traditional SGAP flap **(Fig. 8.18)**.

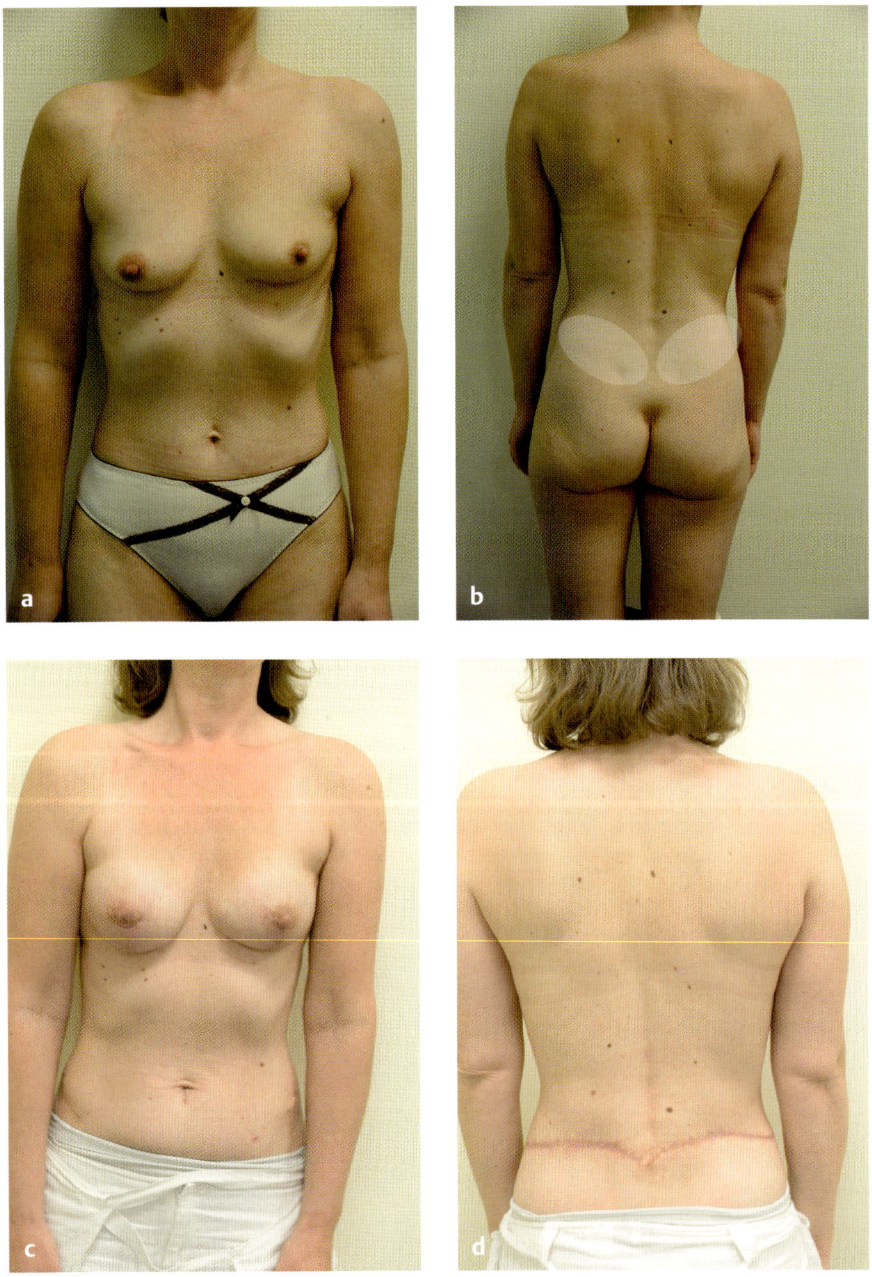

Fig. 8.18 (a) This patient with the *BRCA1* gene mutation is scheduled for a bilateral nipple-sparing mastectomy (NSM) and LAP flap breast reconstruction. **(b)** The highlighted areas show the intended donor site. **(c)** Six months postoperative after bilateral NSM and LAP flap breast reconstruction. **(d)** Bilateral LAP donor site at 6-month follow-up.

Seroma formation and depression of the donor-site scar can be an issue, but they can be prevented by not overdoing the size of the flap and by careful donor-site closure and postoperative treatment. The scar in the lumbar area on top of the buttock is generally well accepted, although sometimes secondary corrections by lipofilling/liposuction are necessary, but they can be combined with the usual secondary corrections of breast reconstruction.

Conclusion

The LAP flap offers a valuable alternative to other autologous breast reconstruction options in selected patients, and should become a part of our armamentarium.

References

1. Allen RJ, Treece P. Deep inferior epigastric perforator flap for breast reconstruction. Ann Plast Surg 1994;32:32–38
2. Blondeel PN. One hundred free DIEP flap breast reconstructions: a personal experience. Br J Plast Surg 1999;52:104–111
3. Allen RJ, Tucker C Jr. Superior gluteal artery perforator free flap for breast reconstruction. Plast Reconstr Surg 1995;95):1207–1212
4. Blondeel PN. The sensate free superior gluteal artery perforator (S-GAP) flap: a valuable alternative in autologous breast reconstruction. Br J Plast Surg 1999;52:185–193
5. Allen RJ, Levine JL, Granzow JW. The in-the-crease inferior gluteal artery perforator flap for breast reconstruction. Plast Reconstr Surg 2006;118:333–339
6. Granzow JW, Levine JL, Chiu ES, Allen RJJ. Breast reconstruction with gluteal artery perforator flaps. J Plast Reconstr Aesthet Surg 2006;59:614–621
7. LoTempio MM, Allen RJ. Breast reconstruction with SGAP and IGAP flaps. Plast Reconstr Surg 2010;126:393–401
8. Arnez ZM, Pogorelec D, Planinsek F, Ahcan U. Breast reconstruction by the free transverse gracilis (TUG) flap. Br J Plast Surg 2004; 57:20–26
9. Wechselberger G, Schoeller T. Transverse upper gracilis flap for breast reconstruction. Plast Reconstr Surg 2012;130:182e–183e, y183e–y184e
10. Allen RJ, Haddock NT, Ahn CY, Sadeghi A. Breast reconstruction with the profunda artery perforator flap. Plast Reconstr Surg 2012;129:16e–23e
11. Saad A, Sadeghi A, Allen RJ. The anatomic basis of the profunda femoris artery perforator flap: a new option for autologous breast reconstruction—a cadaveric and computer tomography angiogram study. J Reconstr Microsurg 2012;28:381–386
12. Tuinder S, Chen CM, Massey MF, Allen RJ Sr, Van der Huist R. Introducing the septocutaneous gluteal artery perforator flap: a simplified approach to microsurgical breast reconstruction. Plast Reconstr Surg 2011;127:489–495
13. Kroll SS, Rosenfield L. Perforator-based flaps for low posterior midline defects. Plast Reconstr Surg 1988;81:561–566
14. Ao M, Mae O, Namba Y, Asagoe K. Perforator-based flap for coverage of lumbosacral defects. Plast Reconstr Surg 1998;101:987–991
15. Arco G, Horch RE, Arkudas A, Dragu A, Bach AD, Kneser U. Double pedicled perforator flap to close flank defects: an alternative for closure of a large lumbar defect after basalioma excision—a case report and review of the literature. Ann Plast Surg 2009;63:422–424
16. de Weerd L, Weum S. The butterfly design: coverage of a large sacral defect with two pedicled lumbar artery perforator flaps. Br J Plast Surg 2002;55:251–253
17. Roche NA, Van Landuyt K, Blondeel PN, Matton G, Monstrey SJ. The use of pedicled perforator flaps for reconstruction of lumbosacral defects. Ann Plast Surg 2000;45:7–14
18. de Weerd L, Elvenes OP, Strandenes E, Weum S. Autologous breast reconstruction with a free lumbar artery perforator flap. Br J Plast Surg 2003;56:180–183
19. Kato H, Hasegawa M, Takada T, Torii S. The lumbar artery perforator based island flap: anatomical study and case reports. Br J Plast Surg 1999;52:541–546
20. Offman SL, Geddes CR, Tang M, Morris SF. The vascular basis of perforator flaps based on the source arteries of the lateral lumbar region. Plast Reconstr Surg 2005;115:1651–1659
21. Lui KW, Hu S, Ahmad N, Tang M. Three-dimensional angiography of the superior gluteal artery and lumbar artery perforator flap. Plast Reconstr Surg 2009;123:79–86
22. Kiil BJ, Rozen WM, Pan WR, et al. The lumbar artery perforators: a cadaveric and clinical anatomical study. Plast Reconstr Surg 2009,123.1229–1238
23. Bissell MB, Greenspun DT, Levine J, et al. The lumbar artery perforator flap: 3D anatomical study and clinical applications. Ann Plast Surg 2015; in press
24. Eberlein TJ, Crespo LD, Smith BL, Hergrueter CA, Douville L, Eriksson E. Prospective evaluation of immediate reconstruction after mastectomy. Ann Surg 1993;218:29–36
25. Yap LH, Whiten SC, Forster A, Stevenson HJ. Sensory recovery in the sensate free transverse rectus abdominis myocutaneous flap. Plast Reconstr Surg 2005;115:1280–1288
26. Yap LH, Whiten SC, Forster A, Stevenson JH. The anatomical and neurophysiological basis of the sensate free TRAM and DIEP flaps. Br J Plast Surg 2002;55:35–45
27. Blondeel PN, Demuynck M, Mete D, et al. Sensory nerve repair in perforator flaps for autologous breast reconstruction: sensational or senseless? Br J Plast Surg 1999;52:37–44

9 Pedicled Lateral Thoracic Flap for Breast Reconstruction

Moustapha Hamdi and Assaf Zeltzer

The microsurgical era evolved from Tansini's work on the pedicled latissimus dorsi (LD) musculocutaneous flap, which has since been a workhorse in reconstructive surgery.[1] It is used extensively as a local flap and as a free flap, providing a large vascularized muscle with or without an overlying skin paddle. The bulk of the flap can be augmented by harvesting it with the surrounding subfascial fat attached to the flap (the extended LD flap), which can especially be useful when dealing with large-size breast reconstructions.[2] The LD flap is the widest muscle in the human body accounting for extension, adduction, transverse extension (also known as horizontal abduction), flexion from an extended position, and internal rotation of the shoulder joint. It also has a synergistic role in extension and lateral flexion of the lumbar spine. Although harvesting this muscle is safe and technically reliable, the donor-site morbidity is not negligible. First, muscle function is lost and has to be taken over by the surrounding muscles. Most patients can function well after a LD muscle harvest but have long-term weakness and in some cases pain at the ipsilateral shoulder.[3,4] Second, almost all patients have a contour deformity at the donor site, which can be highly visible in lean patients. Third, seroma formation at the donor site is a major issue, and considerable attention has been paid to avoiding or reducing it.[5,6]

This long era of sacrificing muscle in reconstructive surgery has finally given way to Taylor's angiosome theory of perforator flaps.[7] Perforator flaps have been one of the major breakthroughs in reconstructive surgery, since the first description of an inferior epigastric artery skin flap without the rectus abdominis muscle in 1989 by Koshima and Soeda.[8] The advantages of perforator flaps have been widely described and proven, and they all are a direct consequence of the principle of sparing the underlying muscle with its motor innervation when harvesting the flap.[9]

In 1995, Angrigiani et al first described the thoracodorsal artery perforator (TDAP) flap as a free flap transferred for cervical burn contracture.[10] Allen et al[11] presented the TDAP flap for breast reconstruction in 1996. Hamdi et al[12] elaborated on pedicled TDAP flaps for breast reconstruction in 2004. As with other perforator flaps, the TDAP flap consists of harvesting a skin paddle with underlying fatty tissue, on a constantly vascularized pedicle, while the underlying LD muscle with its motor innervation is spared. Other flaps have been described in the lateral thoracic region to cover a locoregional defect, such as the intercostal artery perforator (ICAP) flap.[13]

The lateral intercostal artery perforator (LICAP) flap is a good alternative for the TDAP flap for the reconstruction of lateral and inferior defects of the breast. The first description of the lateral intercostal fasciocutaneous flap was by Badran et al[14] in 1984, although the use of a flap based on the intercostal neurovascular bundle had already been described in the 1930s.

This chapter describes the anatomy, surgical technique, flap classifications, and clinical indications of the pedicled perforator flap for breast reconstruction.

Regional Anatomy

The LD and TDAP flap are both based on a reliable and constantly vascularized pedicle that has been widely studied.[15–17]

The major vascular axis supplying the TDAP flap is the same that supplies the LD muscle, namely the thoracodorsal (TD) vessels; the medial and inferior portions of the muscle get its vascular supply from intercostal and paraspinal perforators. After originating from the subscapular vessels, the TD vessels course toward the LD muscle. On reaching the deep surface of the muscle, the TD vessels most commonly divide into two primary muscular

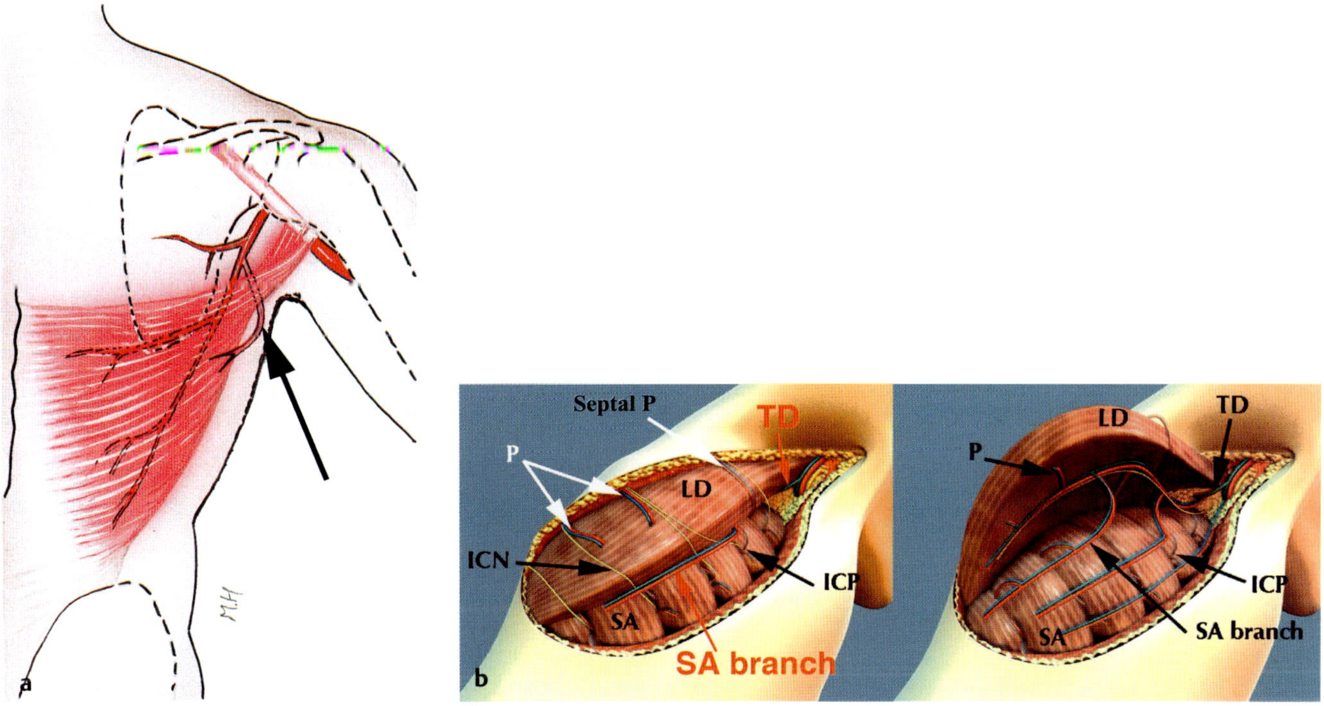

Fig. 9.1 The anatomy of the thoracodorsal (TD) vessels. **(a)** The TD vessels most commonly divide into two primary muscular branches: the transverse branch and the lateral *(arrow)* or vertical branch. A direct branch can also be found that courses anteriorly around the latissimus dorsi (LD) muscle toward the skin. **(b)** Both branches give off musculocutaneous perforators. A septal perforator arises from the direct branch toward the skin. ICN, intercostal nerve; ICP, intercostal perforator; P, posterior; sA, serratus anterior.

branches: the transverse branch and the lateral or vertical branch **(Fig. 9.1a)**. These branches usually diverge at near 45-degree angles to one another. Both travel from the deep surface of the muscle to become intramuscular. The lateral branch courses vertically and at 2 to 3 cm inside the lateral border of the LD. The TD vessel supplies the muscle by its course in the muscle (parallel to its fibers), and supplies the overlying skin by perforators coursing from the TD vessels perpendicularly to the skin surface **(Fig. 9.1b)**. The first perforator is located 6 to 8 cm below the posterior axillary fold and may either be a branch of the distal main TD or arise from its lateral branch. Subsequent perforators, up to a total of three, arise at 1.5- to 4-cm intervals inferiorly off the lateral branch. The first and second perforators are found in most people.[18] Each perforator displays a 3- to 5-cm oblique course through the substance of the muscle, giving off numerous muscular branches before penetrating through the dorsal thoracic fascia to supply the overlying skin and subcutaneous fat layers. Each perforating artery is 0.3 to 0.6 mm in diameter and accompanied by two venae comitantes. Heitmann et al[19] described two rows of perforators arising from the main pedicle at the lateral border of the LD muscle. The lateral row does not pierce the muscle and provides for the direct TDAP perforators **(Fig. 9.1)**. The medial row of perforators courses through the muscle (perforating it) before reaching the skin and subcutaneous tissues.

Various musculocutaneous flaps described by Kerrigan and Daniel[20] can be harvested based on these intercostal vessels. The intercostal vessels form an arcade, between the aorta and the internal mammary vessels, which gives off numerous perforators on which a flap can be designed. Based on the concept of freestyle flap,[21] ICAP flaps can be harvested to cover defects that extend on the trunk from the lower neck to lower abdomen and lumbosacral area.

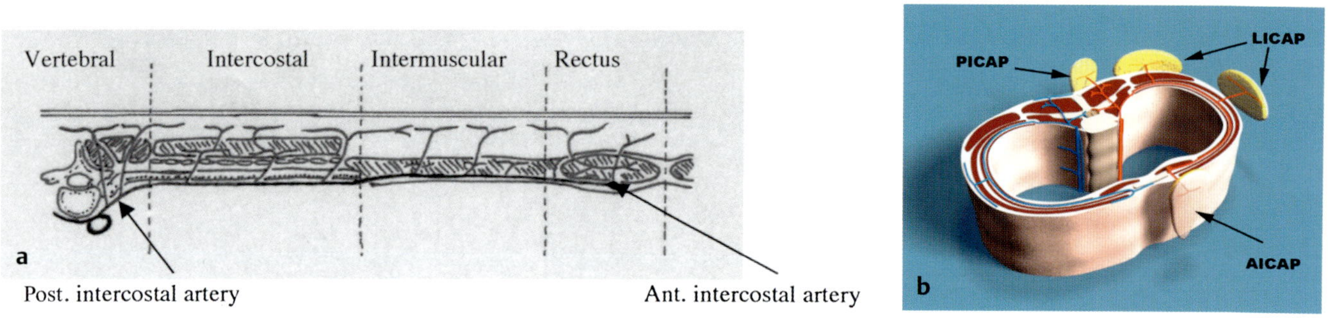

Fig. 9.2 The anatomy of the intercostal perforators. **(a)** The four segments of the intercostal vessels are the vertebral, intercostal, intermuscular, and rectus. **(b)** Intercostal perforator flaps classification: PICAP, posterior intercostal artery perforator; LICAP, lateral intercostal artery perforator; AICAP, anterior intercostal artery perforator.

There are four segments of the intercostal vessels: vertebral, intercostal, intermuscular, and rectus **(Fig. 9.2)**.

The ICAP flaps are classified as follows **(Fig. 9.2b)**:

- The posterior intercostal artery perforator (PICAP) flap, based on perforators originating from the vertebral segment of the intercostal vessels
- The lateral intercostal artery perforator (LICAP) flap, based on perforators arising from the intercostal segment
- The anterior intercostal artery perforator (AICAP) flap, the nutrient perforators of which arise from the muscular or rectus segment

The intercostal segment, which is the longest (12 cm), is very important because it gives off five to seven musculocutaneous perforators, on which flaps can be designed and raised.

The LICAP perforators are found 1 to 3.5 cm anterior to the anterior border of the LD muscle.[22] The largest perforator is most frequently found at the level of the sixth intercostal space (generally between the fourth and eighth intercostal space). The flap can also be harvested with an intercostal nerve, making it sensate.

The serratus anterior artery perforator (SAAP flap) is based on a connection between the thoracodorsal artery branch to the serratus anterior muscle and the intercostal perforators. It is not a constant perforator and is found in only 20% of cases. When an appropriately sized perforator is identified in front of the anterior border of the LD, it can be followed back to the nutrient artery (which in this case is the serratus anterior branch) by dissecting the pedicle within the fascia and the fibers of the aforementioned muscle.

Indications and Clinical Applications of Pedicled Lateral Thoracic Flaps

The TDAP flap has a wide range of indications as a local flap (pedicled) as does its equivalent muscle flap (LD muscle flap). Most patients who could benefit from a pedicled LD flap are good candidates for a TDAP flap. The flap is ideally used for lateral and anterolateral defects of the thorax, and it has an important place in the reconstruction of lateral defects of the breast in partial breast reconstruction both in a primary and in a secondary setting. With the TDAP flap, defects of the two lateral quadrants of the breast can easily be reached. The medial quadrants can sometimes be reached when harvesting a flap that is long enough, but defects of the inferomedial quadrant are difficult to reach with a TDAP flap and are better reconstructed in a different manner.[23] The flap is also useful in implant breast reconstruction for extra coverage of the device without sacrifice of the muscle or as an autoaugmentation flap in post–bariatric surgery patients.[24,25]

The local flap also has applications in the reconstruction of the axilla, shoulder, and upper arm.

The LICAP flap has its main use as a pedicled flap for lateral thoracic defects, superolateral abdominal defects, axillary defects, and supero- or inferolateral breast defects, for which it is most commonly used.

When used as a pedicled flap, dissection of the perforator must be performed far enough to be able to rotate the flap. Dissection in the costal groove is only necessary when harvesting the flap for a free tissue transfer so as to have a longer pedicle with greater diameter of the vessels.

The LICAP flap can also be used for patients after massive weight loss who want to get rid of excessive tissue over the lateral thorax. When performing a mastopexy in these patients, this excess tissue can be used as a pedicled flap to augment the breast (pedicled flap autoaugmentation). Clearly, LICAP flaps have to be harvested bilaterally in these cases.[26]

The indications for the use of lateral thoracic pedicled perforator flaps are as follows:

- Immediate/delayed partial breast reconstruction
- Coverage of thoracic defects after radical excision
- Postmastectomy breast reconstruction (with or without and implant)
- Salvage of major fat necrosis after previous autologous reconstruction
- Autologous breast augmentation (aesthetic, post-bariatric surgery)

Surface Anatomy and Flap Design

Thoracodorsal Artery Perforator Flap

Patients are marked in the standing position before anesthesia for breast surgery. The breast with the defect to reconstruct is marked. The patient is the placed in the lateral decubitus position with the arm abducted 90 degrees from the thorax and the elbow flexed 90 degrees (**Fig. 9.3**). The anterior border of the LD muscle is palpated and marked on the skin. As discussed above, most perforators are found at 8 to 10 cm from the axilla and within 3 cm of the anterior muscle border. At the presumed site of the perforators, a handheld Doppler device is used to identify the exact position of the perforating vessels. More recently, computed tomography (CT) and magnetic resonance imaging (MRI) have been used to preoperatively determine the position of the perforators on the skin.[27,28]

Once the perforator mapping is done, depending on the reconstructive needs, the flap can be designed on the skin. The flap should always extend anteriorly to the anterior muscle edge to be sure to include the vascular hilus. The skin paddle can be designed in every possible direction on a perforator. The vertical design facilitates incorporating good perforators in the flap. When used as pedicled flaps (mostly for breast reconstruction), the design should be done in a horizontal fashion (in the line of the bra) to better hide the scar in the bra, with the scar following the skin lines. This orientation (following the direction of the ribs) also makes it possible to harvest the largest reliable flap possible on a single perforator, in accordance with Taylor's[29] angiosome theory. The actual size of the flap is mostly limited by the requirements for primary closure of the donor defect. Flaps as big as 14 × 25 cm have been raised on a single perforator without any significant complications.

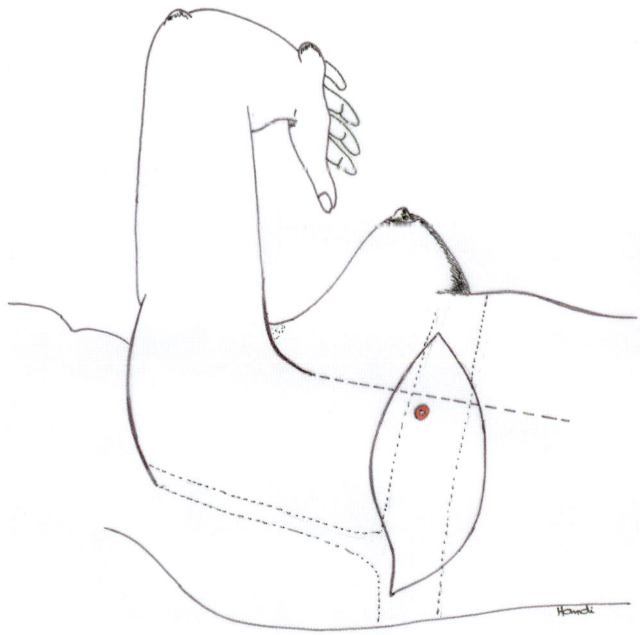

Fig. 9.3 After localizing the perforator, the thoracodorsal artery perforator (TDAP) flap is marked within the bra lines.

Lateral Intercostal Artery Perforator Flap

The LICAP flap is designed on the lateral thorax for small to moderate defects, and when a more extensive flap is necessary the design can reach the posterior thoracic region, up to or almost up to the midline. The flap dimensions can reach a length of 20 to 25 cm, and a width of up to 12 cm can be closed primarily.

Flaps can be raised up to the anterior/posterior midline. Beyond this point the flap will be dependent on a random pattern of vascular supply.

The flap should be designed by using a unidirectional Doppler to map the location of the perforators or using a CT angiogram, as with the TDAP flap.

Flap Dissection

Thoracodorsal Artery Perforator Flap

After the patient is preoperatively marked (**Fig. 9.4a–c**) and the quadrantectomy is performed (**Fig. 9.4d**), the

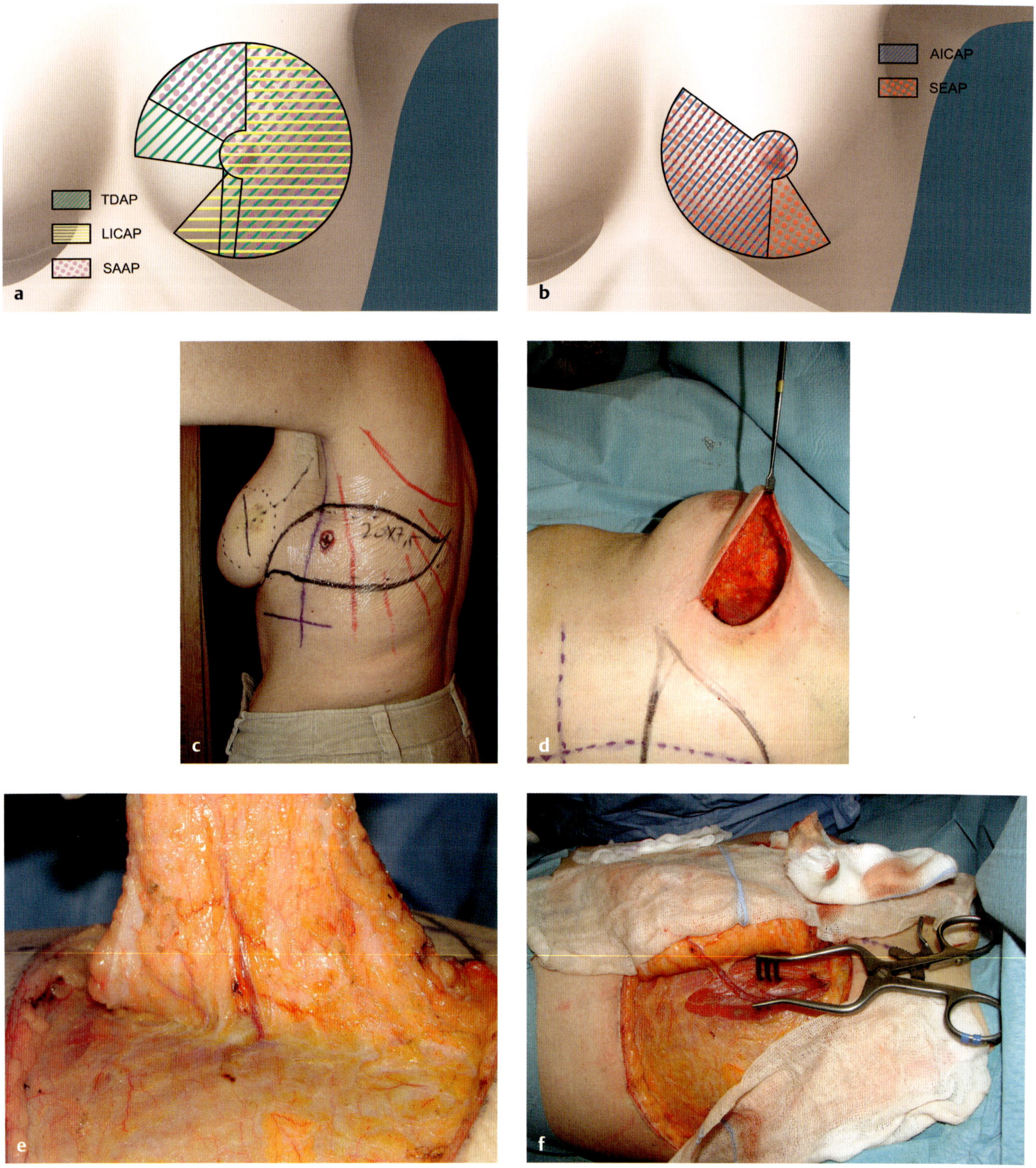

Fig. 9.4 A 49-year-old patient with a ductal carcinoma in the superolateral quadrant of the left breast. The patient was a good candidate for quadrantectomy with axillary dissection and immediate partial breast reconstruction with a TDAP flap. **(a,b)** Preoperative views. **(c)** Flap markings. The perforator was mapped preoperatively using a multidetector row computed tomography (MDCT) scan study. **(d)** The quadrantectomy was performed. **(e)** The flap was harvested with a posterior approach until the marked perforator was found. **(f)** The LD muscle was split and the perforator was freed.

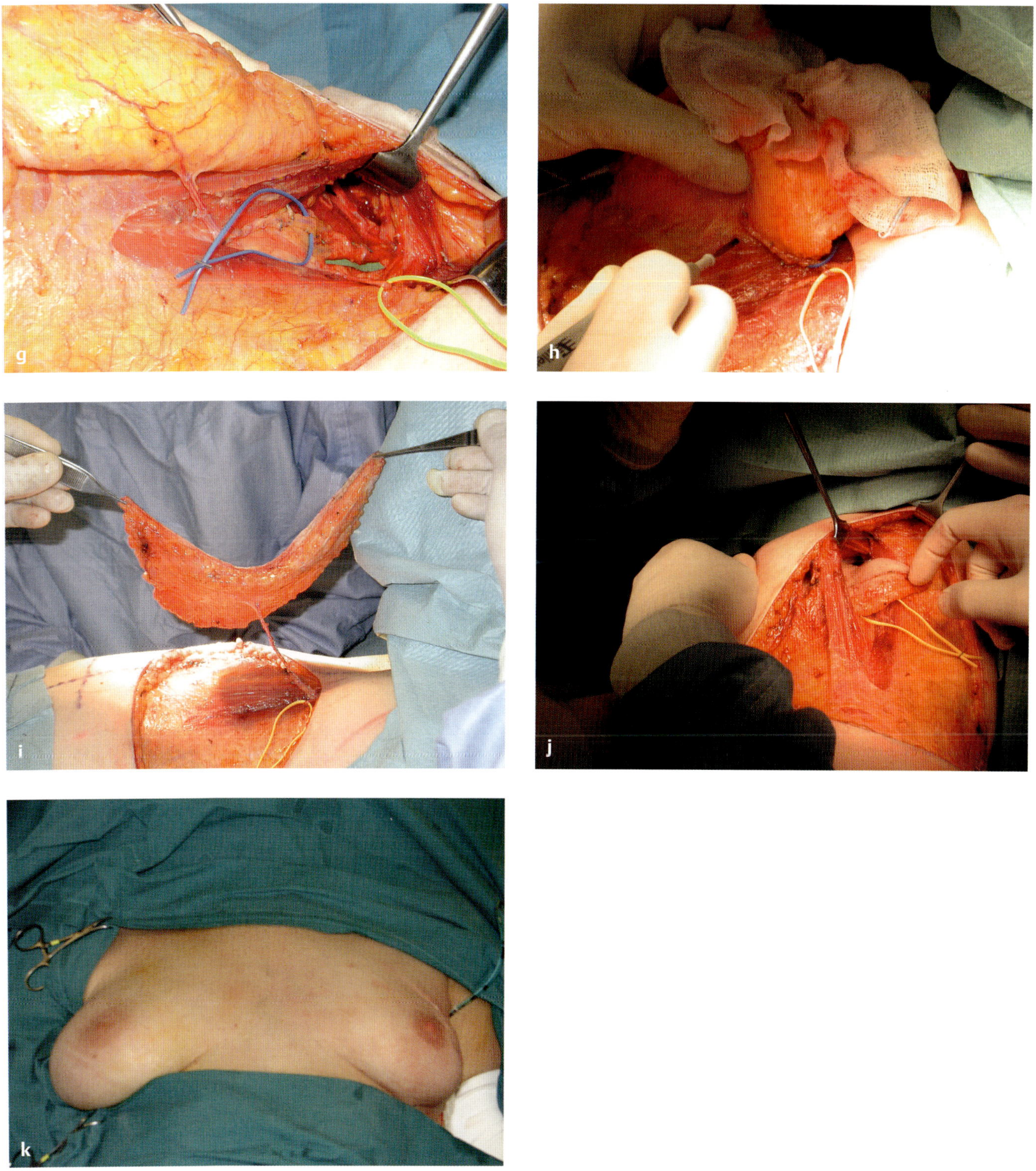

Fig. 9.4 *(Continued)* **(g)** The perforator was dissected through the split LD muscle until the main pedicle. The thoracodorsal nerve was spared. **(h)** When the pedicle is completely dissected and the tunnel under the anterior border of the muscle was made, the posterior side of the perforator was then freed from the muscle fibers. **(i)** The skin paddle, which was based on one perforator, was totally dissected from the LD muscle. **(j)** The skin paddle is passed under the anterior strip of the LD muscle toward the breast defect. **(k)** The patient is repositioned into the supine position for flap shaping.

patient is moved to the lateral position with 90-degree shoulder and elbow abduction. The skin incision is done at the lower and anterior border of the flap. The first step in dissecting a TDAP flap is to look for the anterior border of the LD muscle, as this is the reference line for localization of the perforators. The dissection is then pursued in the loose areolar plane just superficial to the muscular fascia, from lateral to medial and from distal to proximal. A good perforator bundle, including an artery and two venae comitantes, is sought and is visually evaluated for its size and pulsatility **(Fig. 9.4e)**. If the quality of the perforator is in doubt, it is left in place and the dissection is pursued until a final decision can be made. If two (or more) perforators lie on the same line during intramuscular dissection, it is advisable to harvest them together to improve flap perfusion, as this does not cause any extra donor-site morbidity. If the decision is to take only one perforator, the length of the pedicle required for the flap will determine the choice. One should keep in mind that a more distal perforator will give more length to the pedicle but will require longer dissection time. Some of the more distal perforators can originate from the intercostal vessels, and determining whether this is the case is done by elevating the anterior border of the LD and inspecting its deep surface. Once the perforator is chosen, it is further freed from the muscle after opening of the fascia. Dissection is done by splitting of the muscle fibers longitudinally (thus not cutting them) with microscissors, while clipping or coagulating side branches with a bipolar cautery **(Fig. 9.4f)**. Dissection is pursued until the deep surface of the muscle is reached, and dissection is then done by elevating the anterior border of the muscle, further freeing the pedicle 360 degrees. Further dissection proceeds proximally as for a classical thoracodorsal pedicle such as in an LD flap elevation with sparing of the motor nerve branches **(Fig. 9.4g)**. The motor nerves to the LD run on a deeper plane, which enables completely freeing the pedicle without injuring the nerves. The flap then is completely freed from the muscle anteriorly **(Fig. 9.4h)**. The flap based on one perforator is completely dissected **(Fig. 9.4i)**. It is passed under the lateral part of the LD muscle, which makes the pedicle even longer, and finally to the breast defect through the axilla **(Fig. 9.4j)**. The patient then is turned on her back for the flap insertion into the defect to ensure the best breast symmetry **(Fig. 9.4k)**.

Lateral Intercostal Artery Perforator Flap

Similar to the TDAP flap, the patient is marked preoperatively with localization of the perforators **(Fig. 9.5a,b)**. After the quadrantectomy is done **(Fig. 9.5c)**, the patient should be repositioned on the lateral side. The flap is then raised from posterior to anterior to facilitate elevation of the flap. The thoracodorsal perforators are preserved until the intercostal perforator is found **(Fig. 9.5d)**. The flap is elevated from the anterior side. Once the small cutaneous branch is identified, it is followed to encounter the larger anterior branch. If the size of the intercostal perforator is adequate, further dissection is performed within the serratus muscle. Adequate dissection provides enough length of the pedicle to propeller the flap over 180 degrees without twisting the pedicle and without the need for dissecting in the costal groove (with the risk of causing a pneumothorax). The thoracodorsal perforator is then clipped and the flap raised on the intercostal perforator **(Fig. 9.5e)**.

A pedicle length of up to 5 cm can be obtained without dissection in the costal groove. With this length, defects of the superior and lateral parts of the breast can be reached. If more bulk is needed, the flap can be easily folded on itself, yielding an adequate outcome **(Fig. 9.5f)**.

If a longer pedicle is required (for use as a pedicled or free flap), dissection of the pedicle should be performed in the costal groove. This dissection can be performed by retracting both serratus anterior and LD muscles and by splitting their fibers lengthwise, thus reducing donor-site morbidity. The intercostal muscles should then be resected to expose the main pedicle after identifying its junction with the lateral cutaneous branch. When a sensate flap is harvested, the cutaneous nerve can be stripped from the intercostal nerve over the desired length.

Alternatively, a longer pedicle length can be obtained if a connection of the intercostal perforator and the serratus anterior vessels is found, which occurs in only 20% of cases. In these cases, a SAAP flap can be harvested. With a pedicle of 6 to 9 cm, this flap can reach well into the retroareolar region.

Harvesting of a Pedicled Perforator Flap

Flap Orientation

The direction and function of the designed flap are outlined to see if it meets the requirements of the dissection. Longitudinally oriented, the flap can leave a rather wide donor-site scar, although it is partially hidden on the lateral thorax by the arm. In women, the tension of primary closure can temporarily displace the nipple-areola complex laterally. This orientation is mostly used when harvesting a pedicled TDAP flap for distal upper arm, elbow, shoulder, neck, and upper back reconstruction. Transversally oriented, closure takes advantage of the natural skin folds of

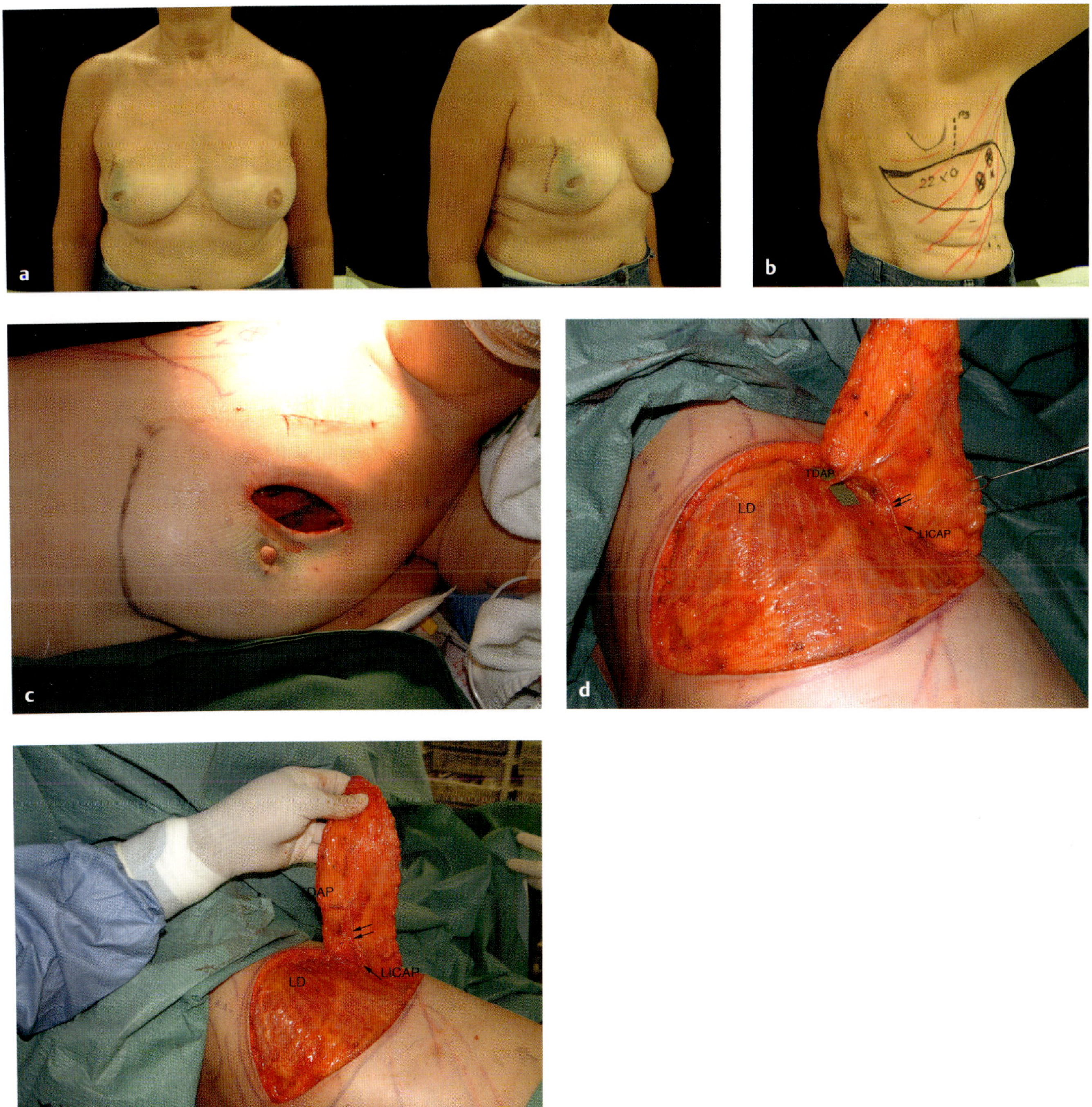

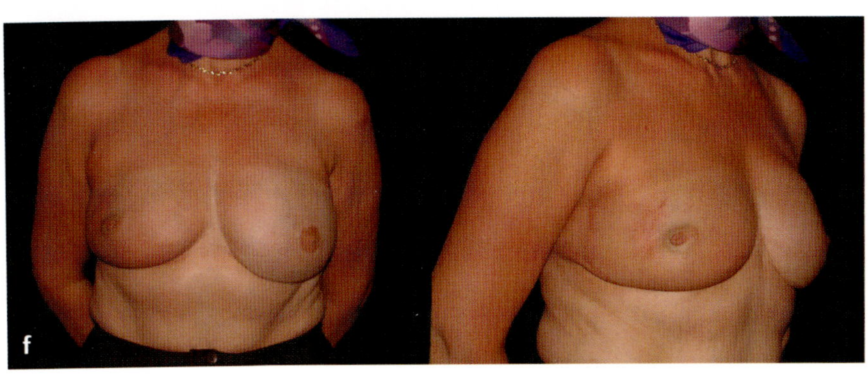

Fig. 9.5 A 59-year-old patient was admitted for quadrantectomy with partial breast reconstruction for right breast cancer located at the superolateral quadrant. **(a)** Preoperative views. **(b)** Flap design with the mapped perforators. **(c)** The defect after the quadrantectomy. **(d)** Perioperative view shows that two perforator were found, one TDAP and one LICAP *(one arrow)*. The intercostal (IC) nerve *(two arrows)* was included in the flap. **(e)** The thoracodorsal perforator was clipped and the flap was based on the ICAP *(one arrow)* and the IC nerve *(two arrows)*. **(f)** Postoperative views.

the back, and the scar can be hidden in the bra, but can still provoke a contour deformity especially if it is unilaterally harvested. But the defect is far less conspicuous than in the traditional musculocutaneous LD flap. The transverse orientation is mostly indicated in reconstructive breast surgery. Another indication is the autologous augmentation in asymmetric breasts or in post–bariatric surgery patients.

Contraindications to Pedicled Perforator Flaps

There are only a few contraindications to using the TDAP flap as a pedicled flap for local defects, mostly for the breast. If the patient has undergone previous radiotherapy or surgery in the axillary region (e.g., axillary clearance, lateral thoracotomy), and thus there is a risk of having a damaged or heavily scarred pedicle and perforator complex, then a TDAP flap is formally contraindicated, as is the case for the traditional LD flap. In those cases, an LICAP flap can often still be harvested for lateral thoracic/breast defects.

Perforator Mapping

The surgeon should use every available radiological method available to map the perforator before surgery. Although the anatomy of the LD muscle is constant, the location of the thoracodorsal and the intercostal perforators is quite variable. Due to the large mobility of the skin at the lateral side of the thorax, the perforator might reach the skin far away from the point where it pierces the underlining muscle. In contrast with other perforator flaps, such as the deep inferior epigastric perforator (DIEP) or superior gluteal artery perforator (SGAP), the TDAP flap has usually one or two large-diameter (clinically usable) perforators.

Safe Harvesting

Searching the mapped perforator progresses from lateral to medial. When no thoracodorsal perforators are found or they are very small, alternative options should be available for reconstruction. An intercostal perforator may be identified and dissected. LICAP flaps have a more restricted arc of rotation because dissecting the pedicle within the periosteum under the rib is technically very difficult. Another alternative is to identify the serratus anterior perforator of a suitable diameter and follow it to the major nutrient artery within the fascia of the serratus anterior muscle. However, in specific situations, converting the TDAP flap to a muscle-sparing TD flap is imperative to avoid major partial necrosis or failure of the flap because of insufficient blood supply through the dissecting perforators. The flap is then harvested, including a very limited segment of the LD muscle. Classification and definition of these flaps are shown in **Table 9.1**. When tiny, but pulsating, perforators are found, a muscle-sparing thoracodorsal (MSTD) type I flap is used, including a 2- to 4-cm piece of LD muscle. In this case, the perforators will be dissected within the split LD muscle but not from that muscular part that is included in the flap, in such a way that the perforators are still attached to the LD segment (**Fig. 9.6**). This means including the muscle under direct visualization of the perforators in order not to damage them during harvesting the muscular segment. Only a small nerve branch to muscle is sacrificed. The MSTD type I enables the surgeon to perform a safer harvesting of the flap in these specific cases. If the perforators are very tiny and nonpulsating, then the flap should be converted to an MSTD type II flap to incorporate a maximum number of perforators within the flap. The nerve that innervates the rest of the LD muscle is always preserved. If most of the LD muscle is harvested, the flap is dissected as an MSTD type III (**Table 9.1**).

Table 9.1 Classification of the Muscle-Sparing Thoracodorsal (MSTD) Flap

Type	Perforators	LD Segment	Goal
MSTD I	Perforator are tiny, but pulsatile; an intramuscular dissection is performed but perforators are left attached to the muscle that is included in the flap.	A small piece of latissimus dorsi (LD) muscle (4 × 2 cm) is incorporated within the flap	To protect the perforators during flap harvesting and transferring, in particular in a pedicled flap
MSTD II	Perforators are tiny and not pulsatile; no dissection is performed within the muscle	A larger segment of up to 5 cm width is designed along the anterior border of the LD muscle	To incorporate the maximum number of the perforators in the flap
MSTD III	No perforator dissection	A larger muscle segment is included	To include more muscle volume for reconstructive purpose

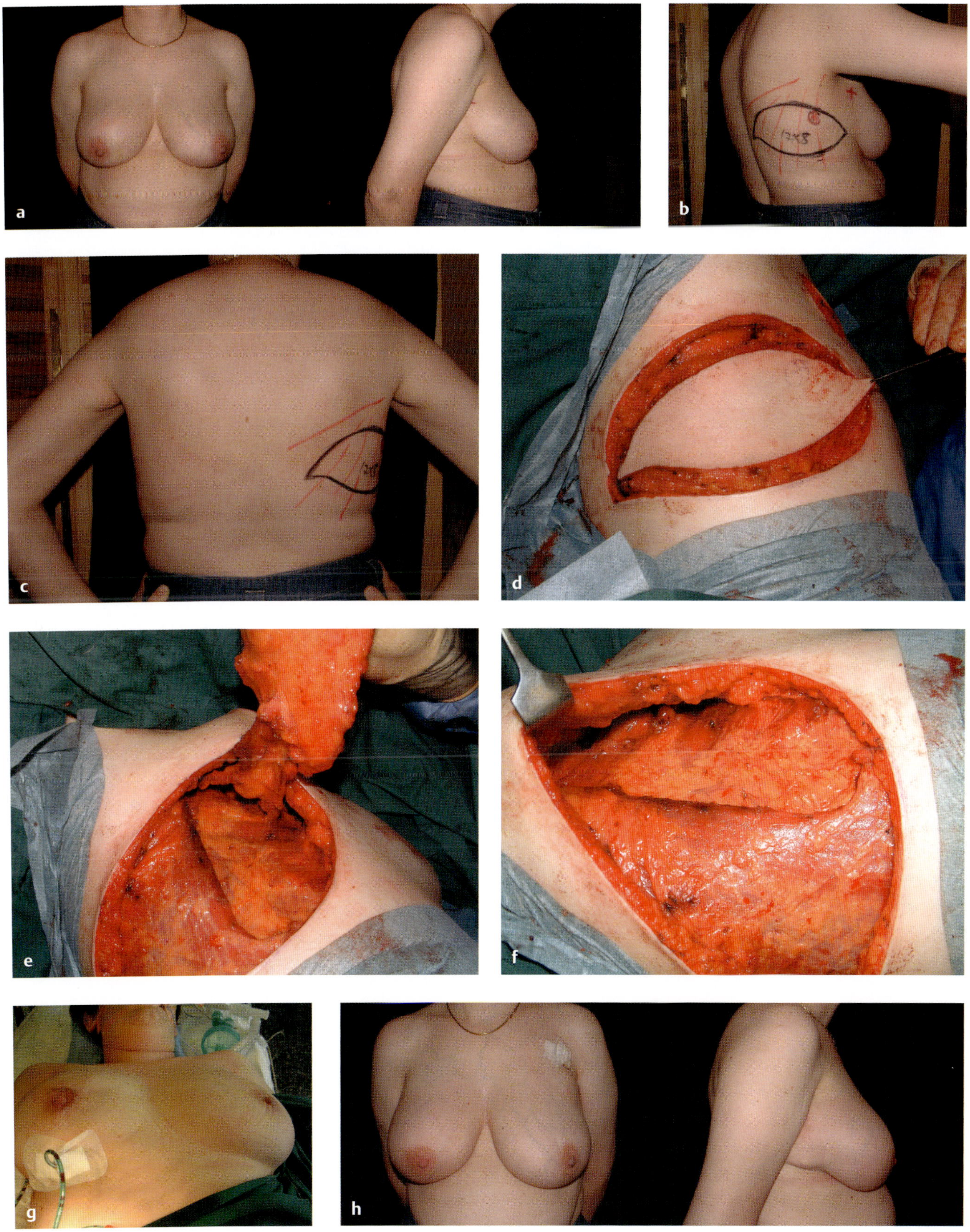

Fig. 9.6 A 39-year-old patient with a ductal carcinoma in the retroareolar area that extended to the superomedial quadrant of the right breast. The patient was scheduled for a quadrantectomy with sentinel lymph node dissection and immediate partial breast reconstruction with a TDAP flap. **(a)** Preoperative views. **(b,c)** Flap markings. **(d)** The flap was dissected. **(e)** To reach the outermost region from the donor site (medial quadrant) a segment of the LD muscle was included to protect the perforator from excessive pull-out. **(f)** The donor site after a 4 cm × 2 cm LD segment harvested within the flap. **(g)** The results at the end of surgery. The defect was filled with the flap through an incision at the medial edge of the areola. **(h)** The results at 1 year postoperatively.

(Continued)

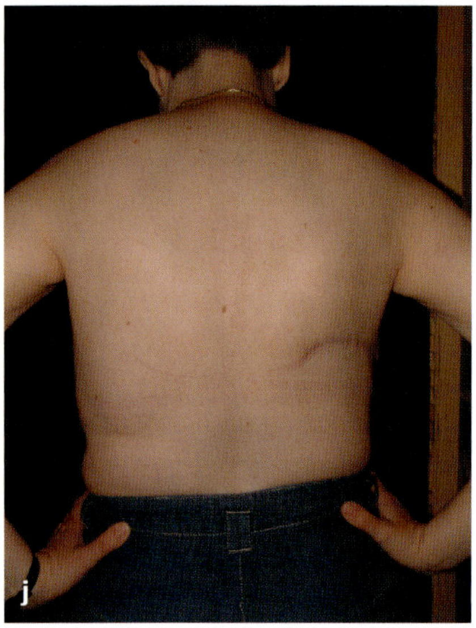

Fig. 9.6 *(Continued)* **(j)** The donor site.

Advantages and Disadvantages of Pedicled Perforator Flaps

The advantages and disadvantages of each flap are summarized in **Table 9.2**. The TDAP flap has all the advantages of perforator flaps, namely muscle preservation with no functional donor-site morbidity. Further, when orienting the flap in a transverse way, the scar can be hidden in the natural folds of the back, which is especially useful in women (hiding the scar in the bra line). The long-term function of the shoulder in terms of mobility and strength do not suffer from the surgery.[30] Another major advantage of the TDAP flap, as compared with its classical muscle flap equivalent (the LD flap), is the elimination of the dead space, thus reducing significantly the risk of seroma formation.[31]

The LICAP flap is a good option for lateral breast defects without sacrificing the thoracodorsal pedicle or the LD muscle. The LICAP flap, being a perforator flap, has the advantage of underlying muscle preservation, thus minimizing donor-site morbidity. Moreover, it avoids the difficult dissection of the costal groove with its potential complication of pneumothorax.

A major advantage of the LICAP harvesting is the preservation of the TDAP and LD for eventual future use. Another advantage is the ease and swiftness of the dissection of the LICAP flap in the hand of the surgeon.

Conclusion

The TDAP flap is a good option for partial (to total) breast reconstructions, preserving the underlying LD and minimizing donor-site morbidity. Perforator mapping is an

Table 9.2 Overview of Advantages/Disadvantages and Indications of Lateral Thoracic Pedicled Perforator Flaps

Pedicled Perforator Flap	Advantages	Disadvantages	Clinical Application
TDAP flap	• Functional muscle preservation • Less seroma formation • Better shoulder mobility/ strength • Scar hidden in bra line	• Inconsistency of perforators (experience necessary) • Doppler perforator mapping misleading • No bulk in thin patients	• Lateral quadrants of breast best • Immediate/delayed breast reconstructions • Full breast reconstruction (with or without implant) in small-moderate size breasts • Thoracic coverage after radical resections
LICAP flap	• Thoracodorsal vessels preserved • LD/intercostal muscles preserved • Fast dissection	• Shorter pedicle • Only lateral quadrants • Potential risk of pneumothorax	• Lateral quadrants of breast • Immediate/delayed breast reconstructions • Autologous breast augmentation (post bariatric corrections) • Lateral thoracic defects
SAAP flap	• Extra pedicle length to LICAP possible	• Connection of intercostal with serratus anterior vessels present in only 20% of cases	• Lateral quadrants of breast, up to retroareolar zone • Immediate/delayed breast reconstructions • Lateral thoracic defects

Abbreviations: LD, latissimus dorsi; LICAP, lateral intercostal artery perforator; SAAP, serratus anterior artery perforator; TDAP, thoracodorsal artery perforator.

essential step in the flap planning to successfully harvest the flap.

The LICAP flap is a perforator flap that can easily be harvested with minimal donor site morbidity, and preservation of future options for other local flaps when necessary. Its main use is in partial breast reconstruction of lateral breast defects.

References

1. Tansini I. Sopra il mio nuovo processo di amputazione della mammella. Gass Med Ital 1906;57:141–143.
2. Marshall DR, Anstee EJ, Stapleton MJ. Soft tissue reconstruction of the breast using an extended composite latissimus dorsi myocutaneous flap. Br J Plast Surg 1984;37:361–368
3. Russell RC, Pribaz J, Zook EG, Leighton WD, Eriksson E, Smith CJ. Functional evaluation of latissimus dorsi donor site. Plast Reconstr Surg 1986;78:336–344
4. Fraulin FO, Louie G, Zorrilla L, Tilley W. Functional evaluation of the shoulder following latissimus dorsi muscle transfer. Ann Plast Surg 1995;35:349–355
5. Randolph LC, Barone J, Angelats J, Dado DV, Vandevender DK, Shoup M. Prediction of postoperative seroma after latissimus dorsi breast reconstruction. Plast Reconstr Surg 2005;116:1287–1290
6. Bailey SH, Oni G, Guevara R, Wong C, Saint-Cyr M. Latissimus dorsi donor-site morbidity: the combination of quilting sutures and fibrin sealant reduce length of drain placement and seroma rate. Ann Plast Surg 2012;68:555–558
7. Taylor GI, Palmer JH. The vascular territories (angiosomes) of the body: experimental study and clinical applications. Br J Plast Surg 1987;40:113–141
8. Koshima I, Soeda S. Inferior epigastric artery skin flaps without rectus abdominis muscle. Br J Plast Surg 1989;42:645–648
9. Allen RJ, Treece P. Deep inferior epigastric perforator flap for breast reconstruction. Ann Plast Surg 1994;32:32–38
10. Angrigiani C, Grill D, Siebert J. Latissimus dorsi musculocutaneous flap without muscle. Plast Reconstr Surg. 1995;96(7):1608–1614.
11. Allen R, Khoobehi K, Montegut W. Abstract: thoracodorsal artery perforator flap for reconstruction. Southern Medical Journal. 90th Annual Scientific Assembly of the Southern Medical Association, Baltimore, Maryland, November 20–24, 1996.
12. Hamdi M, Van Landuyt K, Monstrey S, Blondeel P. Pedicled perforator flaps in breast reconstruction: a new concept. Br J Plast Surg 2004;57:531–539
13. Hamdi M, Van Landuyt K, de Frene B, Roche N, Blondeel P, Monstrey S. The versatility of the inter-costal artery perforator (ICAP) flaps. J Plast Reconstr Aesthet Surg 2006;59:644–652
14. Badran HA, El-Helaly MS, Safe I. The lateral intercostal neurovascular free flap. Plast Reconstr Surg 1984;73:17–26
15. Bartlett SP, May JW Jr, Yaremchuk MJ. The latissimus dorsi muscle: a fresh cadaver study of the primary neurovascular pedicle. Plast Reconstr Surg 1981;67:631–636
16. Rowsell AR, Eisenberg N, Davies DM, Taylor GI. The anatomy of the thoracodorsal artery within the latissimus dorsi muscle. Br J Plast Surg 1986;39:206–209
17. Schaverien M, Saint-Cyr M, Arbique G, Brown SA, Rohrich RJ. Three- and four-dimensional arterial and venous anatomies of the thoracodorsal artery perforator flap. Plast Reconstr Surg 2008;121:1578–1587
18. Lin CT, Huang JS, Yang KC, Hsu KC, Chen JS, Chen LW. Reliability of anatomical landmarks for skin perforators of the thoracodorsal artery perforator flap. Plast Reconstr Surg 2006;118:1376–1386, discussion 1387
19. Heitmann C, Guerra A, Metzinger SW, Levin LS, Allen RJ. The thoracodorsal artery perforator flap: anatomic basis and clinical application. Ann Plast Surg 2003;51:23–29
20. Kerrigan CL, Daniel RK. The intercostal flap: an anatomical and hemodynamic approach. Ann Plast Surg 1979;2:411–421
21. Bravo FG, Schwarze HP. Free-style local perforator flaps: concept and classification system. J Plast Reconstr Aesthet Surg 2009; 62:602–608, discussion 609
22. Hamdi M, Spano A, Van Landuyt K, D'Herde K, Blondeel P, Monstrey S. The lateral intercostal artery perforators: anatomical study and clinical application in breast surgery. Plast Reconstr Surg 2008;121:389–396
23. Hamdi M, Wolfli J, Van Landuyt K. Partial mastectomy reconstruction. Clin Plast Surg 2007;34:51–62, abstract vi
24. Hamdi M, Salgarello M, Barone-Adesi L, Van Landuyt K. Use of the thoracodorsal artery perforator (TDAP) flap with implant in breast reconstruction. Ann Plast Surg 2008;61:143–146
25. Hamdi M, Van Landuyt K. Pedicled perforator flaps in breast reconstruction. In Spear S, ed. Surgery of the Breast, 2nd ed. Philadelphia: Lippincott Williams & Wilkins; 2006:833–846.
26. Hamdi M, Van Landuyt K, Blondeel P, Hijjawi JB, Roche N, Monstrey S. Autologous breast augmentation with the lateral intercostal artery perforator flap in massive weight loss patients. J Plast Reconstr Aesthet Surg 2009;62:65–70
27. Hamdi M, Van Landuyt K, Van Hedent E, Duyck P. Advances in autogenous breast reconstruction: the role of preoperative perforator mapping. Ann Plast Surg 2007;58:18–26
28. Masia J, Clavero JA, Larrañaga JR, Alomar X, Pons G, Serret P. Multidetector-row computed tomography in the planning of abdominal perforator flaps. J Plast Reconstr Aesthet Surg 2006; 59:594–599
29. Taylor GI. The angiosomes of the body and their supply to perforator flaps. Clin Plast Surg 2003;30:331–342, v
30. Hamdi M, Decorte T, Demuynck M, et al. Shoulder function after harvesting a thoracodorsal artery perforator flap. Plast Reconstr Surg 2008;122:1111–1117, discussion 1118–1119
31. Santanelli F, Longo B, Germano S, Rubino C, Laporta R, Hamdi M. Total breast reconstruction using the thoracodorsal artery perforator flap without implant. Plast Reconstr Surg 2014;133:251–254

10 Bipedicled (Double or Stacked) Abdominal Perforator Flap in Unilateral Breast Reconstruction

Julie V. Vasile and Joshua L. Levine

The abdomen remains an ideal choice of donor site for autologous breast reconstruction. In unilateral breast reconstruction, sometimes one hemiabdominal flap, based on the ipsilateral deep inferior epigastric perforator (DIEP) pedicle, does not provide enough volume for a reconstruction that matches the contralateral breast. Adding the contralateral hemiabdomen with its own perforator flap pedicle is an excellent method to increase the volume of perfused fat and skin. The larger, bipedicled flap allows for much greater control in achieving symmetry and ptosis. This surgery is particularly helpful in the radiated or delayed breast reconstruction with a significant skin deficit compared with the contralateral breast. It can also improve success when trying to match a large ptotic breast.

Adding the second hemiabdomen should not be thought of as simply performing another abdominal perforator flap. The addition of the second flap adds to the complexity of the reconstruction for a variety of reasons. Although two flaps are harvested, a midline abdominal incision is not usually made.[1,2] Therefore, the options for approaching the perforators are limited. The second pedicle also has implications with respect to recipient vessel selection and dissection, and if a flap-to-flap anastomoses is to be considered, a suitable branch point off of the primary pedicle must be considered. The increased complexity of the microsurgery influences how the flaps are inset, and postoperative monitoring must be adjusted to take dual perfusion into account. The increased complexity of bipedicled DIEP flap procedures makes them more challenging than a unilateral abdominal perforator flap, but with proper planning, obstacles can be anticipated and overcome, and the bipedicled abdominal perforator flap can be a powerful and rewarding operation for breast reconstruction.

Indications

The bipedicled abdominal perforator flap is considered for unilateral breast reconstruction, especially in thin patients who need a substantial amount of volume to match the contralateral breast. Prior abdominal surgery is not an absolute contraindication, provided that there is enough tissue to reconstruct a breast.

Imaging for Bipedicled Abdominal Perforator Flaps

Preoperative magnetic resonance angiography (MRA) evaluation of the vessels is important for maximizing success and decreasing anesthesia time. The first step is to determine which vessels perfusing each hemiabdomen are best. Most commonly, the DIEP is considered the best vessel because of its larger size and perfusion of thicker fat located along the central lower abdomen. Alternative vessels could be the superficial inferior epigastric pedicle or superficial circumflex iliac pedicle. The second step is to try to determine the ease of connecting one hemiabdominal flap pedicle to the other, and at which locations along the pedicles this may be possible. Each DIEP pedicle is evaluated with respect to its branching pattern. Large branches are compared with the size of the vessels at the cephalad continuation of the pedicle beyond the perforator. If either of these vessel options is robust, flap-to-flap perfusion should be considered. The superficial inferior epigastric arteries are also evaluated.

When evaluating the vascular anatomy, the approach to the dissection should also be considered. If the best perforators are in the medial row of either flap, the microsurgeon must be ready to anticipate the sacrifice of the lateral row, because the medial vessels cannot be viewed via a midline incision.

Donor-Site Dissection

The abdomen is not bisected along the midline. Both hemiabdominal flaps can still be dissected simultaneously, with each surgeon starting laterally or moving from cephalad to caudal. When the lateral perforators are encountered, a vessel is either selected or sacrificed with the knowledge

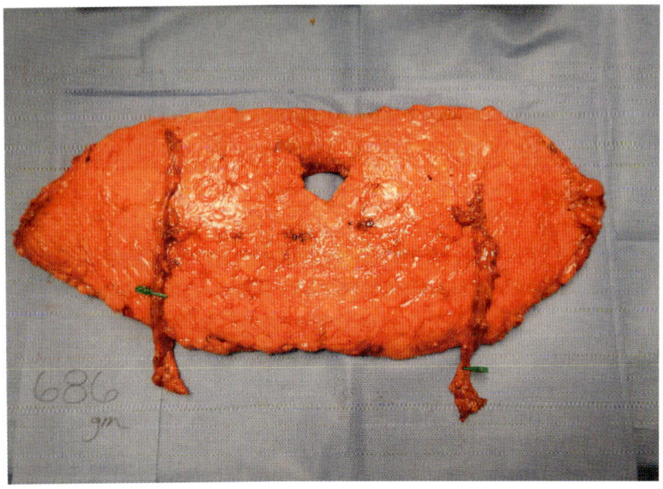

Fig. 10.1 Photograph of DIEP flap turned over on the back table with both pedicles harvested. Lengthy pedicles are advantageous in affording more choices for flap-to-flap anastomoses and insetting after internal mammary (IM) vessel anastomosis.

that a better vessel exists further medial (as seen on MRA). Sometimes lateral perforator options can be preserved while confirming the larger perforators medially. Alternatively, one can learn to trust the MRA image and proceed directly to the perforator of choice, or if one DIEP pedicle dissection is completed first, the pedicle can be transected, and dissection can continue across the midline to approach the second DIEP pedicle medially.

The DIEP pedicle is dissected in the typical manner except for two important points. First, the cephalad continuation and DIEP pedicle branch are dissected for a length adequate for anastomoses if the plan is to connect one pedicle to the other. Second, the DIEP pedicle is dissected caudally until near the external iliac vessels to yield a long pedicle. Dissecting a long pedicle (>8 cm) will aid in decreasing tension on the vessels during microsurgical anastomosis and insetting **(Fig. 10.1)**.

Recipient-Site Dissection

The internal mammary (IM) vessels are typically the recipient vessels chosen. Alternative vessels are the thoracodorsal or lateral thoracic vessels. The IM vessels can be used for both pedicles by providing antegrade and retrograde flow. This can be accommodated by the removal of a 3-cm area of costal cartilage to provide adequate space for the IM dissection and two pedicle anastomoses. The IM vessels are prepared in the standard fashion, except that a longer length of vessels is dissected to enable both pedicles to anastomose to each end of the IM vessels without encumbering one another. Although it can be challenging to do four anastomoses within a narrow area, anastomosing both DIEP pedicles to the IM vessels is frequently advantageous because of the similar arterial and venous caliber match **(Fig. 10.2)**.

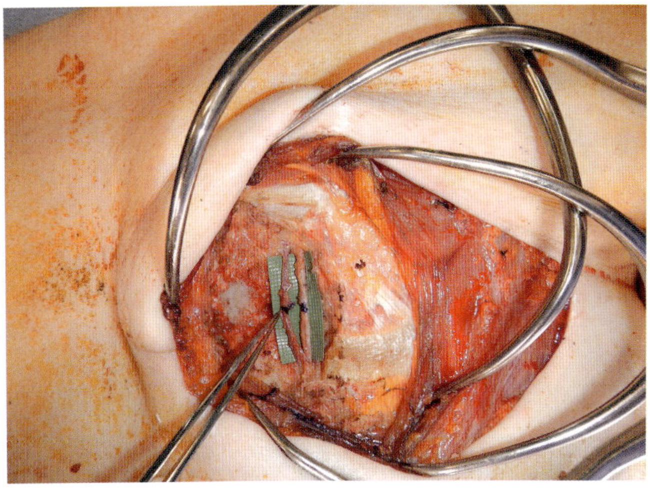

Fig. 10.2 Photograph of the IM vessels prepared after removal of a portion of the third rib cartilage.

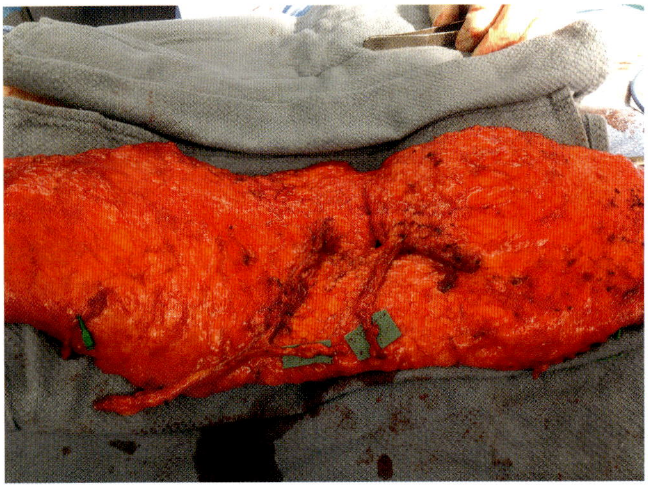

Fig. 10.3 Photograph of the two pedicles brought together and ready for flap-to-flap anastomosis. The green clamp is on a third pedicle, the deep circumflex iliac artery (DCIA), which was harvested as a backup.

Another option is to connect one pedicle to the other. The secondary pedicle can be anastomosed to either a side branch of the main DIEP pedicle or to the superior continuation of the vessels after the perforator branches off of the flap **(Fig. 10.3)**.

Microsurgical Anastomosis

The dissection of each flap should include the harvest of extra length of any suitable side branch, and of the superior continuation of the DIEP pedicle so that there will be several options for a flap-to-flap connection. After removing a portion of medial rib cartilage, the retrograde IM can also be used for the second pedicle, but the decision about which vessels will supply the second flap should only be made after evaluating all reasonable options.

A fortuitous scenario is when the IM artery is flanked by a medial and lateral IM vein because both pedicle veins can be anastomosed to an anterograde IM vein. The retrograde IM vein sometimes has valves,[3] and it is preferable to use antegrade venous outflow from both pedicles if possible. When only one IM vein is present, it is still acceptable to anastomose to a retrograde IM vein once retrograde flow is confirmed by back flushing with heparinized saline. Although a retrograde IM artery has lower pressure than an anterograde artery, it is more than adequate for flap perfusion.

Internal Mammary Anastomoses Antegrade and Retrograde

The order in which the IM vessels are anastomosed to the flap vessels is determined by the orientation of the vessels. In general, the most difficult anastomosis is performed first. The pedicles are draped over the interspace to determine the best orientation for anastomoses **(Fig. 10.4)**. It can be helpful to anastomose the longer pedicle first to the retrograde vessels, and then push the pedicle out of the way to obtain visualization for anastomosis of the shorter pedicle to the anterograde vessels.

If the plan is to anastomose one pedicle to the other, it is best to do this on a prepared sterile side table before connection with the IM vessels. It is helpful to confirm patency by flushing saline through one pedicle artery and visually confirm it flows into the second pedicle artery and back out the pedicle vein.

Insetting and Monitoring

Placing the flaps under the breast skin is very challenging because of the lack of visualization of both pedicles. Extending the incision may improve exposure and decrease tension on the flap during insetting. It is helpful to have a good estimate of the volume needed for the breast reconstruction being performed so that the flap can be trimmed down to size prior to insetting. Once the flap is set in place, it is difficult to remove it for further size tailoring without changing the orientation of the two pedicles.

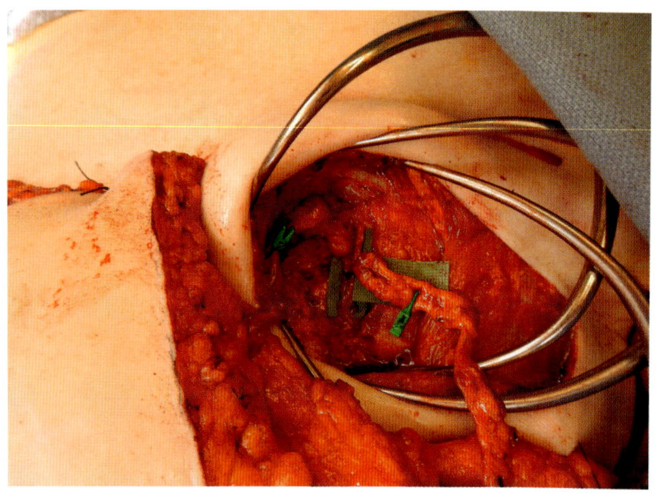

Fig. 10.4 Photograph of the pedicles draped over the interspace to choose the orientation for anastomosis to the IM vessels.

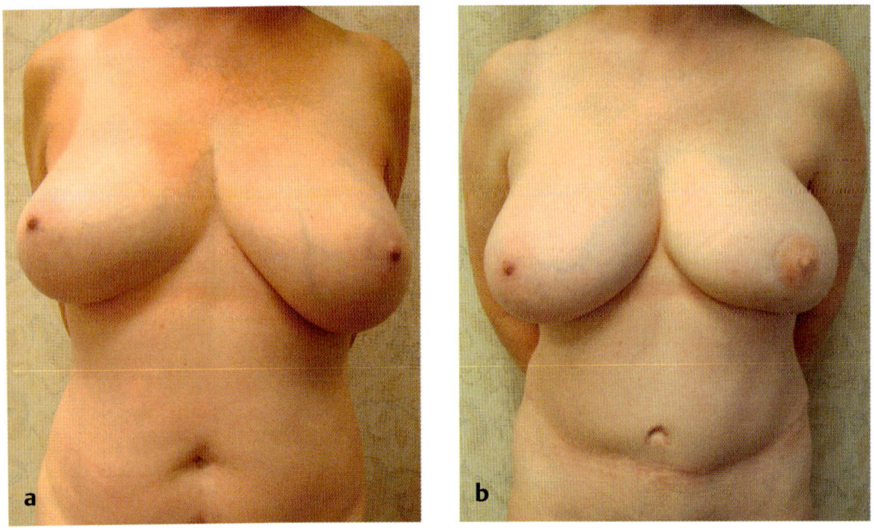

Fig. 10.5 (a) Preoperative photograph of a 58-year-old woman with left ductal breast cancer. She has a depressed lower midline incision from an appendectomy. **(b)** Postoperative photograph 1 year after a left skin-sparing mastectomy and immediate double DIEP flap reconstruction, and 6 months after nipple reconstruction with nipple areola tattooing.

The placement of an internal Doppler is enormously beneficial during flap insetting because the auditory signal confirms patency when visualization of the pedicles is lost. An internal Doppler may also be required for postoperative flap monitoring because it may not be possible to keep a large enough skin island that encompasses the Doppler skin signals of both pedicles, and one of the pedicle Doppler skin signals may be located under the breast skin.

Monitoring

It is important to monitor the flap skin paddle postoperatively for perfusion. Even if an internal Doppler is placed on each pedicle, a skin island should be kept. A large skin paddle accommodates postoperative flap swelling to decrease tension on the anastomoses, and enables accurate assessment of flap venous congestion. A skin island can be removed 2 to 4 weeks after surgery if not needed for the final reconstruction.

Despite the increased complexity, the use of bipedicled or double abdominal perforator flaps for unilateral reconstruction is a very rewarding procedure. It is a reliable technique that provides adequate volume of viable tissue in one stage **(Figs. 10.5** and **10.6)**. Having adequate tissue for unilateral breast reconstruction allows more options for size, shape, and perfusion. The best-perfused tissue can be selected, and the reconstructed breast can be shaped to

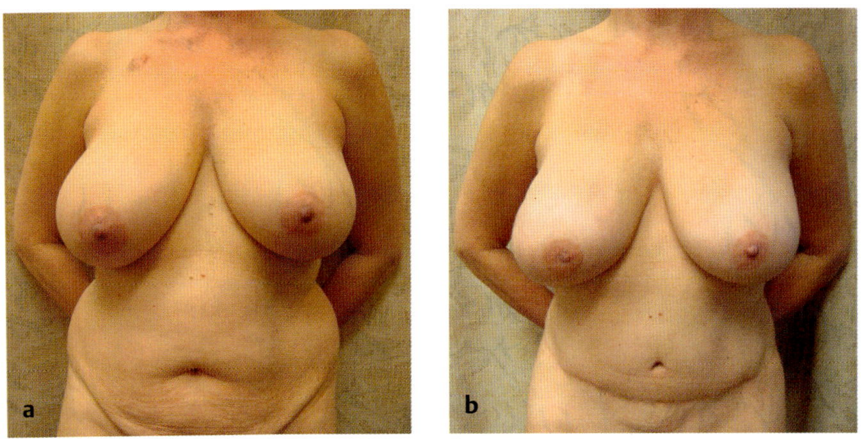

Fig. 10.6 (a) Preoperative photograph of a 50-year-old woman with right breast cancer treated with neoadjuvant chemotherapy. She has a Pfannenstiel incision from a cesarean section. **(b)** Postoperative photograph 6 months after a right nipple-sparing mastectomy with immediate double DIEP flap breast reconstruction.

match the other side, or lifted with a commensurate symmetrizing procedure on the other breast.

References

1. Holm C, Mayr M, Höfter E, Ninkovic M. Perfusion zones of the DIEP flap revisited: a clinical study. Plast Reconstr Surg 2006;117:37–43
2. Wong C, Saint-Cyr M, Mojallal A, et al. Perforasomes of the DIEP flap: vascular anatomy of the lateral versus medial row perforators and clinical implications. Plast Reconstr Surg 2010;125:772–782
3. Mackey SP, Ramsey KW. Exploring the myth of the valveless internal mammary vein—a cadaveric study. J Plast Reconstr Aesthet Surg 2011;64:1174–1179

11 Venous Salvage Procedures in the Deep Inferior Epigastric Perforator Flap for Breast Reconstruction

Thomas Constantinescu and Ming-Huei Cheng

The deep inferior epigastric perforator (DIEP) flap is presently the standard for autologous breast reconstruction. The major advantage of the DIEP flap is decreased donor-site morbidity, as the function of the rectus abdominis muscle is preserved. In a pedicled or free transverse rectus abdominis musculocutaneous (TRAM) flap, this muscle may need to be partially or completely sacrificed. The major disadvantage of the DIEP flap is its associated venous congestion.[1–6] Studies show that venous congestion can limit reliable flap dimensions to a larger extent than arterial inflow.[1,7] As well, the superficial venous system is interrupted in harvest, and is not always compensated well by the deep venous system,[7] which can result in venous congestion. Some authors advocate primary anastomosis of both venous systems, with excellent survival rates.[8]

Venous congestion is defined as a noncompensated mismatch in a flap's ability to drain the blood it requires for adequate perfusion of its entirety. Common etiologies can include an insufficient venous network for the given flap volume, tension at inset, thrombus, and pedicle compression. The incidence of venous congestion in DIEP flaps is reported to be 4 to 20%.[4,9,10] The early sign of venous congestion is flap hyperemia, as the venous system begins to be overwhelmed by arterial inflow. As this discrepancy is not alleviated and persists, capillaries begin to burst as arterial pressure exceeds normal capillary pressure, and the flap begins to look purple. Skin survival is largely compromised at this point, but there is the potential for flap survival and eventual reepithelialization with successful salvage. In our series,[10] venous congestion developed about one third (31%) of the time before pedicle division **(Fig. 11.1)**, and about two thirds (69%) of the time after microsurgical anastomosis **(Fig. 11.2)**, including postoperatively **(Fig. 11.3)**.

Key Anatomy Points

There are important steps in flap harvest that can help prevent venous congestion, as well as help treat it once it is established. The potential venous drainage of the DIEP flap is through the deep system via the deep inferior epigastric vein (DIEV) or veins accompanying the arterial pedicle, and through the superficial system via the superficial inferior epigastric vein (SIEV), located above Scarpa's fascia, 4 to 6 cm lateral to the midline.

Attention must be paid to the SIEV early in flap harvest when it is encountered. After making the inferior incision, the vein should be carefully identified in the subcutaneous fat. In a virgin field, it can be dissected inferiorly to a length of 7 to 10 cm with a diameter of 1 to 3 mm.[10] As the rest of the flap dissection proceeds, the surgeon should take care to identify sizable perforators for use, and to protect the pedicle, including the DIEVs. The maximum length of DIEVs should be harvested, in case additional length is needed for augmentation, or a DIEV would be required as a vein graft to bridge the SIEV to a recipient vein.

Preoperative Management

As with any surgery, patient selection is key. In taking the medical history, it is important to note prior low abdominal scars, whether midline, paramedian, or transverse, in case the SIEV needs to be used. Theoretically, prior scars can also contribute to "delay" of the flap and improved blood supply. A previous transverse cesarean section can sometimes injure both SIEVs, negating their use as lifeboats. In addition, knowing the availability of other potential recipient vessels, such as the thoracodorsal vessels, will assist with intraoperative decision making. Finally, it is important to gather information preoperatively about any clotting issues that may preclude free flap reconstruction.

The patient is asked to sign a specialized informed consent form that specifically includes consent for vein grafting, additional donor-site incisions, and scars in the event that additional recipient veins need to be dissected. We inform the patient that if complications occur the recovery time and the time by which the breast reconstruction will be completed will be delayed. Finally, we routinely discuss the need for potential transfusion perioperatively, especially if needed for nonmicrosurgical decongestion of the flap.

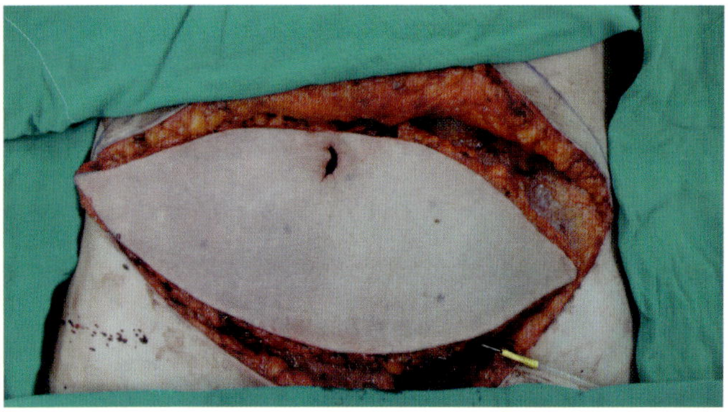

Fig. 11.1 Venous congestion before pedicle division.

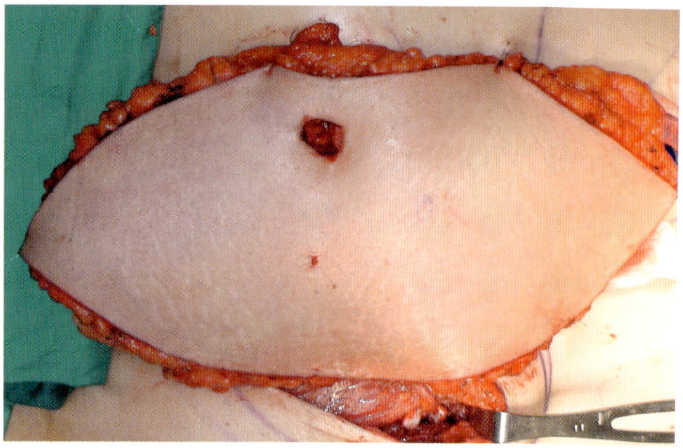

Fig. 11.2 Venous congestion after microsurgical anastomosis.

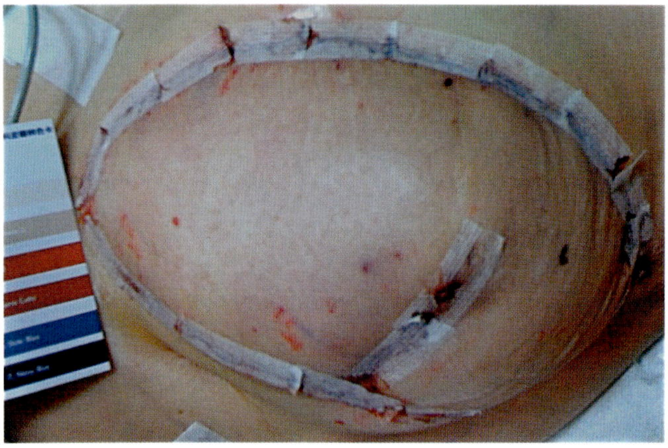

Fig. 11.3 Venous congestion postoperatively.

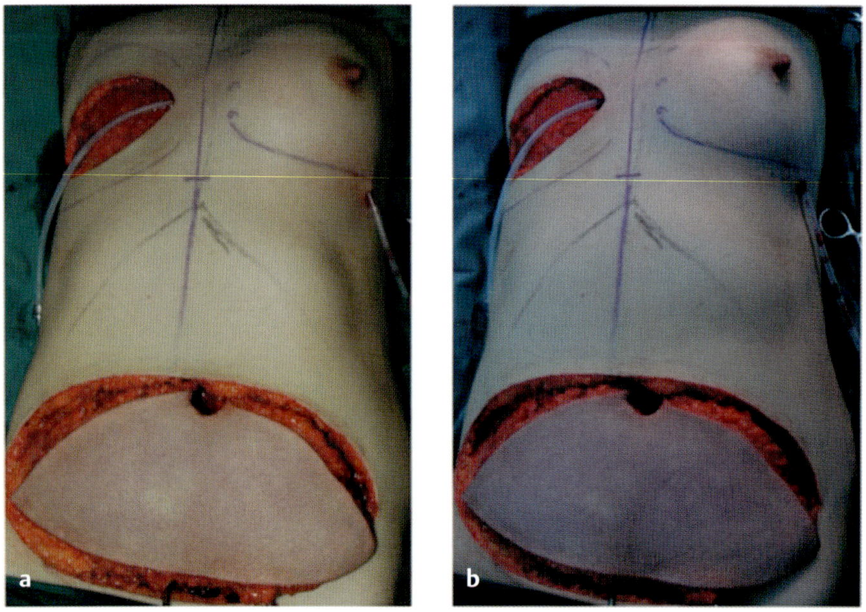

Fig. 11.4 Venous congestion intraoperatively, with **(a)** and without **(b)** operating room lights.

Intraoperative Management

The importance of early diagnosis cannot be overstated. Hypervigilance and early recognition of flap compromise is essential for the microsurgeon, especially because ischemia critically affects transferred tissue. Diagnosis of venous congestion begins intraoperatively. In a study by Dr. Cheng's group,[10] all patients with venous congestion showed intraoperative signs of it (**Fig. 11.4a**). Examination is aided by removing the operative lights from the field (**Fig. 11.4b**). Damaged pedicles during harvest must be recognized and repaired. Veins that drain well must be chosen for anastomosis. This step is especially critical when large DIEP flaps are used, with large angiosomes responsible for draining of substantial amounts of tissue, in the contralateral medial or even contralateral lateral zone.[11] Once the pedicle is skeletonized but not divided, examining the flap for early signs of venous congestion can help alert the surgeon to any need for venous salvage procedures. A step-by-step sequential solution to venous congestion is presented in this chapter.

Microsurgical Salvage

The key issue in assessing venous congestion is the etiology, which is necessary to determine in order to decide on the appropriate treatment. Unless flap compromise is due to a hematologic problem, intraoperative physical exam is crucial to reveal the cause of flap congestion. Because flap congestion is almost always a surgical problem, it requires a surgical solution. The best time to provide the surgical solution is intraoperatively, during the initial surgery. The complication rate is significantly improved with intraoperative salvage versus postoperative reexploration.[10]

Alleviation of Compression

Early hematoma, leading to venous compression and compromise can be detected intraoperatively. Even with closure over drains, hematoma can develop and must be treated. Pedicle compression can occur easily in this setting, when wedged between a heavy DIEP flap and a rigid chest wall, or when limited by tight radiated skin envelope in a delayed reconstruction.

Flap Trimming

Undue tension can cause flap compromise if the flap is too large for the breast footprint and the remaining mastectomy skin flaps. Such a flap should be trimmed and inset again in tension-free fashion. The penumbra zone of the flap can be evaluated clinically or with SPY technology (Novadaq, Bonita Springs, FL). If a portion of the congested flap can be discarded, especially if it is part of zone IV or the contralateral lateral zone, the treatment is excision, which will reduce venous load and may ameliorate circulation of the entire flap.

Pedicle Repair and Repositioning

The anastomosis, although the weakest part of the vessel when it was divided, is often the most rigid part of it after suturing and especially after the stenting effect of coupling. Thus, sometimes the cause of venous failure is far from the anastomosis, as in pedicle injury or kinking. With anastomosis to the internal mammary vessels, a kink can occur at the junction of the pectoralis major and rib periosteum, regardless of whether a rib is removed or not (**Fig. 11.5**). The search for a sharp bend in pedicle should

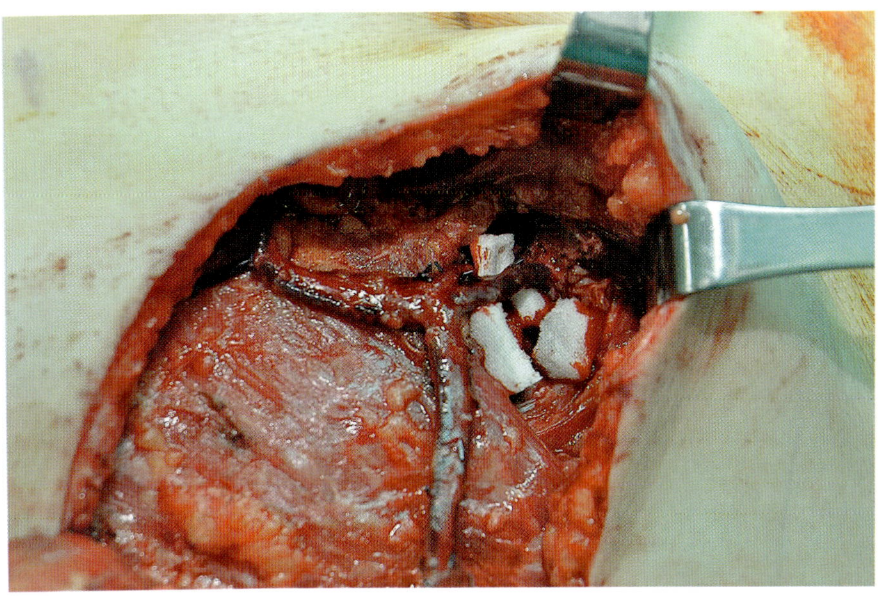

Fig. 11.5 Kinking of the pedicle against chest wall.

include the entire length of the pedicle, as repeated reanastomosis will not treat an unrecognized kink or pedicle injury. Such misdirected efforts will only lead to further ischemia, unresolved problems, and narrowing of the salvage window.

Anastomotic Revision

Flow tests verifying anastomotic patency should be performed proximally and distally, for both veins and arteries. Spasm can often be relieved pharmacologically with lidocaine and papaverine, or surgically with adventitiectomy. These treatments, should be attempted first to allow the flap to recover. Arterial compromise must also be diagnosed and treated. Adequate outflow is irrelevant without adequate inflow. Once spasm and arterial inflow problems have been ruled out, focus should shift to venous congestion related to the anastomosis. If poor venous flow is seen, the anastomosis should be taken down and reanastomosed with or without use of a vein graft. Thrombosis is treated with thrombectomy, which we prefer to do without the assistance of a Fogarty catheter, because we feel that the catheter can injure the intima. Veins can be irrigated with generous amounts of heparinized saline, to dilate the venous tree, and reestablish flow. With an intact arterial inflow, venous outflow must be restored. Once flow is restored, if it is seen to be inadequate, venous augmentation is considered.

Selecting an Alternate Recipient Vein

Selecting an alternate recipient vein adds a new vein to the flap's outflow, promoting venous egress. An algorithm for treating venous congestion in DIEP flaps is provided in **Fig. 11.6** to help visualize options succinctly and streamline intraoperative decision making. Attention should be first directed on establishing the patency or viability of the internal mammary vein (IMV). If the vessel is problematic, performing a pedicled TRAM flap is a possible alternative, which "supercharges" venous outflow by anastomosing the SIEV to an additional recipient vein. **Figs. 11.7** to **11.9** describe options for changing the recipient vein when the IMV is not usable. **Fig. 11.7** shows that using the thoracodorsal vein (TDV) can be an attractive option because it

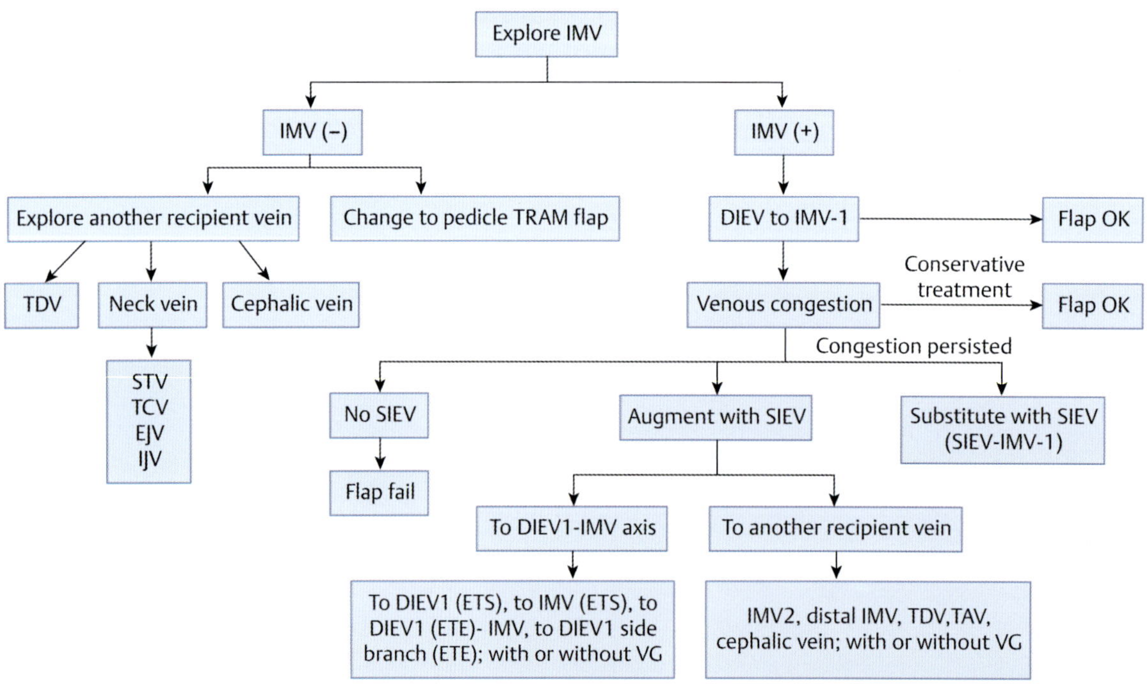

Fig. 11.6 Algorithm for recipient vein options in intraoperative management of venous congestion. DIEA, deep inferior epigastric artery; DIEV, deep inferior epigastric vein; EJV, external jugular vein; IJV, internal jugular vein; IMA, internal mammary artery; IMV, internal mammary vein; SIEA, superficial inferior epigastric artery; SIEV, superficial inferior epigastric vein; STV, superior thyroid vein; TCV, transverse cervical vein; TDV, thoracodorsal vein; TRAM, transverse rectus abdominis musculocutaneous; VG, vein graft.

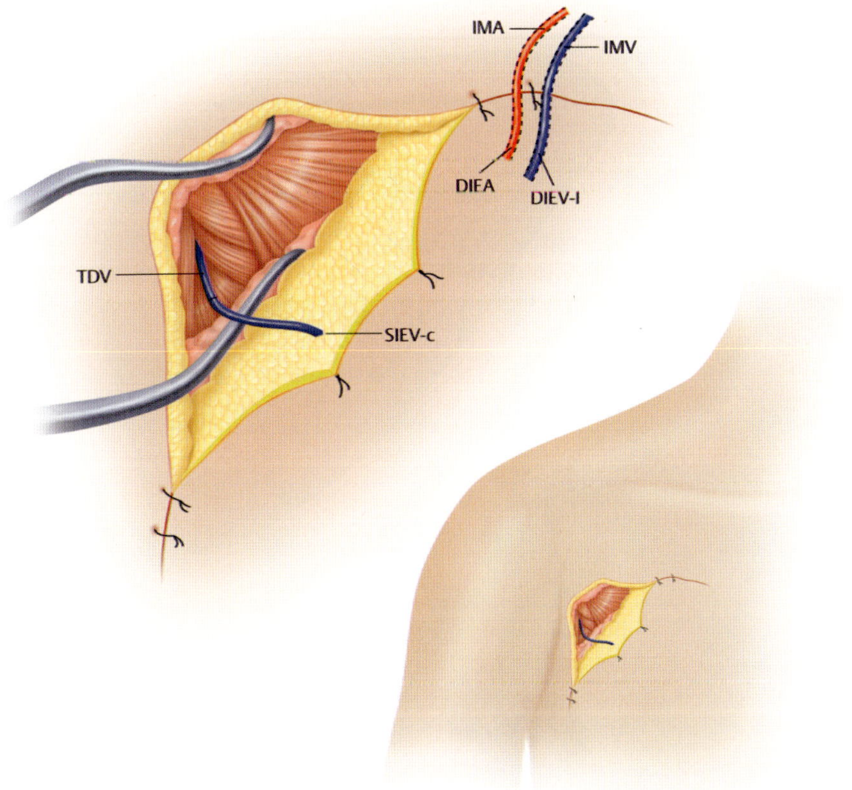

Fig. 11.7 Contralateral superficial inferior epigastric vein anastomosed (SIEV-c) to thoracodorsal vein (TDV).

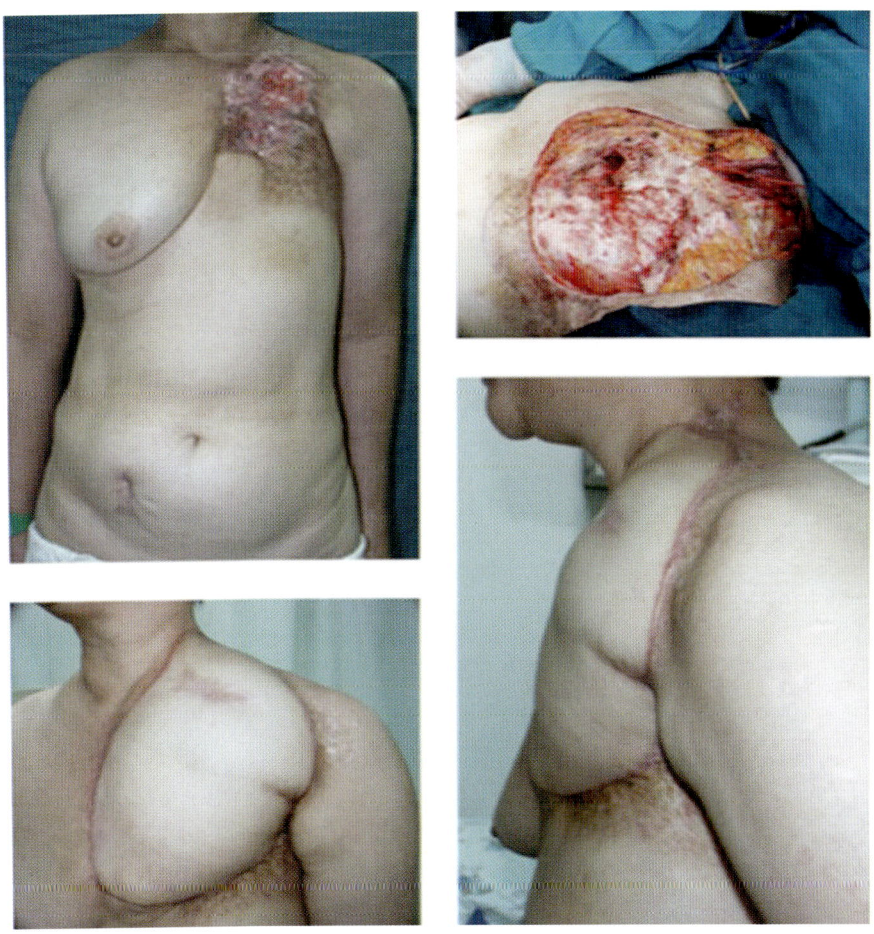

Fig. 11.8 Superficial thyroid artery (STA) and vein (STV) as new recipient vessels after dissection found a poor bed for internal mammary vessel use. One year postoperative photographs: fontal view and lateral view.

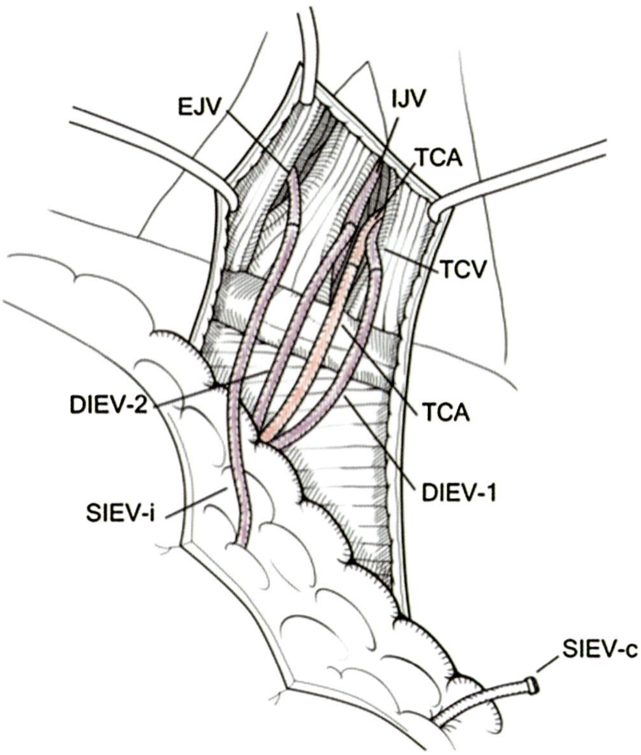

Fig. 11.9 Deep inferior epigastric vein (DIEV-1) anastomosed to the transverse cervical vein (TCV), deep inferior epigastric vein (DIEV-2) anastomosed to internal jugular vein (IJV) end-to-side, ipsilateral superficial inferior epigastric vein (SIEV-i) anastomosed to external jugular vein (EJV).

is near the SIEV when the flap is turned 180 degrees at inset, and does not require a new incision to access. However, committing this vein for augmentation of the DIEP flap precludes its use to drain the latissimus dorsi muscle, which is a common salvage option in breast reconstruction.

Venous Augmentation with the Superficial Inferior Epigastric Vein

In cases where the IMV is functional but insufficient to drain the entire flap, venous augmentation can be obtained with the use of the superficial system. **Figs. 11.10** to **11.13** illustrate possible options, including the use of vein grafts. In this setting, the flap can be drained by both the superficial and deep systems, which is theoretically the best situation for draining the blood from a congested DIEP flap.

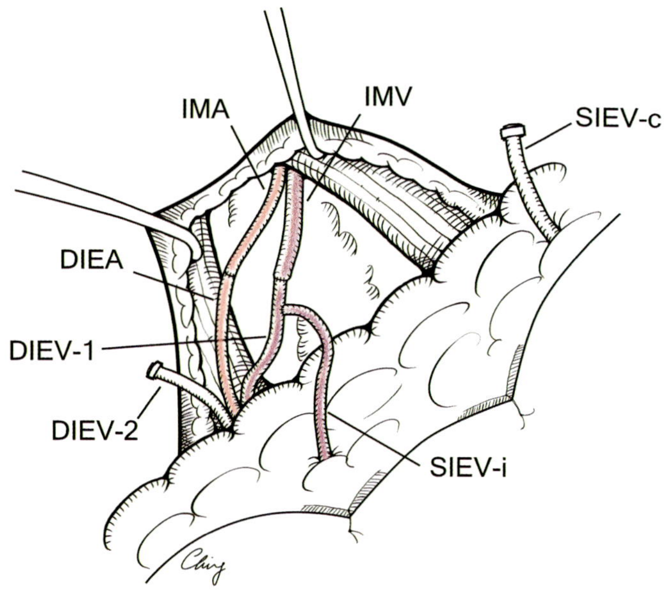

Fig. 11.10 Ipsilateral superficial inferior epigastric vein (SIEV-i) anastomosed to deep inferior epigastric vein (DIEV) in end-to-side fashion.

Venous Substitution with the Superficial Inferior Epigastric Vein

This procedure replaces the venous drainage of the flap through a new donor vein. As surgeons gain experience,

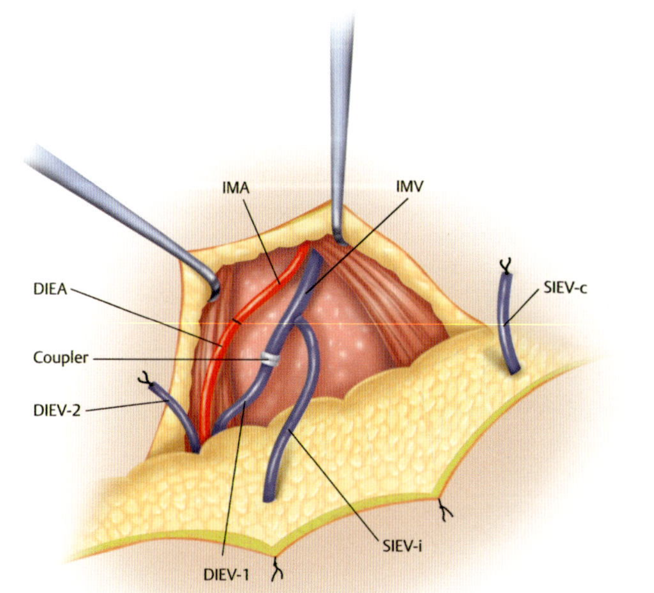

Fig. 11.11 Ipsilateral superficial inferior epigastric vein (SIEV-i) anastomosed to internal mammary vein (IMV) in end-to-side fashion.

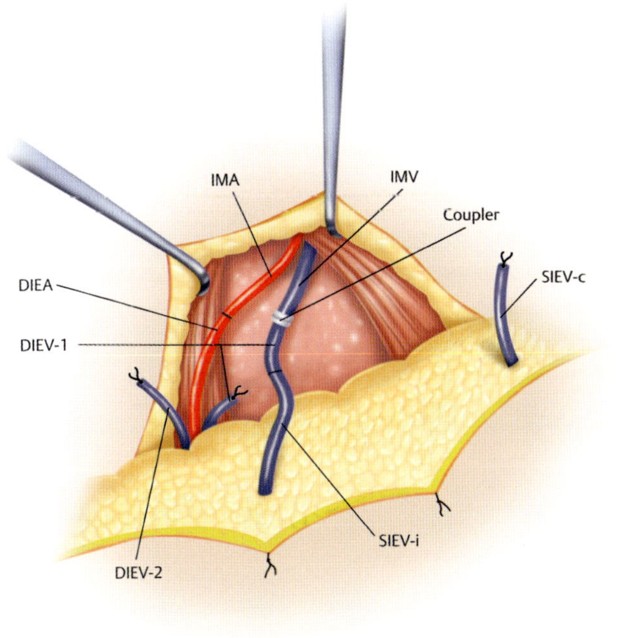

Fig. 11.12 Ipsilateral superficial inferior epigastric vein (SIEV-i) anastomosed to internal mammary vein (IMV) with deep inferior epigastric vein (DIEV-1) used as vein graft.

using the SIEV instead of the DIEV can effectively drain the flap through the superficial system instead of the deep (**Fig. 11.14**). As demonstrated by Cheng's group's[10] study and that of others,[1,2,9,12–16] incorporation of the superficial venous system via the SIEV, instead of a second DIEV draining the deep venous system, appears to be the critical factor in treating venous congestion. We now use the anastomosed DIEV–IMV axis as the recipient vessel for the SIEV, sparing the need for a vein graft or a second recipient vein. We prefer to use the SIEV initially at the venous anastomosis along the DIEV-IMV axis because it accompanies the arterial pedicle, facilitating flap inset.

Nonmicrosurgical Salvage

In cases where microsurgical salvage is ineffective, consideration must be given to nonmicrosurgical salvage techniques before the flap is abandoned. Thrombolysis of the flap is indicated when thrombus is occluding circulation beyond what can be removed with resection of a segment of vessel. Such thrombi can occur to varying degrees up the vascular tree, including into the microcirculation. Furthermore, venous congestion that is allowed to persist long enough will cause arterial compromise, presenting a second diagnosis of flap compromise that requires concomitant treatment of the artery. Key steps must be observed before thrombolysis, because these agents are very powerful. Allergic reactions to the agents must be known, as well as systemic contraindications to their use, which can be verified with past medical history and the anesthetist. The flap should be disconnected from the systemic circulation so that thrombolytic agents do not spread throughout the body. Thrombolytic agents, such as urokinase and streptokinase, should be given via the arterial pedicle and be allowed enough time to act and drain out from the divided venous pedicle, depending on their half-lives. After thrombolysis, the vasculature of the flap should be irrigated to dilute the thrombolytic load prior to reanastomosis.

If flow is partially restored, but venous congestion persists, venous outflow can be improved by de-epithelializing the periphery of the skin paddle. Allowing slow venous egress through the microcirculation can decongest the flap while compensatory angiogenesis occurs over the next week, leading to stable decongestion. In cases where permissive bleeding was allowed from the de-epithelialized flap periphery or via leeches, additional care must be coordinated. Postoperative hourly bedside abrasion of the insensate dermis and applying heparin-soaked gauze sponges promotes continued bleeding by stopping dermal clotting. Another option is to leave a draining vein open, although this maneuver causes significant blood loss and is not routinely recommended. If available and accepted by

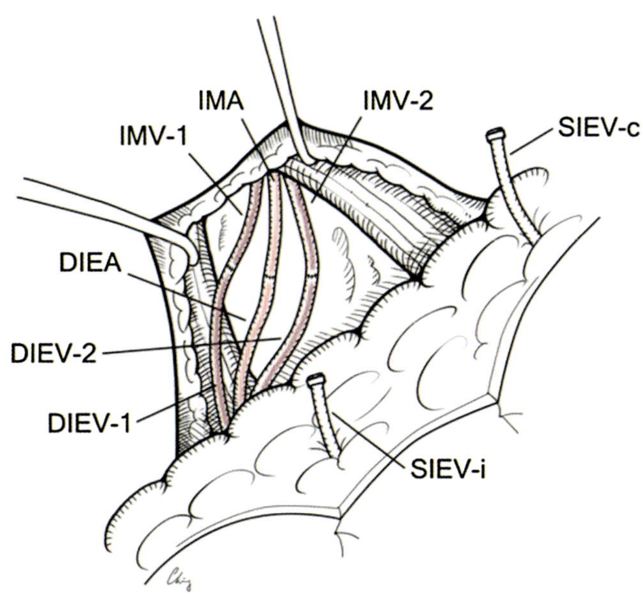

Fig. 11.13 Deep inferior epigastric vein (DIEV-2) anastomosed to internal mammary vein (IMV-2).

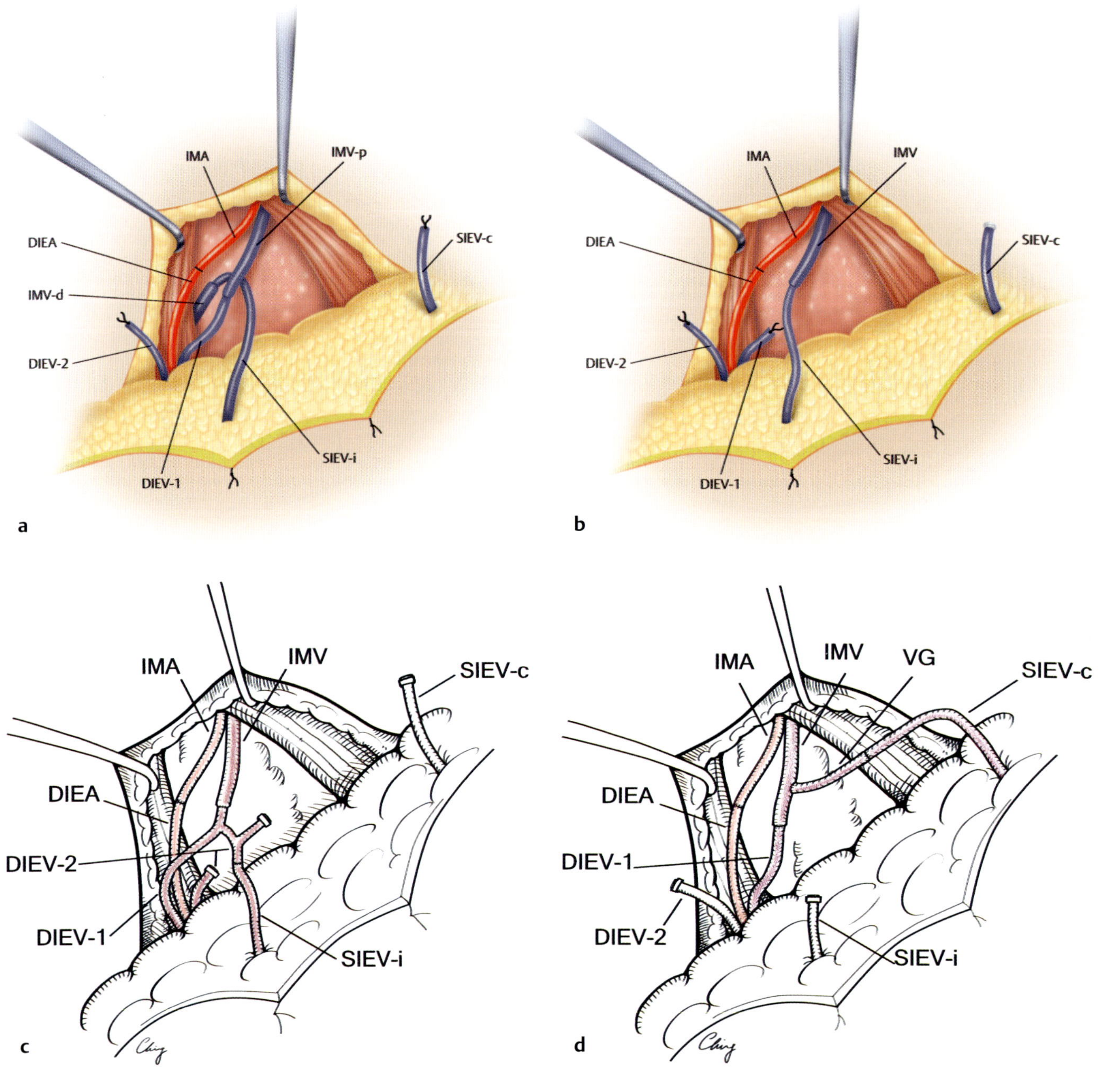

Fig. 11.14 Venous substitution with the SIEV can effectively drain the flap through the superficial system instead of the deep, shown here anastomosed to the internal mammary vein (IMV) in various configurations: **(a)** to the distal end of IMV (IMV-d), **(b)** to the IMV directly if the length is adequate, **(c)** to the DIEV-2 and then to the communicated branch to the DIEV-1 and then to the IMV, **(d)** the contralateral SEIV (SIEV-c) to the IMV with a segment of vein graft.

the patient, leeches, or *Hirudo medicinalis*, applied to the dermis, are useful for drainage of congested flaps. A continuous supply of leeches must be available by the hour to be changed by the nursing personnel, and appropriate antibiotic prophylaxis against *Aeromonas hydrophila* must be instituted, such as ciprofloxacin 500 mg PO/IV b.i.d. throughout the duration of leech application. Blood loss must be anticipated, monitored with daily blood counts, and replaced as indicated. Furthermore, the blood count serves to verify platelet levels and diagnose heparin-induced thrombocytopenia early, especially in such patients with possible venous clotting.

Accepting Flap Loss and Plan B

If the decision is made to abandon a flap, temporary wound management may be considered with a vacuum-assisted closure (VAC) if a second surgery is anticipated in the early postoperative period. Such closure will help prevent wound edge retraction and prevent the defect from enlarging, requiring a larger skin paddle on a subsequent closure attempt. This can be an issue if salvage is planned with a latissimus dorsi flap, which usually does not allow a skin paddle as large as the DIEP flap for direct donor-site closure. In addition, closure can also be obtained with a skin graft from the flap itself, or the contralateral hemiabdominal flap if it is not part of the reconstruction. Otherwise, standard skin graft donor sites may be used. If the thigh is employed, care must be taken not to compress the donor site, as DIEP patients are more prone to DVTs due to the tightness of abdominal closure. A second compression of the venous system, akin to a "double crush," should not be induced in these patients, who do not always mobilize well postoperatively and who are fitted with abdominal binders.

Postoperative Management

Early recognition of venous congestion is important at all times, from isolation of the pedicle, to the anastomoses and throughout the postoperative period. In our practice, we administer pharmacological treatment with heparin for deep venous thrombosis prophylaxis, and continue heparin postoperatively for 7 days when there were issues with the pedicle intraoperatively. Clinically, it is important to detect any potential hematomas and seromas to avoid flap compromise. In addition, it is essential to avoid flap compression when placing dressings and abdominal binders. If venous congestion is suspected, first-line maneuvers include releasing sutures and repositioning the flap and patient. There needs to be a low threshold for postoperative reexploration of a compromised flap. As a rule, the surgeon should not hesitate to return the patient promptly to the operating room if venous congestion is suspected.[17] We find monitoring the flap with serial photographs taken with a smartphone to be very useful in autologous breast reconstruction because any color change in the skin paddle can be readily assessed with a standard color card.[18]

Conclusion

Considerations for venous congestion in DIEP flaps begin with preoperative planning and risk assessment. The DIEP flap is the gold standard for autologous breast reconstruction, but early recognition of venous congestion is critical. If venous congestion is noted, the best time to intervene is intraoperatively, and there should be a low threshold to address any questionable venous outflow prior to leaving the operating room. Both microsurgical and nonmicrosurgical strategies exist to salvage congested flaps, and the choice is guided by the reason for venous congestion. An algorithmic approach to salvage, combined with surgeon experience, makes it possible to optimize venous management so that the DIEP flap may be used for breast reconstruction in a safe and reliable manner.

Key Points

1. Vigilance and patience are key to success in microsurgery.
2. The incidence of venous congestion in DIEP flaps is 4 to 20%.
3. Early intraoperative salvage can significantly decrease the complications of congested DIEP flaps.
4. Although vein grafts are seldom required, the surgeon should anticipate any potential need for a vein graft or additional incisions, and should discuss this issue with the patient preoperatively.
5. Excellent salvage rates can be achieved with early detection and an algorithmic approach to treatment.

References

1. Blondeel PN, Arnstein M, Verstraete K, et al. Venous congestion and blood flow in free transverse rectus abdominis myocutaneous and deep inferior epigastric perforator flaps. Plast Reconstr Surg 2000;106:1295–1299
2. Tran NV, Buchel EW, Convery PA. Microvascular complications of DIEP flaps. Plast Reconstr Surg 2007;119:1397–1405, discussion 1406–1408
3. Nahabedian MY, Momen B, Galdino G, Manson PN. Breast reconstruction with the free TRAM or DIEP flap: patient selection, choice of flap, and outcome. Plast Reconstr Surg 2002;110:466–475, discussion 476–477
4. Hallock GG, Rice DC. Efficacy of venous supercharging of the deep inferior epigastric perforator flap in a rat model. Plast Reconstr Surg 2005;116:551–555, discussion 556
5. Taylor GI. Invited discussion for "The surgically delayed unipedicled TRAM flap for breast reconstruction." Ann Plast Surg 1996;36:238–245
6. Masia J, Clavero JA, Larrañaga JR, Alomar X, Pons G, Serret P. Multidetector-row computed tomography in the planning of abdominal perforator flaps. J Plast Reconstr Aesthet Surg 2006; 59:594–599

7. Schaverien M, Saint-Cyr M, Arbique G, Brown SA. Arterial and venous anatomies of the deep inferior epigastric perforator and superficial inferior epigastric artery flaps. Plast Reconstr Surg 2008;121:1909–1919
8. Boutros SG. Double venous system drainage in deep inferior epigastric perforator flap breast reconstruction: a single-surgeon experience. Plast Reconstr Surg 2013;131:671–676
9. Wechselberger G, Schoeller T, Bauer T, Ninkovic M, Otto A, Ninkovic M. Venous superdrainage in deep inferior epigastric perforator flap breast reconstruction. Plast Reconstr Surg 2001;108:162–166
10. Ali R, Bernier C, Lin YT, et al. Surgical strategies to salvage the venous compromised deep inferior epigastric perforator flap. Ann Plast Surg 2010;65:398–406
11. Henry SL, Cheng MH. A call for clarity in TRAM/DIEP zones. Plast Reconstr Surg 2010;125:210e–211e
12. Mehrara BJ, Santoro T, Smith A, et al. Alternative venous outflow vessels in microvascular breast reconstruction. Plast Reconstr Surg 2003;112:448–455
13. Villafane O, Gahankari D, Webster M. Superficial inferior epigastric vein (SIEV): "lifeboat" for DIEP/TRAM flaps. Br J Plast Surg 1999;52:599
14. Niranjan NS, Khandwala AR, Mackenzie DM. Venous augmentation of the free TRAM flap. Br J Plast Surg 2001;54:335–337
15. Tutor EG, Auba C, Benito A, Rábago G, Kreutler W. Easy venous superdrainage in DIEP flap breast reconstruction through the intercostal branch. J Reconstr Microsurg 2002;18:595–598
16. Liu TS, Ashjian P, Festekjian J. Salvage of congested deep inferior epigastric perforator flap with a reverse flow venous anastomosis. Ann Plast Surg 2007;59:214–217
17. Vasconez L. 2005 Jurkiewicz Lecture. Ann Plast Surg 2006;56: 1–8
18. Engel H, Huang JJ, Tsao CK, et al. Remote real-time monitoring of free flaps via smartphone photography and 3G wireless Internet: a prospective study evidencing diagnostic accuracy. Microsurgery 2011;31:589–595

12 Imaging for Perforator Flap Breast Reconstruction

Julie V. Vasile

Magnetic resonance angiography (MRA) is an extremely useful preoperative imaging test for evaluation of the vasculature of donor tissue to be used in autologous breast reconstruction. MRA has sufficient spacial resolution to reliably visualize 1-mm perforating vessels and to accurately locate vessels in reference to a patient's anatomic landmarks without exposing the patient to ionizing radiation or iodinated contrast. The use of a blood pool contrast agent and the lack of radiation exposure allow multiple studies of multiple anatomic regions in one examination. This chapter discusses the MRA protocol developed with the radiologists at our center and provides examples that illustrate the utility of MRA in perforator flap breast reconstruction.

Preoperative Imaging

Preoperative anatomic imaging of the vasculature markedly enhances the ability of the surgeon to devise a surgical strategy before going to the operating room. Prior to the era of preoperative perforator imaging, a surgeon had little knowledge of the patient's vascular anatomy until surgery was well underway. As a result, perforator selection could be a complicated decision process taking place in the operating room at the expense of operating time and prolonged anesthesia time.

Doppler

As technology has advanced, surgeons have favored varying modalities for preoperative imaging. Initially, a handheld Doppler ultrasound was solely used to attempt to locate perforating vessels. A Doppler ultrasound is portable and simple to use but cannot differentiate perforating vessels from superficial and deep axial vessels, or robust perforators from minuscule ones, cannot accurately determine the location where perforators exit the fascia, and cannot provide information on the anatomic course of a vessel.[1,2] In comparison, color Duplex sonography provides more detailed information about the anatomy of the vessels, but requires highly trained technicians with knowledge of perforator anatomy, and it is time-consuming to perform.[2] The technique's most crucial drawback is an inability to produce anatomic images in a format that a surgeon can easily and independently view.

Computed Tomographic Angiography

Computed tomographic angiography (CTA) is a modality that can demonstrate vessel anatomy, assess vessel caliber, accurately locate perforators, and produce anatomic images in a format that a surgeon can easily and independently view. Although CTA can be performed quickly in as little as 15 minutes,[1,2] patients must be exposed to ionizing radiation. Radiation exposure precludes multiple imaging studies in one examination. Articles in the medical literature and the lay press warn that physicians may be exposing patients to excessive and potentially unnecessary radiation.[3–6] Patients with breast cancer may have a heightened concern about any modality that can potentially increase the risk of developing a second cancer and may perceive the risks of radiation exposure even more negatively. Patients with breast cancer gene *(BRCA)* mutations, which confer an increased risk of developing both breast and ovarian cancer, are especially concerned about receiving radiation to the abdomen. An addition drawback of CTA is that the iodinated contrast that is needed to enhance vessels for CTA can be associated with a small but real risk of anaphylaxis and nephrotoxicity.[7,8]

Magnetic Resonance Angiography

Magnetic resonance imaging (MRI) uses a magnetic field to uniformly align the spin of hydrogen atoms in tissue.

The subsequent application of a radiofrequency pulse results in the release of energy as hydrogen atoms return to their relaxed state. MRI coils detect the released energy, and computer software processes the data into anatomic images. Exposure to a magnetic field or radiofrequency pulse with MRI has not been linked to the development of cancer.[9] A paramagnetic contrast agent (gadolinium-containing) is injected to enhance vessel imaging our group reported demonstrated that MRA accurately locates perforating vessel branches and shows vessel anatomy in a format that is easily viewed by a surgeon.[10–13] However, because MRI does not use radiation, this modality has an important advantage over CTA, in that it enables obtaining multiple series of images of the patient in the supine and prone position.

The disadvantages of MRA is that it is contraindicated in patients with a cardiac pacemaker and in very claustrophobic patients. Most patients with claustrophobia can tolerate an MRI if an anxiolytic is prescribed. Continuing advances in MRA have decreased the procedure time for a single donor site to as little as 20 minutes, and decreased the actual acquisition scan time to 20 seconds.[11,13–15] However, the examination time could be as long as 40 minutes for multiple donor-site studies.

Magnetic Resonance Angiography Contrast Agents

Gadolinium-containing contrast agents used for MRA have several distinct advantages over iodinated contrast agents used for CTA. The incidence of an acute allergic reaction to iodinated contrast is 3%, which is orders of magnitude higher than the 0.07% incidence of allergic reaction to gadolinium contrast.[7,16] Unlike gadolinium contrast agents, iodinated CT contrast agents can induce renal insufficiency even in patients with normal renal function.[8,17] Gadolinium contrast agents can potentially induce nephrogenic systemic fibrosis (NSF), also called nephrogenic fibrosing dermopathy. However, reports of NSF have been limited to patients with impaired renal function.[18–20] Patients with an acute kidney injury or chronic severe renal disease (glomerular filtration rate < 30 mL/min/1.73 m^2) are considered most at risk.[18] NSF is a very rare disease, with 380 cases reported worldwide.[19,20] Although patients undergoing elective microsurgical free flap are generally healthy and thus are not at significant risk of developing NSF, a creatinine level is drawn preoperatively in patients with a history of hypertension, diabetes, renal disease, or any other indication that renal function may be impaired.

Advances in gadolinium contrast agents with blood pool contrast agents have resulted in a decreased amount of contrast required and improved MR images, and have increased even further the number of donor sites that can be imaged in one study. The MRA protocol developed with the radiologists at our center uses 10 mL of gadofosveset trisodium, a blood pool MRI contrast agent. Prior to using this blood pool agent, 20 mL (instead of 10 mL) of gadolinium contrast (gadobenate dimeglumine) was required. Gadofosveset trisodium is a gadolinium chelate that reversibly binds to serum albumin with 90% binding fraction, and effectively stays within the blood pool with a redistribution half-life of 28 minutes.[21] It also demonstrates greater T1 relaxivity that enables administration of a fourfold lower molecular dose while still conferring greater vascular enhancement compared with most other gadolinium chelates. This virtually eliminates the risk of NSF.[22]

Gadofosveset improves the vessel-to-muscle contrast ratio and vessel sharpness, mainly due to preferential enhancement of vessels compared with muscle derived from the blood pool distribution of gadofosveset.[23] This results in significantly improved images of the intramuscular course of perforating vessels, which gives valuable information for choosing the best perforating vessel, avoiding transection of muscle, deciding on the feasibility of a flap with more than one perforator, and planning for double flaps to make one breast.

Because blood pool contrast agents are bound to albumin, with a redistribution half life of 28 minutes, there is a significantly increased amount of time to acquire images.[24] This affords the opportunity to assess many donor sites for autologous breast reconstruction in a single examination, with the patient turning from the prone to supine positions to image the posterior (thigh, buttock, back) and anterior (abdomen) donor sites, respectively. In addition, flap volume estimates can be more accurately determined at both anterior and posterior donor sites because the imaging is acquired with the patient in the supine and prone positions, respectively, so that the tissue is not compressed. For example, buttock flap volumes are calculated with the patient in the prone position and abdominal deep inferior epigastric perforator (DIEP) flap volumes are calculated with the patient in the supine position. Once the surgeon has acquired the imaging findings regarding the vessels and flap volume at each donor site, the selection of the most suitable flap donor sites can be discussed with the patient. Moreover, a patient who is found not to be a candidate for an abdominal perforator flap based on imaging findings, who suddenly changes her donor-site preference, or who has a flap failure and requires another perforator flap reconstruction will not require further studies.

Magnetic Resonance Angiography Protocol

Magnetic resonance angiography is performed on a long-bore, self-shielded 1.5-tesla (T) scanner (GE Signa 14.0, Waukesha, WI) using an eight-channel phased array coil. The field of view is individualized, but usually extends from 5 cm above the umbilicus to the upper thigh, and transversely is set to match the width of the patient. After acquiring a three-plane localizer, axial and coronal T2-weighted, single-shot, fast spin echo images are acquired to screen for unexpected pathology and to help characterize any lesions detected on postgadolinium scans. Because most of these patients have a history of breast cancer, metastatic disease is detected occasionally. This sequence is also helpful in confirming the central position of the umbilicus in the prone position. A transverse pre- and postcontrast arterial-phase three-dimensional (3D) liver accelerated volume acquisition (LAVA) sequence is acquired with the following imaging parameters: TR/TE/flip = 3.9/1.9/15; bandwidth = 125 kHz; slice thickness = 3 mm reconstructed at 1.5-mm intervals using twofold zero interpolation (ZIP 2); matrix = 512 × 128–256; parallel acceleration factor = 2. Precontrast imaging is important to determine the adequacy of fat suppression. Central frequency and shim field of view can be adjusted as necessary to ensure effective fat suppression over the subcutaneous tissues of interest if Dixon fat-water separation is not available.

The arterial-phase imaging is bolus tracked by automated triggering (SmartPrep, GE Healthcare), and scanning is initiated after the contrast arrives in the suprarenal aorta; 10 mL of gadofosveset trisodium blood pool MRI contrast agent is injected, followed by 20 mL of normal saline at a rate of 1 mL/s. Hand injection is preferred, especially if there is a tenuous intravenous (IV) line, because approximately one third of patients may experience some sensation at the injection site or in the pelvis related to the ionic contrast agent.[24] The k-space is mapped sequentially, with the absolute center of k-space collected in the middle of the scan, which is ~ 20 seconds after bolus detection, for a 35-second scan duration and a 5-second pause for breath holding instruction. This is important to provide time for the contrast to reach and fill perforating arteries. However, only the largest perforator arterial/vein bundles are adequately seen on this sequence. This is followed by equilibrium phase transverse 3D LAVA at higher resolution without parallel imaging using the following parameters: TR/TE/flip = 4/1.9/15; matrix = 512 × 512 × (172–240); bandwidth = 125 kHz; slice thickness = 3 mm reconstructed at 1.5-mm intervals using ZIP2 slice interpolation. Phase encoding is set to the right-left direction. This is the primary sequence utilized to generate reconstructions and create reports and also serves as a reference for the plastic surgeons. It is acquired with free breathing and typically requires 3- to 5-minute acquisition duration with 0.9 × 0.9 × 3 mm acquired voxel dimension and 0.9 × 0.9 × 1.5 mm reconstructed voxel dimensions. Thereafter, a lower resolution coronal and sagittal plane LAVA is acquired with acquisition matrix of 512 × 256 and 512 × 224, respectively, in a single breath hold and parallel acceleration factor of 2 to evaluate internal organs.

The planned donor site is imaged first, followed by single high spatial resolution equilibrium phase imaging of other potential donor sites using the free-breathing 3D LAVA sequence described above. A typical complete perforator flap MR examination, including abdomen, buttocks, and upper thigh, can take 45 minutes.

After screening axial and coronal single-shot fast spin echo images for unexpected pathologies, the arterial-phase images are reviewed to determine the number of perforators available and to look for any enhancing lesions. High spatial resolution equilibrium phase images are used for final perforator evaluation, as perforators are best visualized on these images. The equilibrium phase series is loaded on a computer workstation (GE Advantage Windows 4.4, Milwaukee, WI) for postprocessing. Coronal, sagittal, and surface-rendered reformatted images are generated. The reference point and each candidate perforator artery/vein bundle are identified. The diameter and perforator exit location at the point where the vessel pierces the superficial fascia and enters into subcutaneous fat are noted. The cephalad/caudal and right/left distances of each perforator exit site relative to the reference point are calculated to create a perforator location coordinate. The intramuscular course and length of each perforator is measured to predict the vascular pedicle length. Finally, a predicted flap volume is calculated on the same workstation assuming an elliptical geometry on a slice-by-slice basis.

Coordinates identifying the location of the perforating arteries on the axial images are superimposed and displayed on volume-rendered 3D reconstructed images and coronal 3D minimum intensity projection (MIP) images. These images are especially helpful to locate the perforator vessels during preoperative surface marking and then intraoperatively.

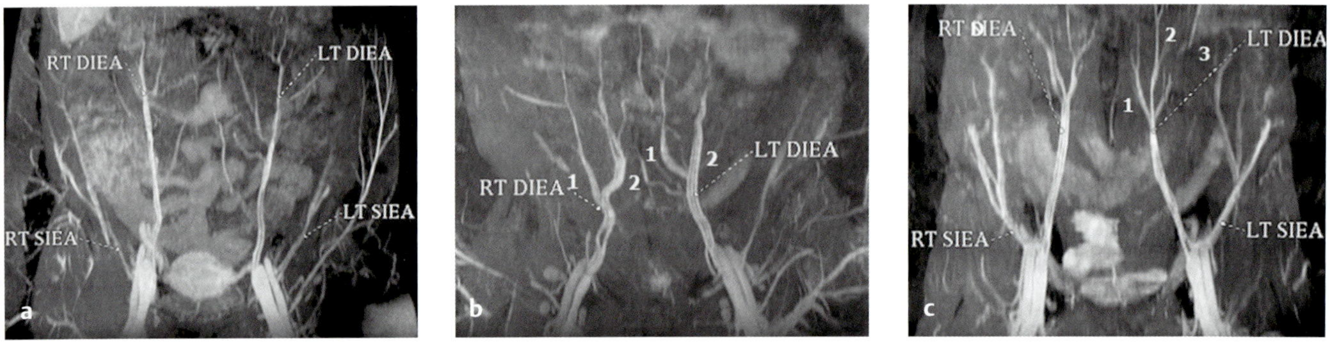

Fig. 12.1 Coronal minimum intensity projection (MIP) magnetic resonance angiography (MRA) abdomen. **(a)** Type 1 deep inferior epigastric branching pattern. **(b)** Type 2 deep inferior epigastric branching pattern on both sides of the abdomen with a medial and lateral branch denoted by *1* and *2*. **(c)** Type 3 deep inferior epigastric branching pattern with *1*, *2*, and *3* denoting multiple branches from the left deep inferior epigastric. DIEA, deep inferior epigastric artery; LT, left; RT, right; SIEA, superficial inferior epigastric artery.

Magnetic Resonance Angiography and Perforator Selection

Vessel caliber in conjunction with a centralized location on the flap are the most important factors for optimal perforator selection at every donor site. Caliber measurements are uniformly performed at the point where a vessel exits the superficial fascia. Location measurements are performed in reference to a landmark at each donor site.

Abdomen

First, the deep inferior epigastric vessel branching pattern is identified on each hemiabdomen. A coronal MIP image **(Fig. 12.1)** best illustrates the branching pattern and is included in the report. This image is helpful for anticipating the direction of dissection, for confirming vessel patency, and for planning when a double flap to reconstruct one breast is anticipated. Next, the location of the largest DIEP is identified at the point of exit from the anterior rectus fascia, and is measured in reference to the center of the base of the umbilical stalk **(Fig. 12.2)**. Vessel caliber measurements are also performed just above the anterior fascia level.

Finally, the intramuscular course or paramuscular (septocutaneous) course is examined **(Fig. 12.3).** The vessel course provides information that tells the surgeon to anticipate either a complicated or a straightforward dissection. The improved visualization of intramuscular perforator course on MRA enables preoperative decision making on harvesting more than one perforator. It also enhances the ability of a surgeon to plan for double flaps used to make one breast, in which one flap vessel pedicle can be connected to a second flap vessel pedicle at a branching point or at the cephalad continuation of the pedicle beyond the perforator **(Fig. 12.4).**

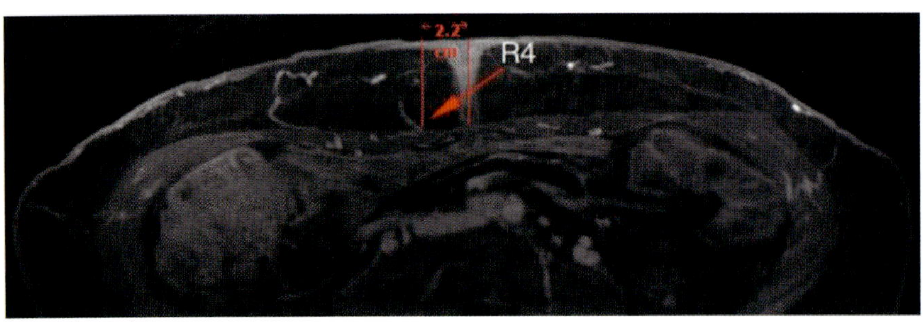

Fig. 12.2 Axial MRA abdomen. Deep inferior epigastric perforator (DIEP) location is measured at the anterior rectus fascia in relation to the center of the umbilicus at the fascia level.

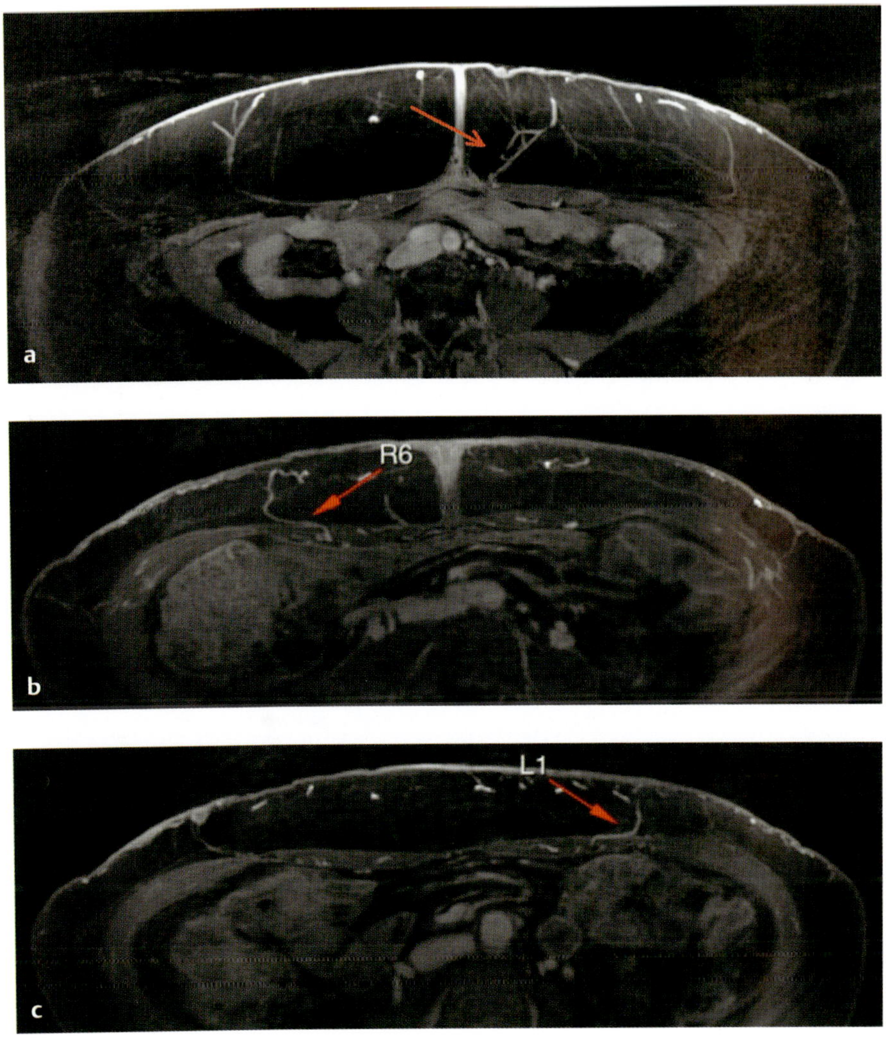

Fig. 12.3 Axial MRA abdomen. **(a)** Left paramuscular (septocutaneous) DIEP *(arrow)*. **(b)** Right DIEP with short intramuscular (IM) course *(arrow)*. **(c)** DIEP with a longer intramuscular course *(arrow)*, and MRA provides helpful information that the perforator has a medial course before it courses caudal.

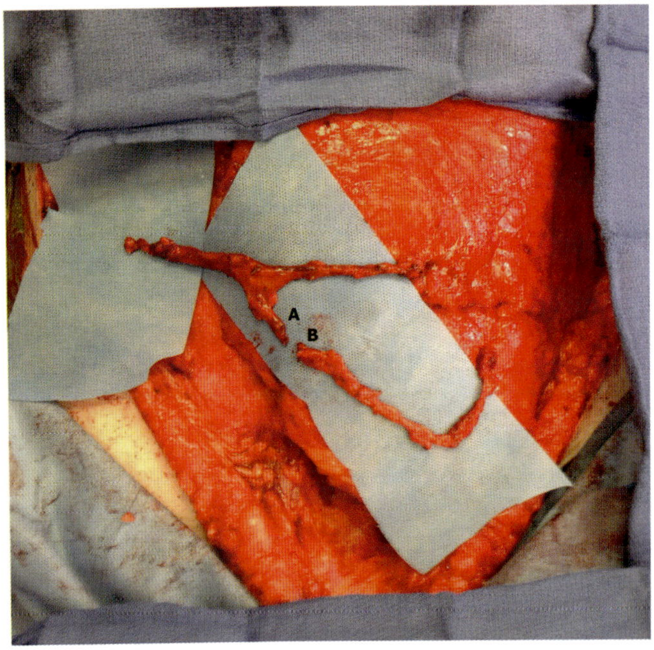

Fig. 12.4 Photograph of a DIEP pedicle lateral branch *(A)* adjacent to the origin of a second DIEP pedicle *(B)* in preparation for microsurgical anastomosis, in which one DIEP flap will perfuse the second DIEP flap (flow-through flap).

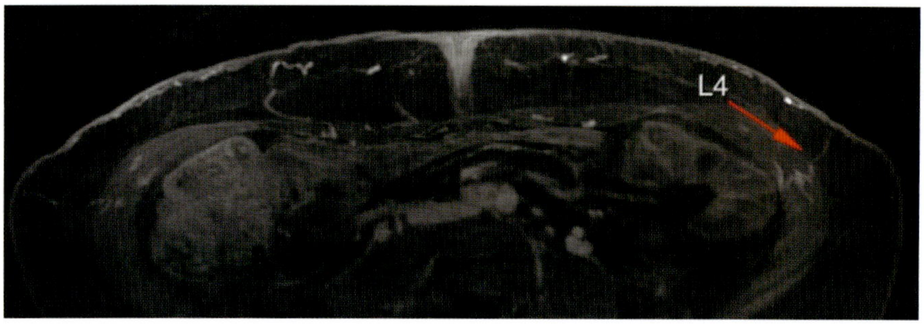

Fig. 12.5 Axial MRA abdomen. The left DCIA is shown (arrow).

The location of the largest deep circumflex iliac artery (DCIA) perforators may also be identified, and they are measured in reference to the umbilicus **(Fig. 12.5)**. The perforator locations and course are then superimposed onto a volume-rendered 3D reconstructed image, and this image is included in the report **(Fig. 12.6)**.

If the superficial inferior epigastric artery is prominent, then this is noted in the radiology report, and whether the superficial inferior epigastric artery shares a common origin with the superficial circumflex iliac vessels is also noted, as this will result in a larger caliber vessel for anastomosis.

A clinical example of the utility of MRA in planning bilateral breast reconstruction using an abdominal perforator flap in a patient with a midline and two right paramedian scars from several bowel surgery operations as an infant and an adult is shown in **Fig. 12.7**.

Spiral imaging may be employed by the radiologist to subtract venous flow to view only the superficial inferior epigastric artery (SIEA) **(Fig. 12.8)**, but this is not routinely done. The largest superficial inferior epigastric vein is identified on each hemiabdomen, and the location is measured from the umbilicus at 12 cm inferior to the umbilicus.

Other helpful information to consider when viewing MRA images is the branching pattern of the DIEP within the subcutaneous fat. The two-point Dixon method for fat/water signal separation at 1.5 T and LAVA Flex at 3 T are methods used by radiologists to suppress the fat signal, resulting in clearer images of DIEP arborization into the fat **(Fig. 12.9)**. In a unilateral reconstruction, it is helpful to

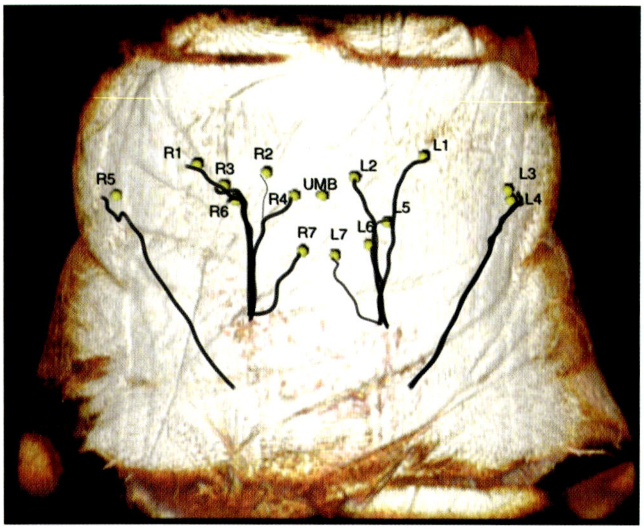

Fig. 12.6 Three-dimensional (3D) volume-rendered MRA of the abdomen with the DIEP, deep circumflex iliac artery (DCIA), umbilicus location, and vessel courses superimposed.

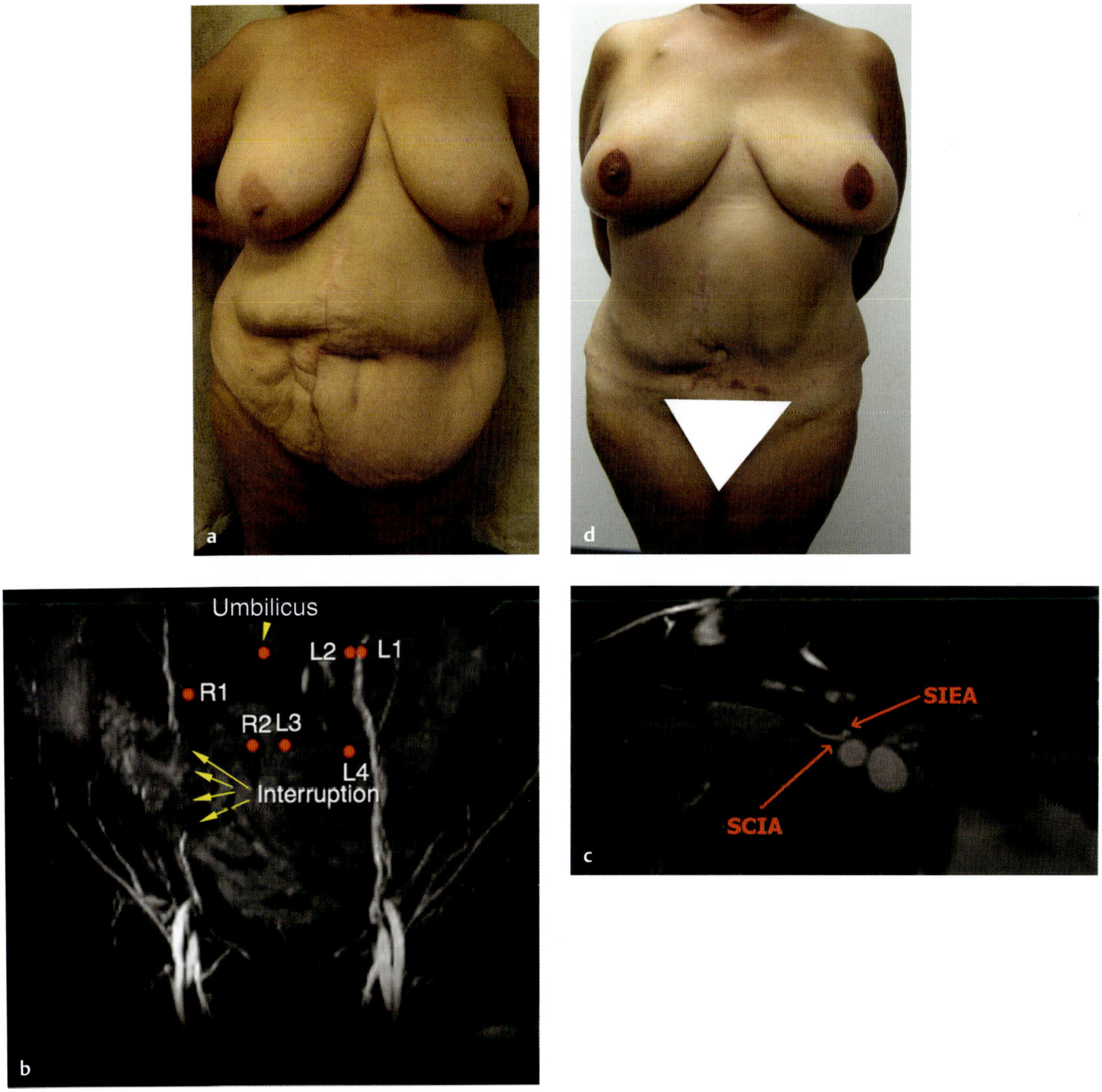

Fig. 12.7 (a) Photograph of a patient scheduled for a bilateral breast reconstruction with a midline and two right paramedian scars from several bowel surgery operations. She requested that the abdomen be the donor site. The estimated hemiabdominal flap volume was 1,000 g and estimated thigh flap volume was 325 g. **(b)** Coronal MRA abdomen. An interruption in contrast in the right deep inferior epigastric perforator (DIEP) pedicle secondary to previous abdominal surgery is shown *(arrows)*. **(c)** MRA abdomen. Common origin of superficial inferior epigastric artery (SIEA) and superficial circumflex iliac artery (SCIA) measures 2.2 mm. **(d)** Postoperative photograph of patient with successful bilateral reconstruction with abdominal tissue (left breast SIEA flap and right breast DIEP flap).

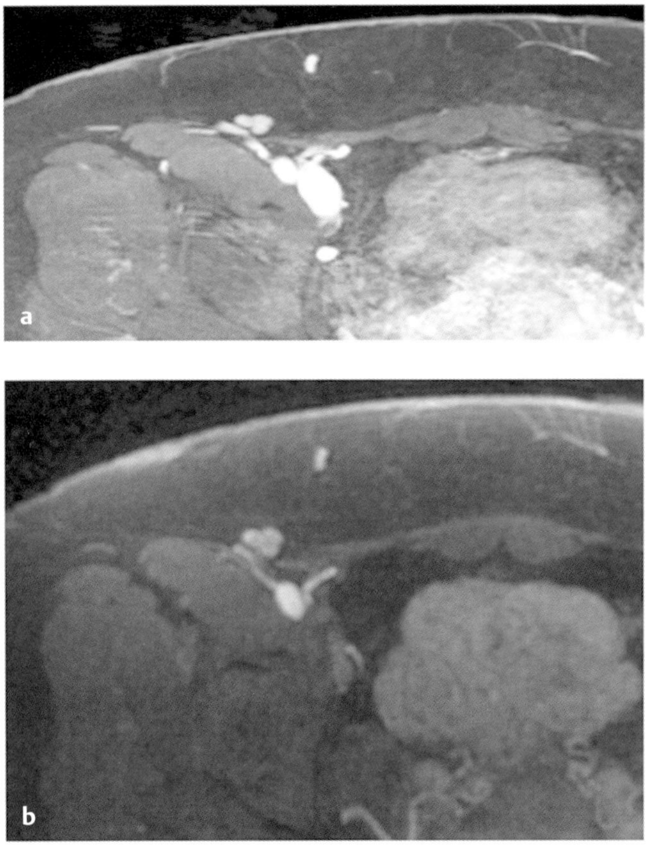

Fig. 12.8 MRA of the abdomen. **(a)** Arterial and venous vessels enhanced. **(b)** Venous vessel enhancement subtracted.

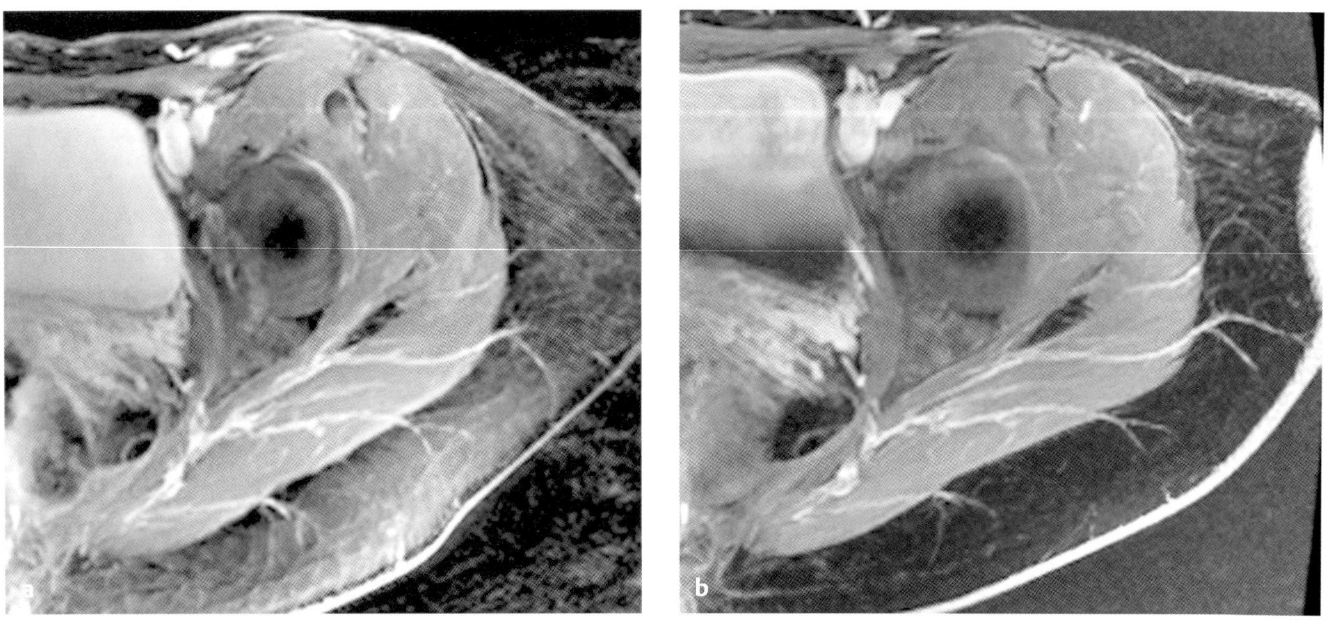

Fig. 12.9 Axial MRA of the abdomen. **(a)** Inhomogeneous fat suppression. **(b)** Liver accelerated volume acquisition (LAVA) Flex used on a 3-tesla image, resulting in improved visualization of deep inferior epigastric perforator (DIEP) arborization into the fat.

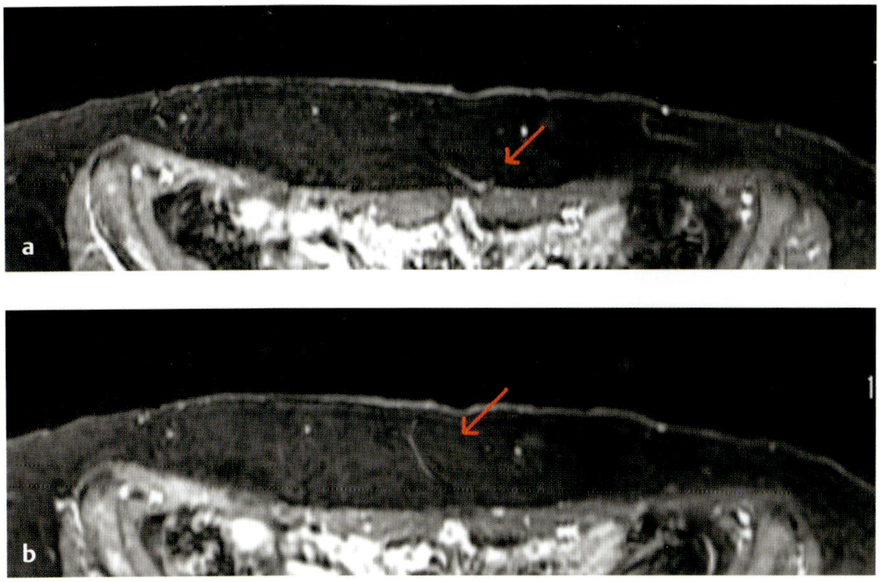

Fig. 12.10 Sequential axial MRA cuts with arrow showing branches of a perforator crossing the midline.

see a medial row DIEP with branches crossing into the subcutaneous fat on the contralateral abdomen because zone III is more likely to be well perfused. **Figs. 12.10** and **12.11** show a DIEP with a very lateral course into the subcutaneous fat and a corresponding photograph of a patient with inadequate venous drainage of the medial tissue. A different perforator selection or indocyanine green injection would have prevented this. Usually DIEP branches can be visualized in close proximity with superficial inferior epigastric venous branches, which may theoretically provide improved venous drainage through connections (**Fig. 12.12**).

Postprocessing software is used by the radiologist to calculate projected abdominal flap volume (**Fig. 12.13**). To increase the accuracy of the estimated flap volume, the radiologist must be experienced in dealing with the typical markings and dimensions of an abdominal flap.

Buttock

A vitamin E capsule is placed on the skin surface at the top of the gluteal crease as a reference point from which the perforator locations are measured. The largest of perforators from the superior gluteal artery perforator (SGAP) and the inferior gluteal artery perforator (IGAP) are identified. The locations of the perforators are calculated at the point of exiting the superficial fascia, and this point is transposed onto the skin surface. Then, the distance of the perforator from the reference point is measured along the curved skin contour of the buttock (**Fig. 12.14**). These measurements are taken with the patient in the prone position for increased accuracy because of the compliance of the gluteal tissue. Then the perforator locations and reference points are superimposed onto a volume-rendered 3D reconstruction of

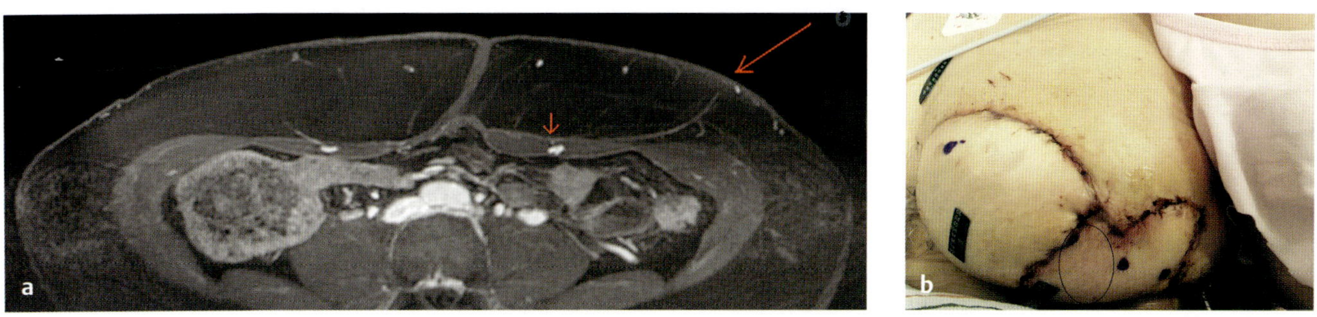

Fig. 12.11 (a) Axial MRA abdomen. The location of the deep inferior epigastric perforator (DIEP) exiting anterior rectus fascia is shown *(short arrow)*. The approximate location that the DIEP arborizes into the subdermal plexus is shown *(long arrow)*. Note the very oblique course laterally. **(b)** Photograph on postoperative day 5 after double DIEP flap in a patient with a midline abdominal scar. The medial flap has decreased venous drainage *(circle)*. A lateral DIEP with very oblique lateral arborization was used.

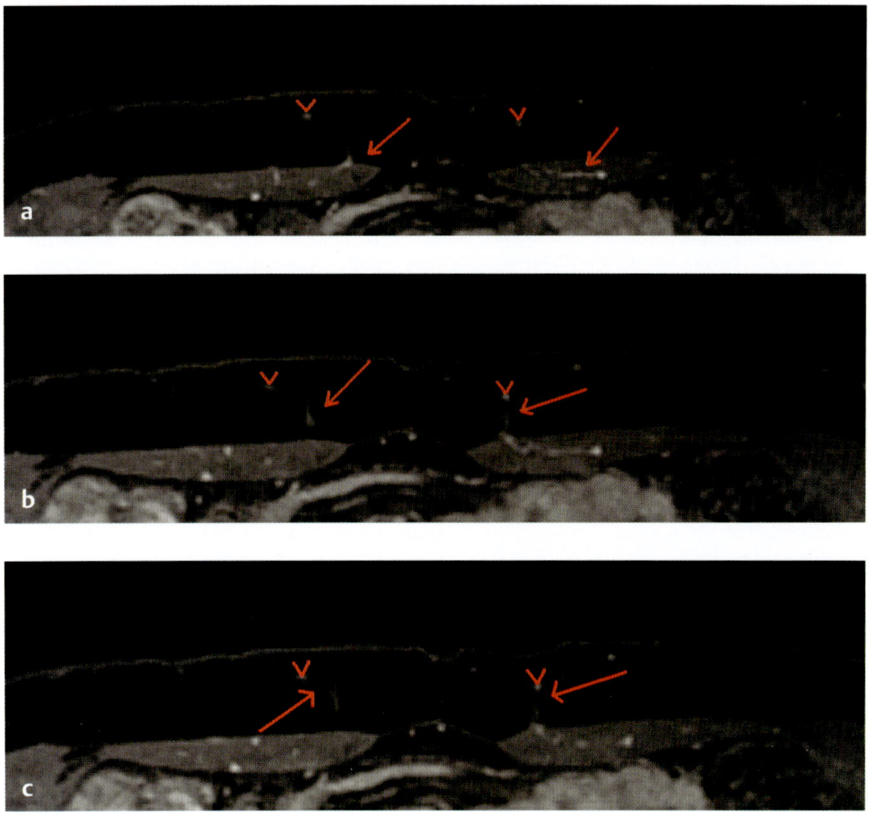

Fig. 12.12 Axial MRA of the abdomen. Superficial inferior epigastric vein (SIEV) *(V)*; bilateral deep inferior epigastric perforators (DIEPs) *(arrows)*. **(a)** Axial MRA. **(b)** Left DIEP meeting the SIEV. **(c)** Right DIEP branch also meeting the SIEV.

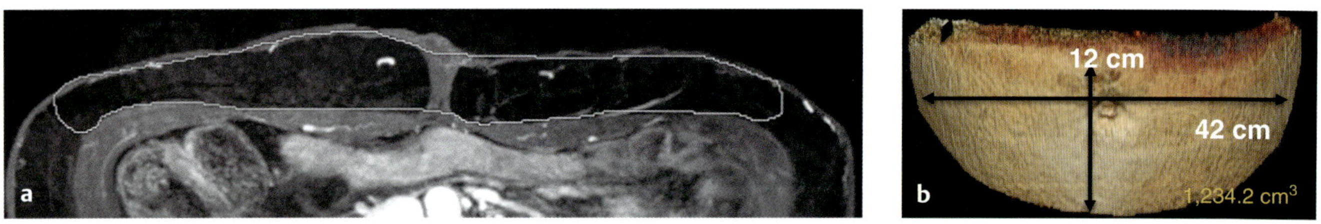

Fig. 12.13 (a) Axial MRA of the abdomen with subcutaneous fat manually outlined to calculate the abdominal flap volume. **(b)** The 3D volume-rendered abdominal flap.

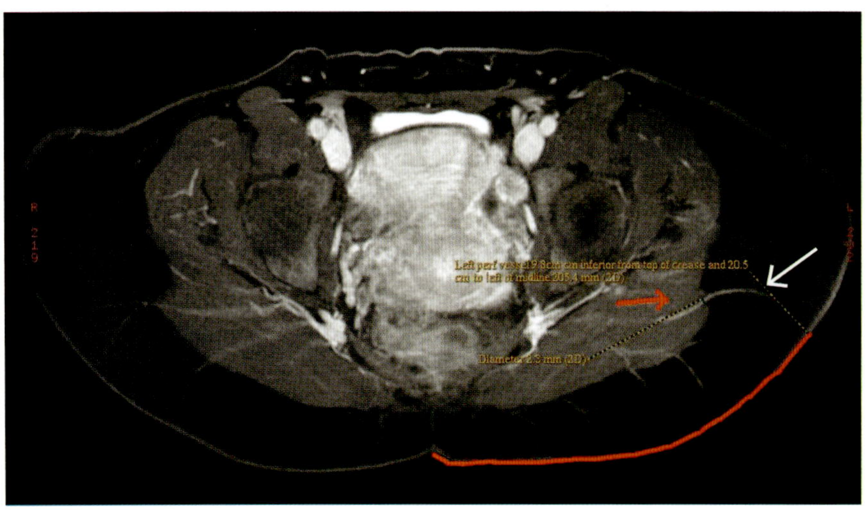

Fig. 12.14 Axial MRA of the buttock showing the gluteal perforator *(arrow)*. The distance from the midline reference point is calculated by measuring the distance along the curved skin surface with the patient in the prone position to increase accuracy. Vessel caliber is calculated at the superficial fascia exit point.

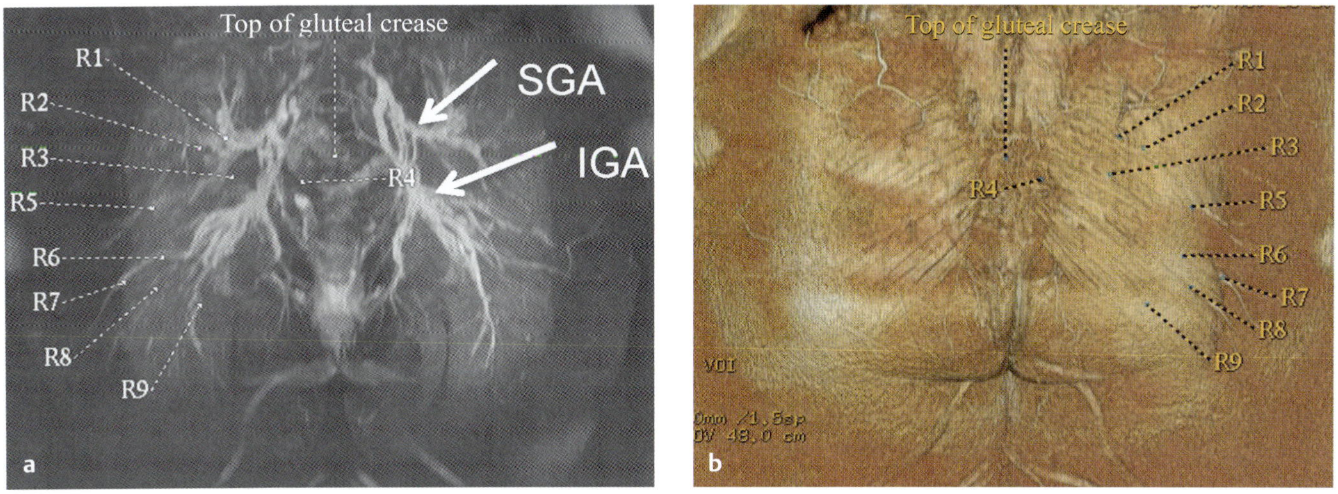

Fig. 12.15 (a) Coronal MRA of the buttock with the superior gluteal artery (SGA) and inferior gluteal artery (IGA) perforator locations and reference point locations marked. **(b)** A 3D volume-rendered MRA of the buttock with the perforator locations and reference points superimposed.

the buttock with the patient in the prone position so that the perforator location markings can be replicated preoperatively **(Fig. 12.15)**.

The placement of the buttock flap skin paddle is significantly influenced by the optimal perforator location. The goal is to design a flap that incorporates the optimal perforator and a backup option. Because there are usually many large-caliber perforator options in the buttock, vessel location is an important determining factor in selecting the optimal vessel. Laterally positioned perforators will result in a longer pedicle, which is advantageous for flap insetting **(Fig. 12.16)**. In addition, more lateral flaps may spare the central aesthetic unit in superior buttock flaps or the medial cushioning fat in lower buttock flaps. In bilateral flaps, an attempt is made to design flaps that will result in symmetrical scars by locating large perforators at a similar position bilaterally. As the radiologist becomes increasingly familiar with typical flap dimensions, predicted upper and buttock flap volumes can be calculated. Generally, an elliptical designed pattern measuring 6 cm in vertical dimension by 20 cm in transverse dimension is used by the radiologist.

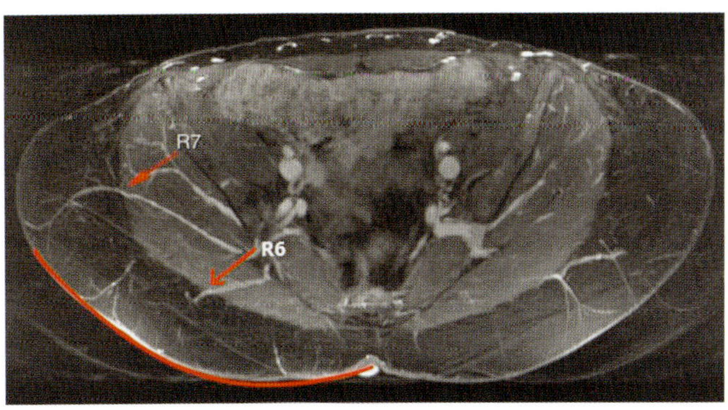

Fig. 12.16 Axial MRA of the buttock showing two superior gluteal perforators. R7 is located more lateral than R6 and has a longer intramuscular course, yielding a longer pedicle.

Thigh

The upper thigh is imaged from the mid-gluteal region to the midthigh (~ 12 cm caudal to the inferior gluteal crease). A transversely oriented upper thigh flap is designed from medial to predominantly posterior thigh tissue to avoid the more anteriorly located lymphatic channels. A typical elliptical flap design for calculating thigh volume is 6 × 20 cm. The reference point from which the perforator locations are measured is the skin surface along the midline at the bottom of the gluteal crease. The locations of profunda artery perforators (for the PAP flap) are calculated at the point of exiting the superficial fascia. The perforators are also located in reference to the distance posterior from the posterior edge of the gracilis muscle, to facilitate intraoperative identification of the perforator **(Fig. 12.17)**. Similar to gluteal artery perforators, the best profunda artery perforators have an oblique course through the adductor magnus to yield a longer pedicle. Perforators that course more laterally adjacent to the femoral bone and then course cephalad into the gluteal vessels may be mistaken for profunda artery perforators. As the surgery is

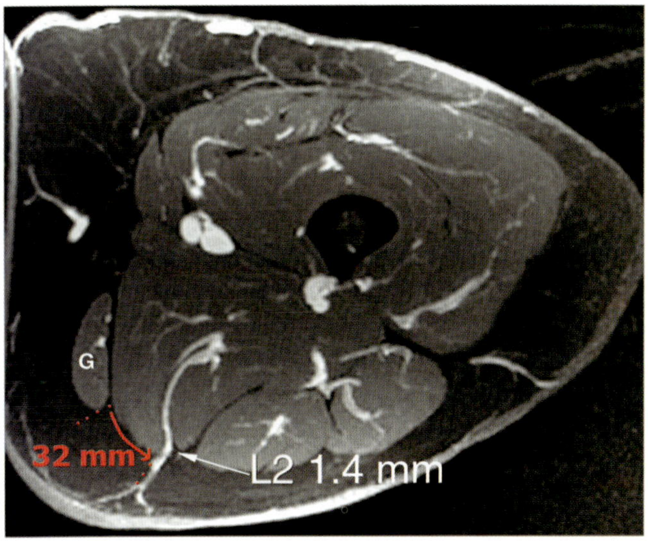

Fig. 12.17 Axial MRA of the left thigh in the supine position showing the profunda femoral artery perforator *(arrow)*, and distance from the posterior edge of the gracilis muscle *(G)* is measured.

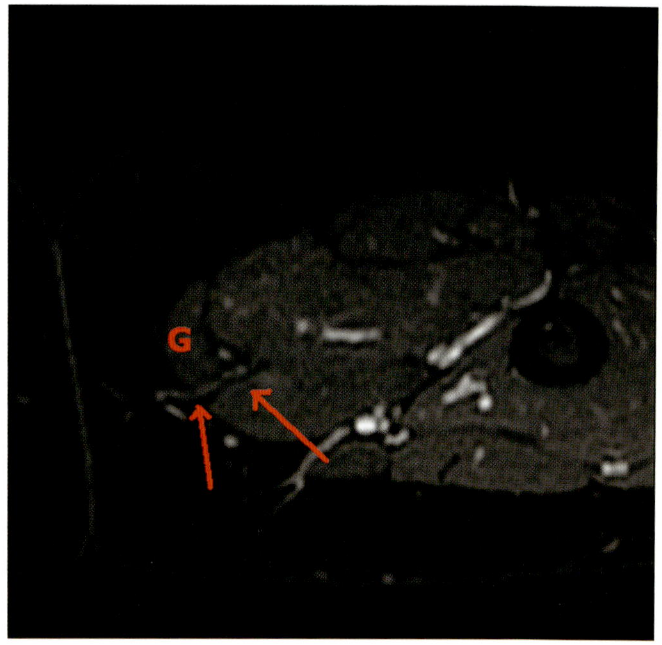

Fig. 12.18 Axial MRA left thigh in the supine position showing a septocutaneous medial circumflex femoral perforator *(arrows)* that courses around the gracilis muscle *(G)*.

performed with the patient in the supine position, these gluteal perforators result in a difficult dissection with difficult exposure to yield adequate caliber and length pedicles. Occasionally, there is a large medial circumflex vessel perforating through the gracilis muscle or a paramuscular (septocutaneous) medial circumflex vessel that courses around the gracilis muscle **(Fig. 12.18)**. Perforator locations and courses and reference point are transposed onto the skin surface **(Fig. 12.19)**.

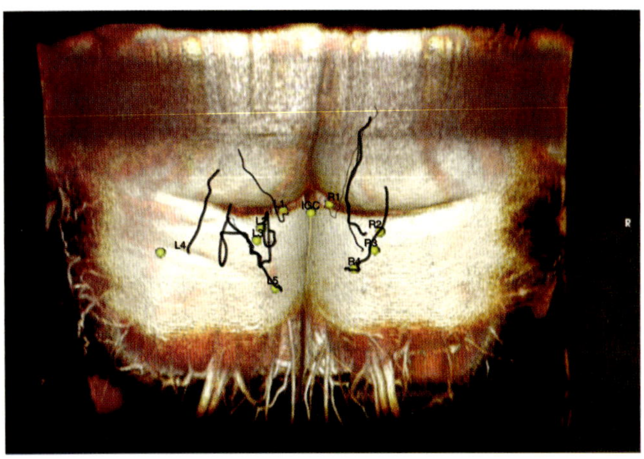

Fig. 12.19 A 3D volume-rendered MRA of the thigh with perforator locations and course and reference point at the inferior gluteal crease *(IGC)* superimposed.

Sometimes the lateral upper thigh has a favorable fat deposition. A septocutaneous (paramuscular) lateral circumflex femoral artery perforators coursing around the tensor fasciae latae is measured in reference to the umbilicus **(Fig. 12.20)**. The anterior superior iliac spine (ASIS) was initially used as a reference point, but it can be difficult to palpate on some patients and thus can lead to inaccuracies.

Lower Back

Lumbar artery perforators (for the LAP flap) are measured in reference to the midline upper gluteal crease. The limiting factor of this flap is the short pedicle length **(Fig. 12.21)**. Sometimes lumbar artery perforators have an oblique course to yield a slightly longer pedicle. In general, these flaps are used as a backup option when the abdomen cannot be used, and the body habitus is not favorable for thigh or buttock flaps.

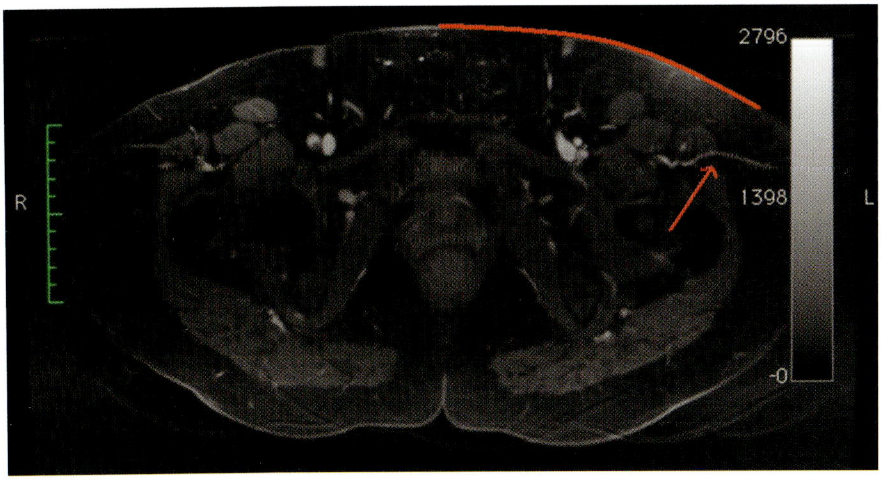

Fig. 12.20 Axial MRA of the pelvis showing the left septocutaneous lateral circumflex femoral perforator *(arrow)*.

Lateral Thorax

The chest is initially imaged with the patient in the supine position and the arms abducted to avoid compression of the lateral chest soft tissue. In patients scheduled for bilateral reconstruction who have a large body mass, each side can be imaged separately so that one arm can be abducted at a time. It may be necessary for patients with a greater volume of upper arm fat to raise their arms and rest their hands on their head. Images should also be obtained of patients in the lateral decubitus position with the arm raised. Most radiology technicians are not aware that patients are positioned in the lateral decubitus position for the surgical reconstruction and part of the preoperative marking, and are not accustomed to scanning patients in this position. Measurements change significantly with the patient's position and arm position. Thus, it is crucial for the radiologist to communicate the patient's position in the series from which the measurements are taken. The radiologist should be aware that preoperatively a patient may need to be turned to the lateral decubitus position to mark posteriorly located perforators, and thus this series should be used for posteriorly located perforator measurements. The reference point is the skin surface at the sternal notch. The locations of thoracodorsal and internal mammary artery perforators are measured from a

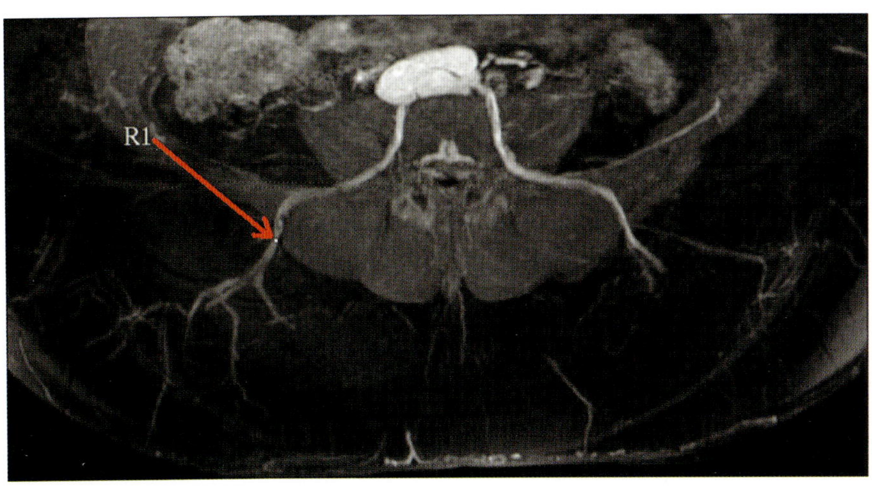

Fig. 12.21 Axial MRA of the back showing the right lumbar perforator *(arrow)*.

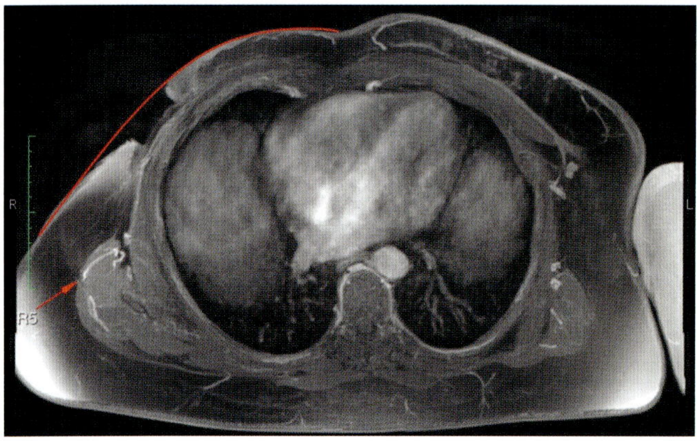

Fig. 12.22 Axial MRA of the chest in a patient with a radiated open left chest wound showing the large thoracodorsal artery perforator *(arrow)*. Emerging through the anterior edge of the latissimus.

reference point at the sternal notch skin surface **(Fig. 12.22)** and transposed onto the skin surface **(Fig. 12.23)**. Thoracodorsal artery perforators usually yield a longer pedicle than inter-costal perforators which is advantageous for insetting the flap.

Conclusion

The tremendous anatomic variability in the vascular system can make perforator flap breast reconstruction challenging for surgeons at all experience levels. Accurate preoperative anatomic vascular imaging enables optimal perforator selection and improves flap design. Shifting the brunt of the perforator selection process preoperatively improves operating efficiency, which can result in reduced operating time, reduced general anesthesia requirements, and potentially increased flap success.[10,11,13] MRA is currently the preoperative method of choice due to the absence of radiation exposure or iodinated contrast agents, and the ability of performing serial imaging acquisitions to visualize multiple donor sites with the patient in different positions in one examination.

Acknowledgments

I would like to thank the radiologists at our center, led by Martin Prince, and his dedicated fellows Nanda Deepa Thimmappa, Jin Ah Kim, and Mukta Agrawal. Weill Cornell Imaging at New York-Presbyterian.

References

1. Masia J, Clavero JA, Larrañaga JR, Alomar X, Pons G, Serret P. Multidetector-row computed tomography in the planning of abdominal perforator flaps. J Plast Reconstr Aesthet Surg 2006;59:594–599
2. Rozen WM, Phillips TJ, Ashton MW, Stella DL, Gibson RN, Taylor GI. Preoperative imaging for DIEA perforator flaps: a comparative study of computed tomographic angiography and Doppler ultrasound. Plast Reconstr Surg 2008;121:9–16
3. Brenner DJ, Hall EJ. Computed tomography—an increasing source of radiation exposure. N Engl J Med 2007;357:2277–2284
4. Stein R. Too much of a good thing? The growing use of CT scans fuel medical concerns regarding radiation exposure. Washington Post, January 15, 2008, p. F1.
5. Safety in medical imaging. American College Radiology Radiological Society North America, Inc. www.radiologyinfo.org/en/safety/index.cfm?pg=sfty_xray&bhcp=1. Accessed September 27, 2010
6. Varnholt H. Computed tomography and radiation exposure. N Engl J Med 2008;358:852–853, author reply 852–853
7. Katayama H, Yamaguchi K, Kozuka T, Takashima T, Seez P, Matsuura K. Adverse reactions to ionic and nonionic contrast media. A report

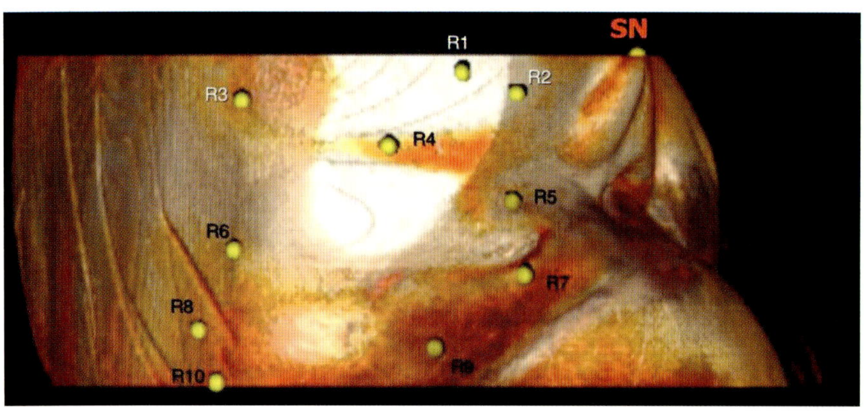

Fig. 12.23 A 3D volume-rendered MRA of the right chest lateral with perforator locations and the reference point at the sternal notch *(SN)* marked.

from the Japanese Committee on the Safety of Contrast Media. Radiology 1990;175:621–628
8. Parfrey P. The clinical epidemiology of contrast-induced nephropathy. Cardiovasc Intervent Radiol 2005;28(Suppl 2):S3–S11
9. Shellock FG, Crues JV. MR procedures: biologic effects, safety, and patient care. Radiology 2004;232:635–652
10. Vasile JV, Newman T, Rusch DG, et al. Anatomic imaging of gluteal perforator flaps without ionizing radiation: Seeing is believing with MRA. J Reconstr Microsurg 2010;26:45–57
11. Greenspun D, Vasile J, Levine JL, et al. Anatomic imaging of abdominal perforator flaps without ionizing radiation: Seeing is believing with MRA. J Reconstr Microsurg 2010;26:37–44
12. Newman TM, Vasile J, Levine JL, et al. Perforator flap magnetic resonance angiography: a review of 25 deep inferior epigastric and gluteal perforator artery flap patients. J Magn Reson Imaging 2010;31:1176–1184
13. Vasile JV, Newman TM, Prince MR, et al. Contrast-enhanced magnetic resonance angiography. Clin Plast Surg 2011;38:263–275
14. Neil-Dwyer JG, Ludman CN, Schaverien M, McCulley SJ, Perks AG. Magnetic resonance angiography in preoperative planning of deep inferior epigastric artery perforator flaps. J Plast Reconstr Aesthet Surg 2009;62:1661–1665
15. Masia J, Kosutic D, Cervelli D, Clavero JA, Monill JM, Pons G. In search of the ideal method in perforator mapping: noncontrast magnetic resonance imaging. J Reconstr Microsurg 2010;26:29–35
16. Dillman JR, Ellis JH, Cohan RH, Strouse PJ, Jan SC. Frequency and severity of acute allergic-like reactions to gadolinium-containing i.v. contrast media in children and adults. AJR Am J Roentgenol 2007;189:1533–1538
17. Niendorf HP, Alhassan A, Geens VR, Clauss W. Safety review of gadopentetate dimeglumine. Extended clinical experience after more than five million applications. Invest Radiol 1994;29(Suppl 2):S179–S182
18. U.S. Food and Drug Administration. FDA drug safety communication: new warnings for using gadolinium-based contrast agents in patients with kidney dysfunction. http://www.fda.gov/drugs/drugsafety/ucm223966.htm. Accessed September 21, 2010
19. Cowper SE. Nephrogenic fibrosing dermopathy [International Center for Nephrogenic Systemic Fibrosis Website]. 2001–2014. http://www.icnfdr.org. Accessed April 24, 2015
20. Scheinfeld NS, Cowper SE. Nephrogenic fibrosing dermopathy. 2008. http://www.emedicine.com/derm/topic934.htm. Accessed August 7, 2008
21. Lauffer RB, Parmelee DJ, Dunham SU, et al. MS-325: albumin-targeted contrast agent for MR angiography. Radiology 1998; 207:529–538
22. Ersoy H, Jacobs P, Kent CK, Prince MR. Blood pool MR angiography of aortic stent-graft endoleak. AJR Am J Roentgenol 2004;182: 1181–1186
23. Zou Z, Kate Lee H, Levine JL, et al. Gadofosveset trisodium-enhanced abdominal perforator MRA. J Magn Reson Imaging 2012;35:711–716
24. Agrawal MD, Thimmappa ND, Vasile JV, et al. Autologous breast reconstruction: preoperative MRA for perforator flap vessel mapping. J Reconstr Microsurg 2015;31:1–11

13 Lateral Thigh Perforator Flap (Septocutaneous Tensor Fasciae Latae Perforator Flap)

Stephania Tuinder, Arno Lataster, and Rene Remmelt Willie Johan van der Hulst

Although the deep inferior epigastric perforator (DIEP) flap is the first choice in autologous breast reconstruction, the abdomen cannot be used as a donor site in some patients. The main advantage of the septocutaneous tensor fasciae latae (sc-TFL) flap is that the upper lateral thigh region usually has sufficient fat tissue to reconstruct a breast, even in very thin patients. The other advantage is that the dissection of the pedicle is septocutaneous between the gluteal muscles and tensor fascia latae muscle, and thus can be more straightforward.

Topographical and Functional Anatomy

The tensor fasciae latae (TFL) muscle is located in a connective tissue compartment consisting of a superficial and deep layer of the fascia lata **(Fig. 13.1)**. TFL muscle fibers attach only to the deep layer of the TFL compartment, not to the superficial one. TFL muscle fibers end approximately at the junction of the proximal one third and the distal two thirds of the thigh. At this point, the superficial and deep TFL compartment layers fuse into a longitudinal thick part of the fascia lata, the iliotibial tract. From posteriorly and laterally, the tendinous lamina from the gluteus maximus muscle continues over the greater trochanter into the iliotibial tract.[1]

The TFL compartment arises from the outer edge of the iliac crest, between the lateral surface of the anterior superior iliac spine (ASIS) and the iliac tubercle. The TFL compartment is lined by the gluteus medius/minimus compartment posteriorly and by the rectus femoris/vastus lateralis compartment anteriorly. The joined borders between these three compartments are the posterior and the anterior intermuscular septum **(Fig. 13.1)**.[2]

The lateral femoral cutaneous nerve (LFCN) emerges in the subcutaneous layer near the ASIS. LFCN anterior and posterior branches supply the skin on the anterolateral and lateral side of the thigh and can have a variable course.[3]

The TFL muscle is innervated by the superior gluteal nerve (L4 and L5) and vascularized by vessels from the superior gluteal artery (SGA) and from the ascending branch of the lateral circumflex femoral artery (LCFA).

The TFL perforators have been studied by anatomic dissection, cross-sectional imaging, and clinical studies.[2,4–12] Septocutaneous perforators may run in the anterior or posterior intermuscular septum. Due to the anatomic variability of the vasculature, confusion arose in the past about blood vessel and flap terminology. The TFL perforator flaps can be divided into three categories based on the location of the perforators from the ascending branch of the LCFA **(Fig. 13.2)**:

- Type 1: flaps based on septocutaneous perforators running in the anterior septum of the TFL (between the TFL and the rectus femoris/vastus lateralis muscles)
- Type 2: musculocutaneous perforators running through the TFL
- Type 3: flaps based on septocutaneous perforators running in the posterior septum of the TFL (between the TFL and the gluteus medius/minimus muscles)

The anatomy of the LCFA and its branches is quite variable.[4,13,14] However, a septocutaneous perforator originating from the LFCA is always present in the posterior septum between the TFL muscle and the gluteus medius/minimus muscles[2] (type 3 flap). The type 3 flap, named the lateral thigh perforator (LTP)* flap or septocutaneous (sc)-TFL flap for simplicity, is advantageous for reconstruction because of its straightforward dissection and usually large-caliber vessels. The preoperative planning and the operative dissection are described in the following sections.

Editor's note: The "lateral thigh perforator flap" is a simple name for this flap, and also the initials of Linda Truluk Perry, who continues to inspire the work of one of the editors.

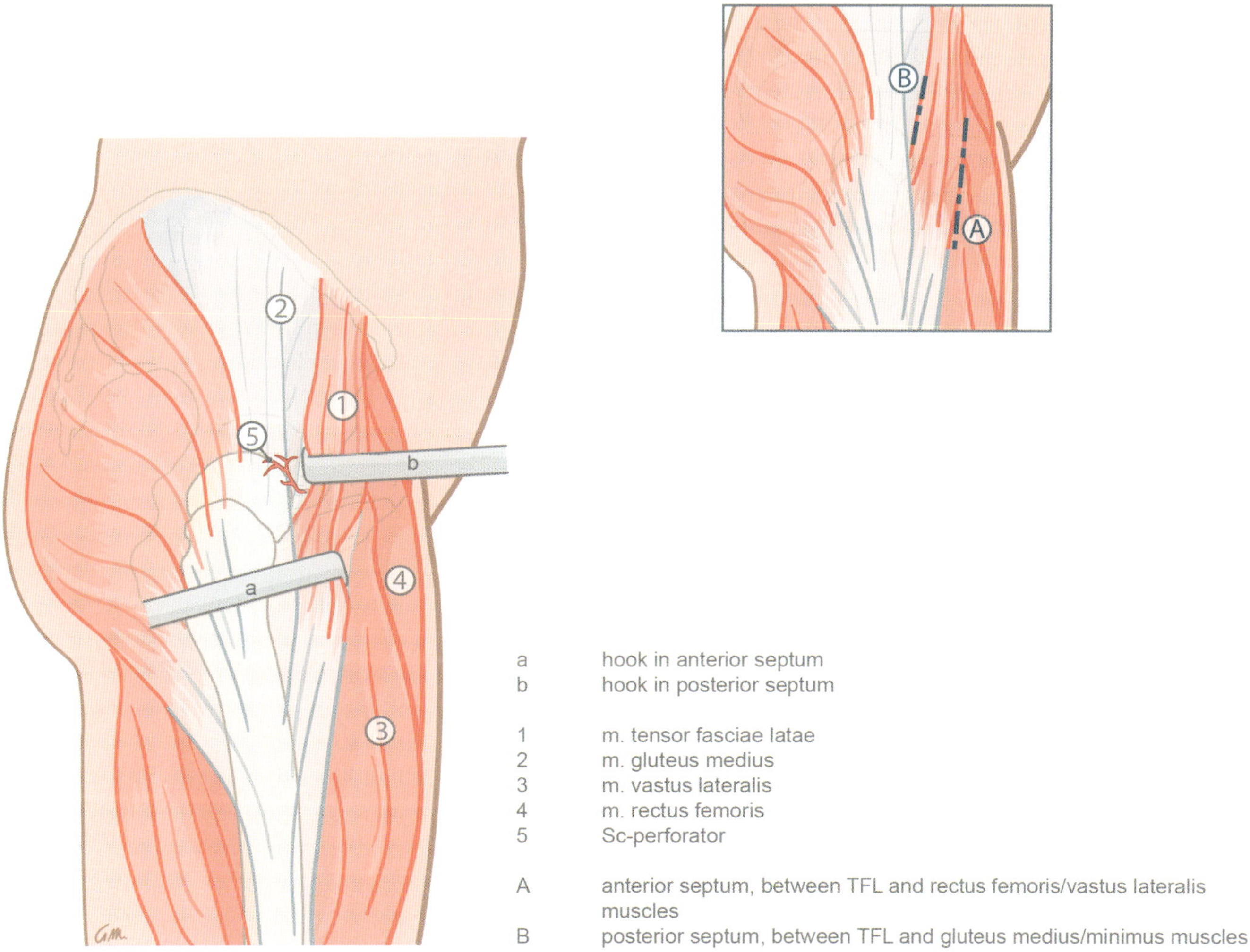

Fig. 13.1 Illustration of the lateral thigh anatomy. TFL, tensor fasciae latae muscle. (© 2015 by Greet Mommen. www.greetmommen.be.)

Preoperative Planning

Every patient undergoes preoperative imaging with magnetic resonance angiography (MRA) using the protocol previously described.[15] The septocutaneous perforators are identified **(Fig. 13.3)**. The distance, in a sagittal plane, of the perforators from the ASIS or pubic tubercle is measured. A handheld Doppler is used to confirm perforator locations, and which are marked on the skin surface.

A skin island is drawn around the perforator. In contrast to the TFL flap described by Deiler et al,[10] the flap is not drawn along the longest axis of the TFL. Usually the perforator is located peripherally and not in the center of the flap. Alternative drawings of the flap are possible depending on its shape and on the preference of the patient **(Fig. 13.4)**. The flap can be oriented just above the lateral upper part of the gluteal region. In this case, most of the scar will be hidden under the underwear but no major modification of the saddlebags occurs (type 1 skin flap design). If the flap will be oriented toward the infragluteal fold (type 2 skin flap design), the scar will probably not be hidden by standard underwear, but a correction of the saddlebags will occur. Typical flap dimensions are as follows: 5 to 8 cm in width by 18 to 22 cm in length. Fat can be beveled for additional volume, but may result in a

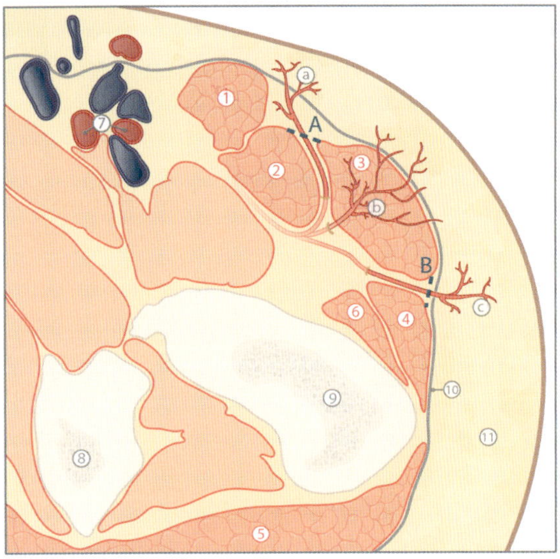

1. m. sartorius
2. m. rectus femoris
3. m. tensor fasciae latae
4. m. gluteus medius
5. m. gluteus maximus
6. m. gluteus minimus
7. a. femoralis
8. ischium
9. greater trochanter
10. fascia lata
11. subcutis

a. septocutaneous perforator in anterior septum
b. musculocutaneous perforator through TFL
c. septocutaneous perforator in posterior septum

A. anterior septum, between TFL and rectus femoris/vastus lateralis muscles
B. posterior septum, between TFL and gluteus medius/minimus muscles

Fig. 13.2 Illustration of a cross section of the tensor fascia muscle with anterior septocutaneous, musculocutaneous, and posterior septocutaneous perforators from the lateral circumflex femoral artery (LCFA). (© 2015 by Greet Mommen. www.greetmommen.be.)

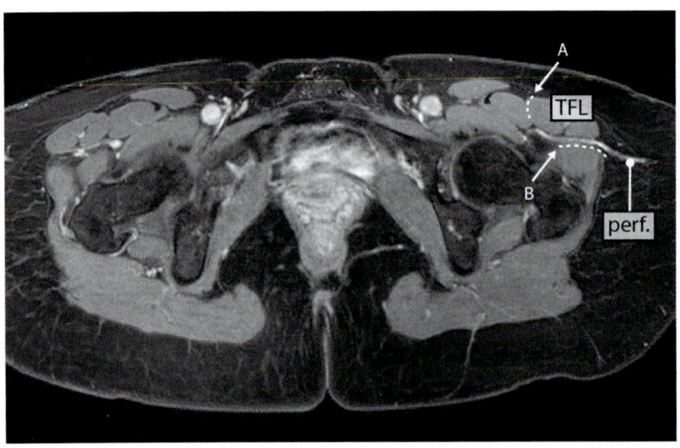

Fig. 13.3 Magnetic resonance angiography (MRA) axial view. A, anterior septum; B, posterior septum; TFL, tensor fasciae latae muscle; perf, posterior septocutaneous perforator.

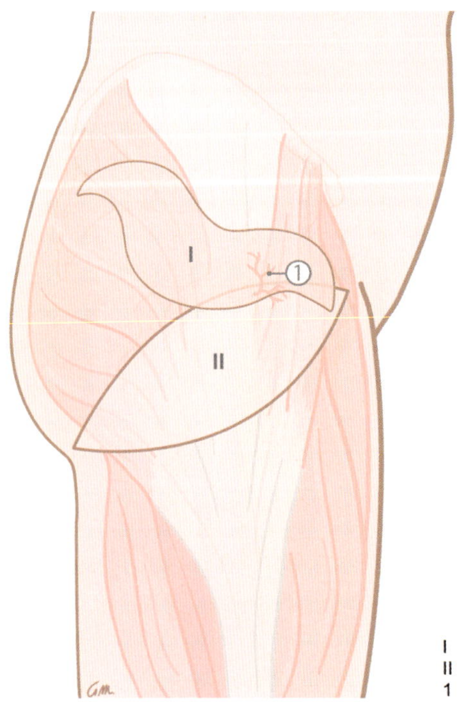

I skin flap (Type I)
II skin flap (Type II)
1 Sc-perforator

Fig. 13.4 Illustration of two skin flap designs. (© 2015 by Greet Mommen. www.greetmommen.be.)

contour deformity along the donor area, requiring correction during a second-stage procedure. An example of patient markings is shown in **Figure 13.5**.

Surgical Technique

The patient is placed in the supine position. The lateral position should be avoided because it results in excessive tension on the TFL. The lateral position causes the leg to be more adducted, exerting more tension along the septum, and resulting in a more difficult dissection in the septum. Mobilization of the leg can sometimes help to identify the septum because the fascia above the gluteus medius is less tight than the fascia of the TFL. The incision starts proximally and anteriorly. The lateral femoral cutaneous nerve is avoided unless a sensate flap is required.

The posterior septum between the TFL and the gluteus medius/minimus is found proximally and opened. The perforator is identified and dissected. Usually a small piece of fascia lata is left around the perforator to avoid damage. With the help of a fine hook, blunt dissection of the perforator in the posterior septum of the TFL is performed **(Fig. 13.6)**. The dissection proceeds initially between the TFL and the gluteus medius/minimus. The muscular branches to those muscles are identified and ligated. Sometimes a branch of the femoral nerve can be identified in the most proximal part of the pedicle and dissected. The

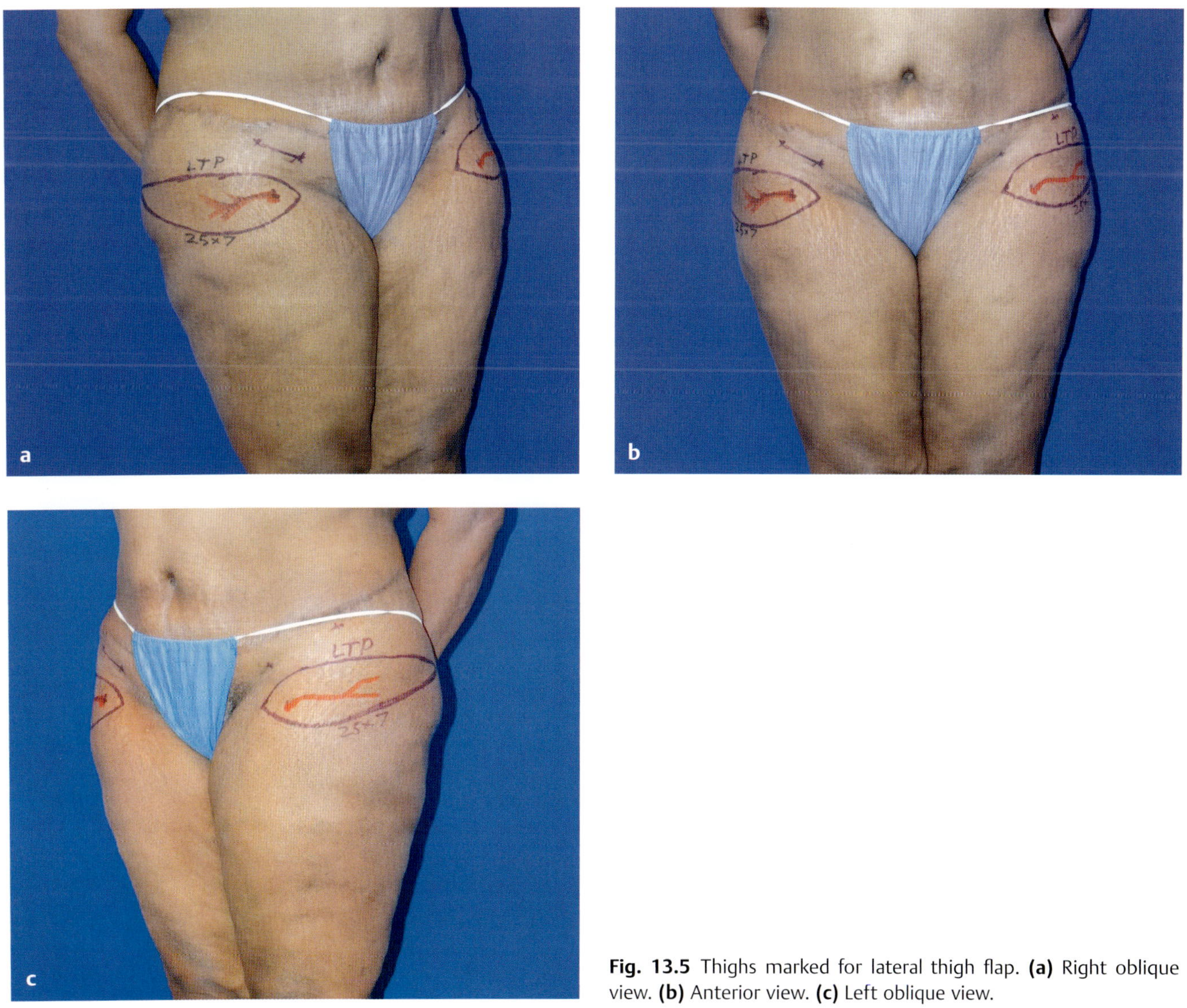

Fig. 13.5 Thighs marked for lateral thigh flap. **(a)** Right oblique view. **(b)** Anterior view. **(c)** Left oblique view.

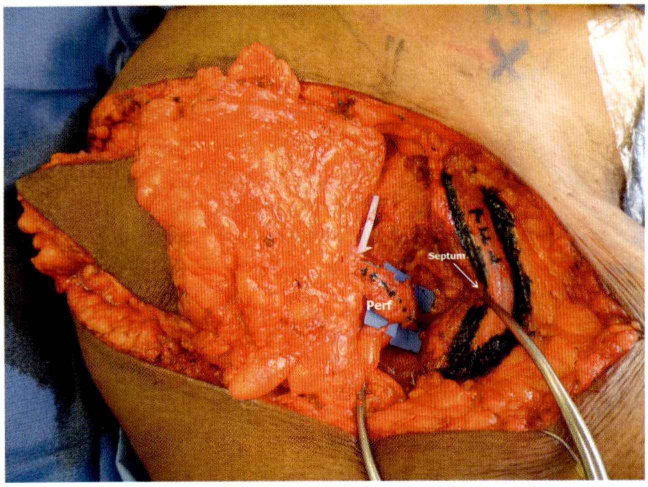

Fig. 13.6 Intraoperative photograph. TFL, tensor fasciae latae muscle; Septum, posterior septum; Perf, posterior septocutaneous perforator.

perforator is dissected to its origin from the ascending branch of the LCFA **(Fig. 13.7)**. The mean length of the pedicle is 8 cm.[16]

At times, a large septocutaneous perforator is identified in the anterior septum of the TFL (type 1 flap). An anterior septum perforator can be dissected between the TFL and the rectus femoris/vastus lateralis muscles. Usually the dissection is easier because the anterior fascia is less tight. The downside is that the perforator will be located more peripherally in the flap and the pedicle will be shorter, with a mean length of 6 cm.

Microsurgical Anastomosis

Usually an end-to-end anastomosis with the internal mammary vessels is performed for the artery and the vein. The caliber of the vein is usually 2 to 2.5 mm, which matches well with the mammary vein. The caliber of the artery is usually 2 to 2.4 mm and also matches well with the mammary artery.

Flap Insetting

Care should be directed toward the orientation of the pedicle during insetting. It is similar to a gluteal flap in that the pedicle is shorter than a typical DIEP flap and the septocutaneous perforator pedicle may be surrounded by a greater amount of fibrotic and fatty tissue. Malposition resulting in kinking of the pedicle can occur.

If the flap design is S-shaped or a type 1 skin flap design (usually with a flap designed along the upper gluteal region), it is easier to fold the flap on itself, similar to a profunda artery perforator (PAP) flap. If the flap design is a type 2 (usually along the infragluteal region), it may be more difficult to fold the flap, and DIEP flap positioning techniques can be employed. **Figs. 13.8 and 13.9** are photographs of patients reconstructed with a type 1 and a type 2 skin flap design, respectively.

The lateral thigh perforator flap or septocutaneous tensor fasciae latae flap is an excellent option for autologous tissue breast reconstruction. It consistently has a septocutaneous perforator to spare the muscle and yields sufficient tissue even in thin patients.

Acknowledgments

We acknowledge the help provided by Greet Mommen for the drawings explaining our work.

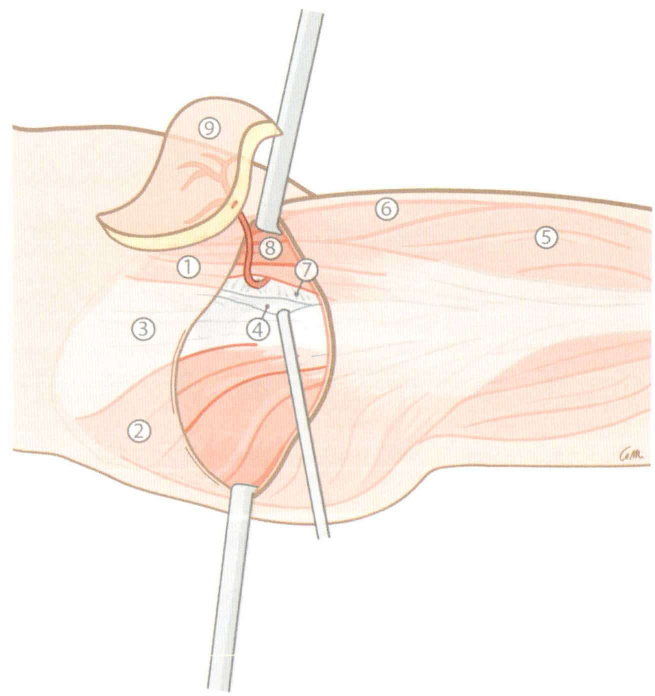

1 m. tensor fasciae latae
2 m. gluteus maximus
3 m. gluteus medius
4 m. gluteus minimus
5 m. vastus lateralis
6 m. rectus femoris
7 posterior septum, between TFL and gluteus medius/minimus muscles
8 Sc-perforator
9 skin flap

Fig. 13.7 Illustration of septocutaneous LTP flap islanded on perforator. (© 2015 by Greet Mommen. www.greetmommen.be.)

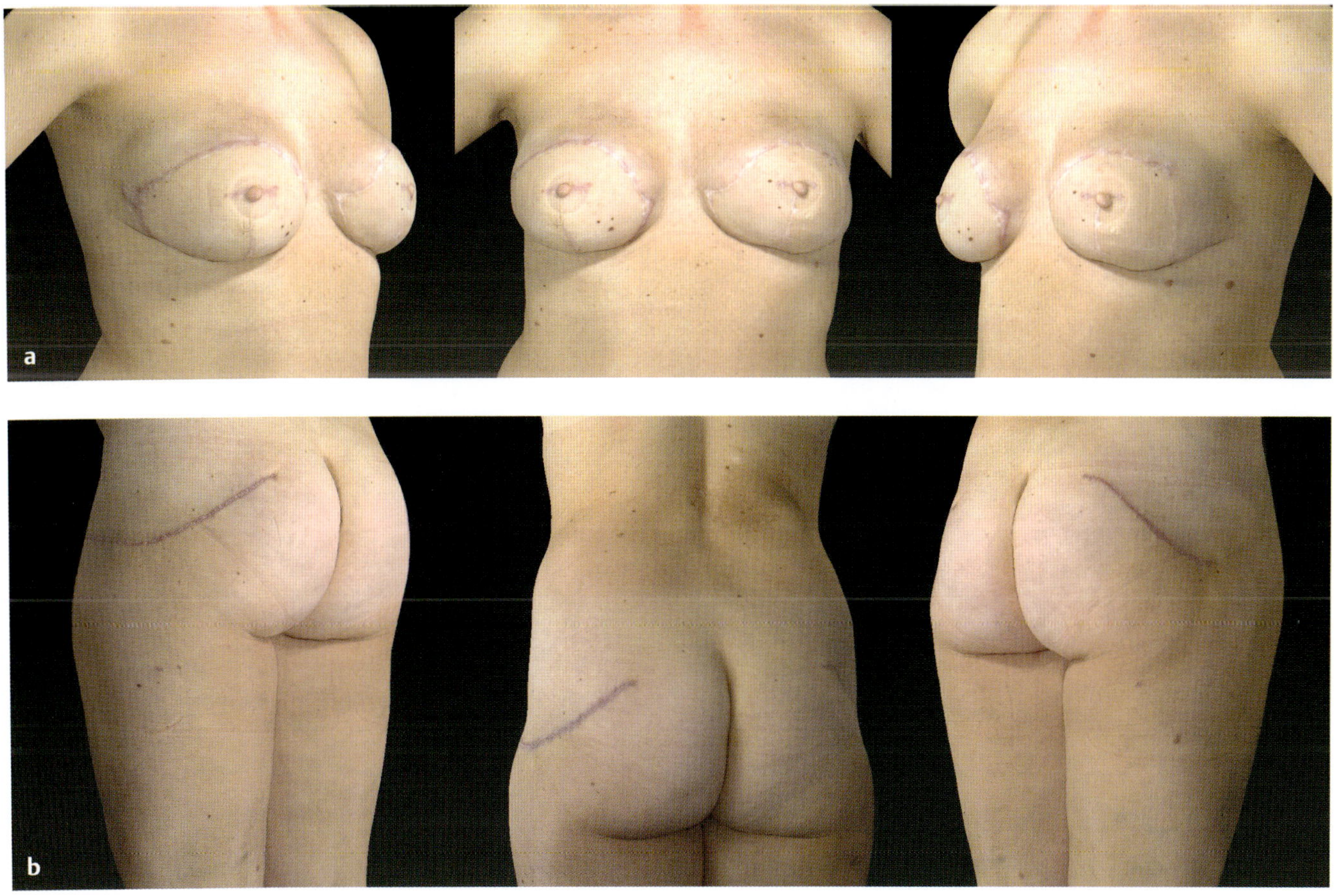

Fig. 13.8 (a) Postoperative photograph of bilateral breast reconstruction with bilateral septocutaneous lateral thigh perforator (LTP) flaps. **(b)** Postoperative photograph of donor site when a type 1 skin design was used.

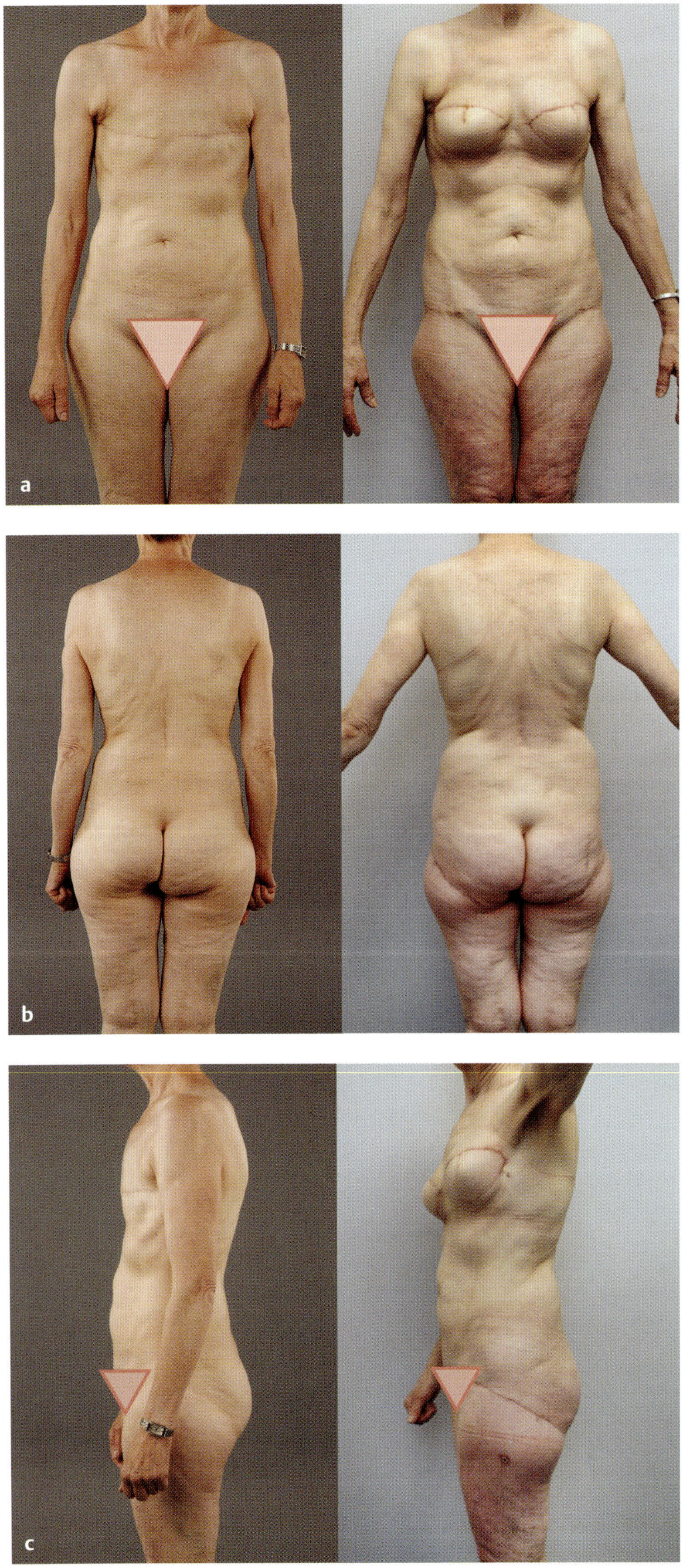

Fig. 13.9 (a) Preoperative and 6-week postoperative photograph of patient with bilateral reconstruction with LTP flaps. **(b)** Preoperative and 6-week postoperative photograph of donor site when a type 2 skin design was used (posterior view). **(c)** Preoperative and 6-week postoperative photograph (lateral view).

References

1. Warwick R, Williams PL. Gray's Anatomy, 35th ed. Edinburgh: Longman Group; 1973
2. Vegas MR, Martin-Hervas C. The superolateral thigh flap: cadaver and computed tomographic angiography studies with a clinical series. Plast Reconstr Surg 2013;131:310–322
3. Patijn J, Mekhail N, Hayek S, Lataster A, van Kleef M, Van Zundert J. Meralgia paresthetica. Pain Pract 2011;11:302–308
4. Hubmer MG, Schwaiger N, Windisch G, et al. The vascular anatomy of the tensor fasciae latae perforator flap. Plast Reconstr Surg 2009;124:181–189
5. Hubmer MG, Justich I, Haas FM, et al. Clinical experience with a tensor fasciae latae perforator flap based on septocutaneous perforators. J Plast Reconstr Aesthet Surg 2011;64:782–789
6. Kimura N, Satoh K. Consideration of a thin flap as an entity and clinical applications of the thin anterolateral thigh flap. Plast Reconstr Surg 1996;97:985–992
7. Ishida LH, Munhoz AM, Montag E, et al. Tensor fasciae latae perforator flap: minimizing donor-site morbidity in the treatment of trochanteric pressure sores. Plast Reconstr Surg 2005;116:1346–1352
8. Koshima I, Urushibara K, Inagawa K, Moriguchi T. Free tensor fasciae latae perforator flap for the reconstruction of defects in the extremities. Plast Reconstr Surg 2001;107:1759–1765
9. Kind GM, Foster RD. Breast reconstruction using the lateral femoral circumflex artery perforator flap. J Reconstr Microsurg 2011;27:427–432
10. Deiler S, Pfadenhauer A, Widmann J, Stützle H, Kanz KG, Stock W. Tensor fasciae latae perforator flap for reconstruction of composite Achilles tendon defects with skin and vascularized fascia. Plast Reconstr Surg 2000;106:342–349
11. Coskunfirat OK, Ozkan O. Free tensor fascia lata perforator flap as a backup procedure for head and neck reconstruction. Ann Plast Surg 2006;57:159–163
12. Hsieh CH, Yang JC, Chen CC, Kuo YR, Jeng SF. Alternative reconstructive choices for anterolateral thigh flap dissection in cases in which no sizable skin perforator is available. Head Neck 2009;31:571–575
13. Saadeh FA, Haikal FA, Abdel-Hamid FA. Blood supply of the tensor fasciae latae muscle. Clin Anat 1998;11:236–238
14. Lakhiani C, Lee MR, Saint-Cyr M. Vascular anatomy of the anterolateral thigh flap: a systematic review. Plast Reconstr Surg 2012;130:1254–1268
15. Vasile JV, Newman TM, Prince MR, et al. Contrast-enhanced magnetic resonance angiography. Clin Plast Surg 2011;38:263–275
16. Tuinder S, Baetens T, De Haan MW, et al. Septocutaneous tensor fasciae latae perforator flap for breast reconstruction: radiological considerations and clinical cases. J Plast Reconstr Aesthet Surg 2014;67:1248–1256

14 Stacked DIEP/PAP Flap Breast Reconstruction

James L. Mayo and Robert J. Allen, Sr.

Stacking free flaps when a single flap would fall short in providing adequate volume has proven to be a safe and effective option for breast reconstruction.[1–7] Several flap combinations can offer the desired volume. However, as perforator-based free flap breast reconstruction evolves, so too does the quest for the most aesthetically pleasing reconstruction. To create the natural breast shape, the surgeon must construct a breast with both lower pole projection and width that gradually tapers into the superior pole, maintaining appropriate superior pole fullness. When stacking flaps from the same donor site, molding the natural breast shape can be challenging.

The combination of the deep inferior epigastric perforator (DIEP) and profunda artery perforator (PAP) flaps can be inset in such a way that the thicker PAP flap is inset in the inframammary fold, providing ideal projection and base width, while the DIEP flap reconstructs the superior pole, providing fullness and a likeness to the natural axillary tail at its apex **(Fig. 14.1)**. This combination is most commonly utilized in four-flap breast reconstruction when the abdominal tissue provides too little reconstructive volume but can also be considered when the hemiabdomen is contraindicated due to previous surgery.[8]

Technique

Preoperative magnetic resonance angiography (MRA) or computed tomography angiography (CTA) is utilized to locate and follow the course of favorable perforators. Patients are seen and marked in the office setting the day prior to surgery **(Fig. 14.2)**. The next day, in the operating room, the patient is placed in the supine position with bilateral arms and legs prepped into the surgical field. The legs are placed in a frog-legged position. A two-team approach is used to simultaneously raise the DIEP and PAP flaps. The surgeon who completes flap harvest first will then harvest the internal mammary vessels.

Typically, the PAP flap is anastomosed to the antegrade internal mammary vessels and the DIEP flap to the retrograde internal mammary vessels. In our experience, the retrograde vessels are consistently favorable recipient vessels, which spare the thoracodorsal system. The PAP flap is then coned and inset inferiorly. The DIEP flap is inset superiorly, providing upper pole fullness that tapers into a pseudo-axillary tail. The pedicles rest without tension in a crisscrossed fashion within the breast pocket **(Fig. 14.3)**. The flaps are then de-epithelialized and secured as appropriate to the chest wall. Skin paddles are utilized for monitoring of flaps.

Discussion

With an increased armamentarium of flaps for breast reconstruction and a foundation of proven safety and efficacy, perforator-based free flap breast reconstruction can now offer an increased level of breast reconstruction aesthetics. This is no more obvious than in the patient who needs greater volume breast reconstruction than one donor site can offer. Numerous options exist, all providing good results. Stacked DIEP and PAP flaps both provide adequate volume with favorable donor sites.[1,7] Stacked superior gluteal artery perforator (SGAP) flaps, although providing adequate volume, necessitate a change in patient positioning and can be a more technically demanding harvest. An extended DIEP can offer additional volume but may fall short, offering only an additional 16% in volume.[9]

The DIEP/PAP flap combination very closely replicates the natural breast shape **(Fig. 14.4)**. For a unilateral reconstruction, this combination may be bypassed, given the need for two donor sites, but it should be considered when harvest of a hemiabdomen is not possible. When bilateral reconstruction is necessary, this combination is ideal. The patient remains in the supine position while both microsurgeons are able to harvest the flaps simultaneously. Review of our series of patients shows acceptable operating times and complication rates. Overall, this stacked flap combination at present is our preferred choice for four-flap

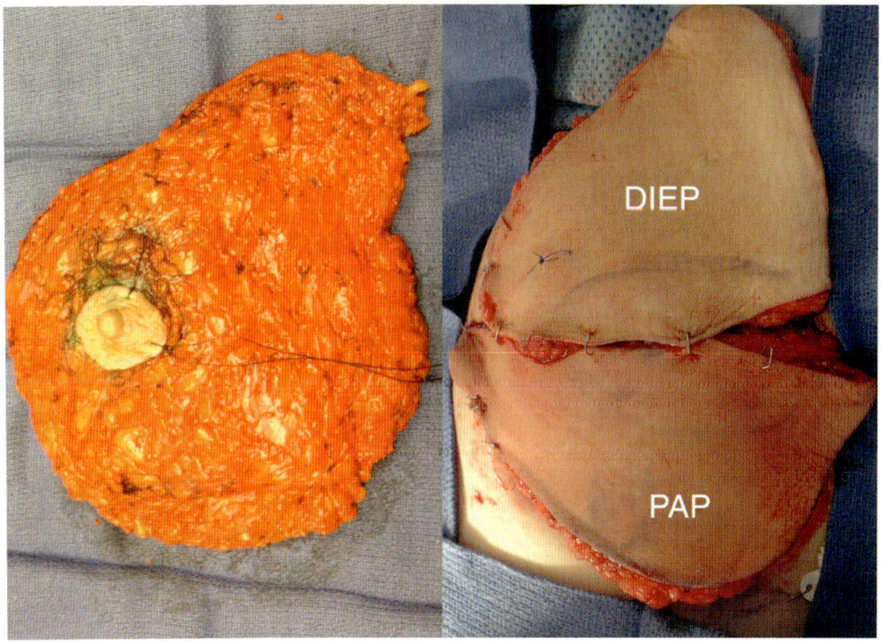

Fig. 14.1 The combination of the deep inferior epigastric perforator (DIEP) and profunda artery perforator (PAP) flaps closely resembles the shape of a natural breast, providing both lower pole projection and superior pole volume.

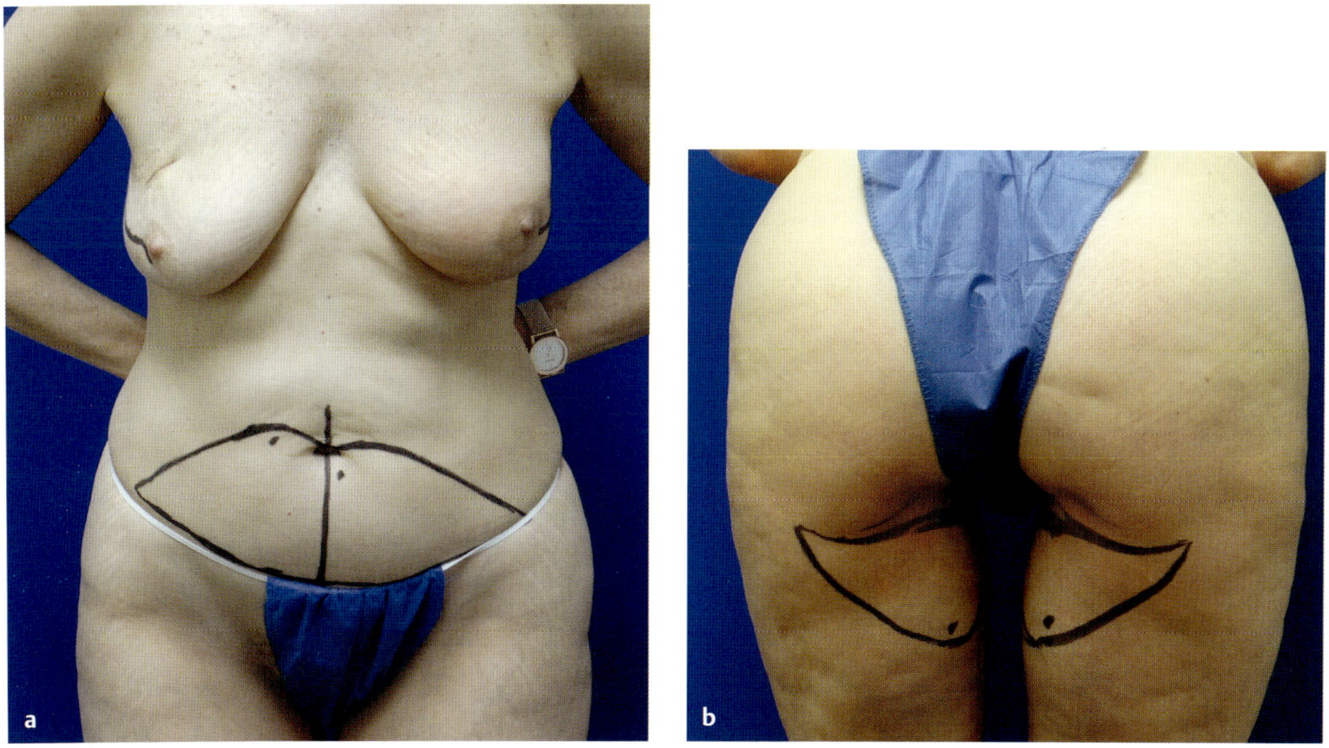

Fig. 14.2 Preoperative markings for both the **(a)** DIEP and **(b)** PAP flaps are made in the office the day prior to surgery. Key perforators, identified on preoperative imaging, are identified with a handheld Doppler and marked.

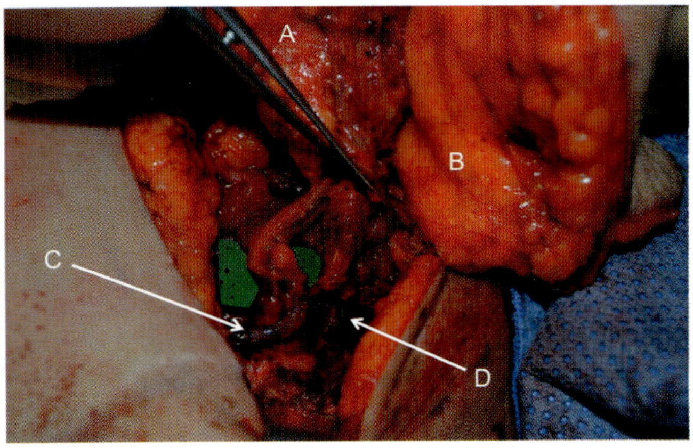

Fig. 14.3 The recipient vessels most commonly used are the antegrade and retrograde internal mammary vessels. The PAP flap *(A)*, which is inset inferiorly is anastomosed to the antegrade vessels *(D)*, and the DIEP flap *(B)*, inset superiorly, is anastomosed to the retrograde vessels *(C)*. creating a crisscrossed pattern.

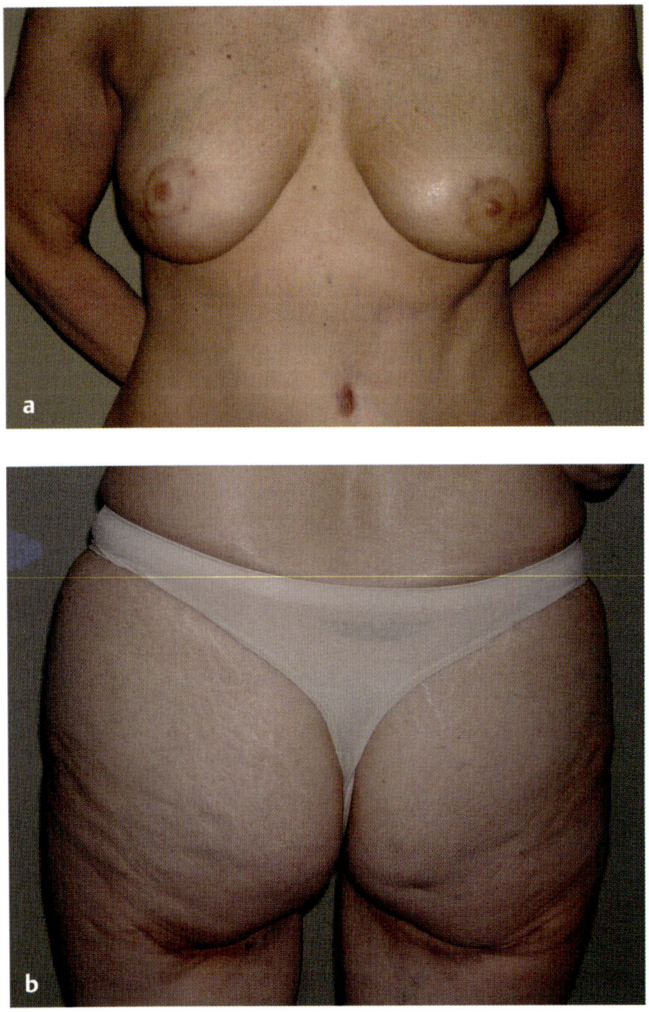

Fig. 14.4 (a) Postoperative view of a patient status post–bilateral mastectomy and bilateral DIEP/PAP flap breast reconstruction. **(b)** The PAP flap donor site seen from the posterior view after complete healing.

breast reconstruction and unilateral reconstruction in the appropriate setting.

Conclusion

Stacked DIEP/PAP flaps should be considered for bilateral breast reconstruction in the setting of single flap volume inadequacy. In select settings, the combination can also be utilized for unilateral breast reconstruction. The procedure has been shown to be safe and efficient. It allows the potential of aesthetic breast reconstruction to be further realized.

References

1. Ali RS, Garrido A, Ramakrishnan V. Stacked free hemi-DIEP flaps: a method of autologous breast reconstruction in a patient with midline abdominal scarring. Br J Plast Surg 2002;55:351–353
2. Arnez ZM, Scamp T. The bipedicled free TRAM flap. Br J Plast Surg 1992;45:214–218
3. Pennington DG, Nettle WJS, Lam P. Microvascular augmentation of the blood supply of the contralateral side of the free transverse rectus abdominis musculocutaneous flap. Ann Plast Surg 1993;31:123–126, discussion 126–127
4. Agarwal JP, Gottlieb LJ. Double pedicle deep inferior epigastric perforator/muscle-sparing TRAM flaps for unilateral breast reconstruction. Ann Plast Surg 2007;58:359–363
5. Figus A, Fioramonti P, Ramakrishnan V. Letter to the editor: stacked free SIEA/DIEP flap for unilateral breast reconstruction in a thin patient with an abdominal vertical midline scar. J Reconstr Microsurg 2007;23(8):523–525.
6. Hamdi M, Khuthaila DK, Van Landuyt K, Roche N, Monstrey S. Double-pedicle abdominal perforator free flaps for unilateral breast reconstruction: new horizons in microsurgical tissue transfer to the breast. J Plast Reconstr Aesthet Surg 2007;60:904–912, discussion 913–914
7. Blechman KM, Broer PN, Tanna N, Ireton JE, Ahn CY, Allen RJ. Stacked profunda artery perforator flaps for unilateral breast reconstruction: a case report. J Reconstr Microsurg 2013;29:631–634 http://www.ncbi.nlm.nih.gov/pubmed/23784788 [Internet]
8. Mayo JL, Allen RJ, Sadeghi A. Four-flap breast reconstruction: bilateral stacked DIEP and PAP Flaps. Plast Reconstr Surg Glob Open 2015;3:e383
9. Shafighi M, Constantinescu MA, Huemer GM, et al. The extended DIEP flap: extending the possibilities for breast reconstruction with tissue from the lower abdomen. Microsurgery 2013;33:24–31

15 Deep Circumflex Iliac Artery Perforator Flap for Breast Reconstruction

Edward Buchel

Autologous breast reconstruction using abdomen-based perforator flaps continues to be a highly successful means of reconstructing partial and complete breast defects. Much has been learned about the perfusion characteristics associated with the deep inferior epigastric perforator (DIEP) flap and the superficial inferior epigastric artery (SIEA) flaps. The SIEA flap routinely perfuses an ipsilateral hemiabdomen, whereas the DIEP flap reliably perfuses the ipsilateral and occasionally portions of the contralateral anterior abdominal tissue. Neither reliably perfuses tissue posterior to the anterior axillary line. This tissue, the flanks or "love handle" area, is frequently abundant and in fact is one of the most common areas of the trunk that undergoes secondary revision surgical contouring after abdomen-based breast reconstruction ("dog-ear" excision). This flank tissue is of significant value, either on its own or in conjunction with the anterior abdominal wall, for patients in whom the anterior abdominal wall has been already harvested, or the volume of tissue is inadequate for breast volume replacement, respectively. The deep circumflex iliac artery perforator perfuses lateral abdominal and hip tissue reliably and has proven to be an excellent adjunct to abdomen-based perforator breast reconstruction. Secondarily, it further improves the abdominal aesthetics by contouring the flanks as an extended "dog-ear" excision.

Anatomy

Taylor et al[1] first described the deep circumflex iliac artery (DCIA) as the supply for the groin flap in 1979. The preliminary reports documented an arterial diameter greater the 2 mm at the origin of the external iliac just lateral to the deep inferior epigastric artery. It reliably has two venae traveling with it varying in size from 1.5 to 2.5 mm. Starting from the external iliac artery origin, the artery travels laterally along the medial surface of the ilium and then superficially where it pierces the transversalis fascia. At this position it gives off musculocutaneous perforators and nutrient perforators to the iliac crest. At a point just superior and lateral to the anterior superior iliac spine (ASIS), the DCIA frequently gives off an ascending branch supplying the inferior lateral peritoneum and muscle of the abdominal wall.[2] The pedicle then continues as the lateral branch, supplying the iliac crest and the overlying skin after piercing the internal and external oblique muscles. In most cases the vascular bundle travels for 1 to 2 cm obliquely between the muscle layers before piercing the next most superficial muscle layer. The main perforator artery has an average diameter of 0.7 mm with an average of 1.6 DCIA perforators found on cadaveric injection studies.[3] Perforators were located 5 to 11 cm posterior to the ASIS, and 1 to 35 mm superior to the iliac crest, resulting in a perforator zone of 31 cm.[3] In clinical cases the dominant perforator has been found 1 to 2 cm superior and 1 to 4 cm lateral to the ASIS. The skin territory reliably supplied is superior to the iliac crest for 10 to 15 cm, and 10 to 15 cm horizontally in each direction from the entry point of the perforator into the flap.

Indications

Anterior abdominal wall tissue is always the first choice when considering autologous breast reconstruction. When the anterior abdomen tissue does not provide sufficient volume or has been previously resected, the flank tissue should be considered. Tissue lateral to the ASIS and superior to the iliac crest typically has thicker associated fat than is appreciated at first. Skin laxity on the flanks is variable, and will determine the maximum width of the flap that can be harvested and still allow for easy closure of the donor site. In general, the DCIA perforator flap is harvested alone when the anterior abdominal tissue has been previously resected, and as a combined flap with the ipsilateral DIEP or SIEA when a traditional hemiabdomen flap provides insufficient volume. In both situations, the donor site needs to be assessed to ensure that it has adequate fat and skin laxity. Closure of the donor site can provide a markedly improved abdominal contour, especially around the waist, but aggressive flap harvest can present difficulties in wound closure and prolonged wound healing. In general, the maximum vertical harvest dimensions of the DCIA flap

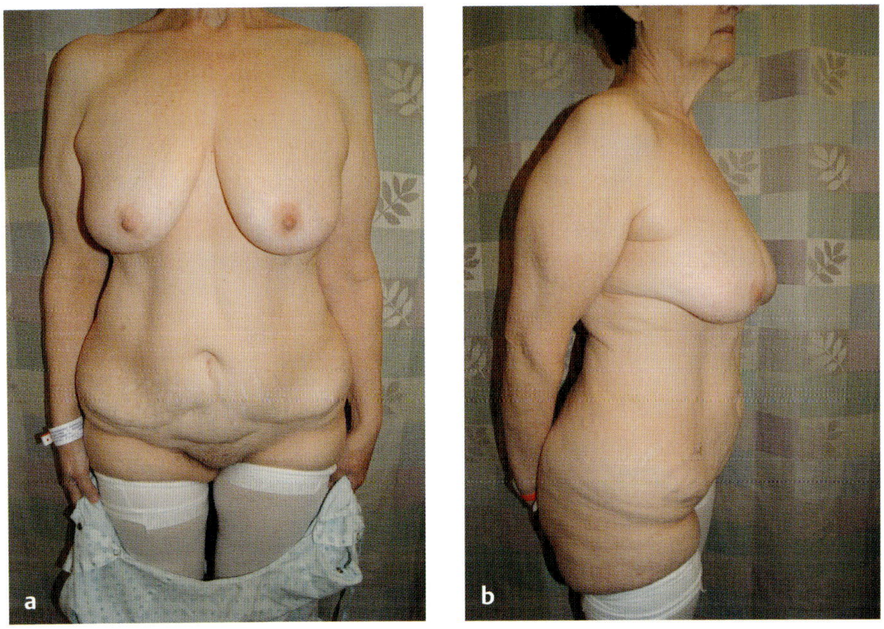

Fig. 15.1 (a) Preoperative view of a patient with a history of abdominal skin resection. Lateral abdominal tissue can still be harvested for breast reconstruction based on the deep circumflex iliac artery (DCIA) vessels. **(b)** Lateral view.

are determined in the same way as they would be for a body-lift cosmetic procedure. Thus, the donor-site closure will result in a similarly improved aesthetic result.

Technique

Markings

The DCIA flap is designed to be centered on the DCIA perforator. The use of the DCIA flap by itself or in conjunction with the DIEP or SIEA flap will determine the harvesting dimensions on the anterior abdominal wall. If the DCIA is used by itself, as is the case when the anterior abdominal wall has been resected previously **(Fig. 15.1)**, an inferior horizontal skin mark is made just lateral to the ASIS, extending posteriorly to include the excess tissue, or "dog ear." The corresponding superior horizontal skin mark is made by pinching the skin at this level to determine the maximum amount of excess skin that can be harvested. This will define the dimensions of the DCIA flap. The DCIA perforator will be located just superior and lateral to the ASIS **(Fig. 15.2)**. The upper and lower incision lines are

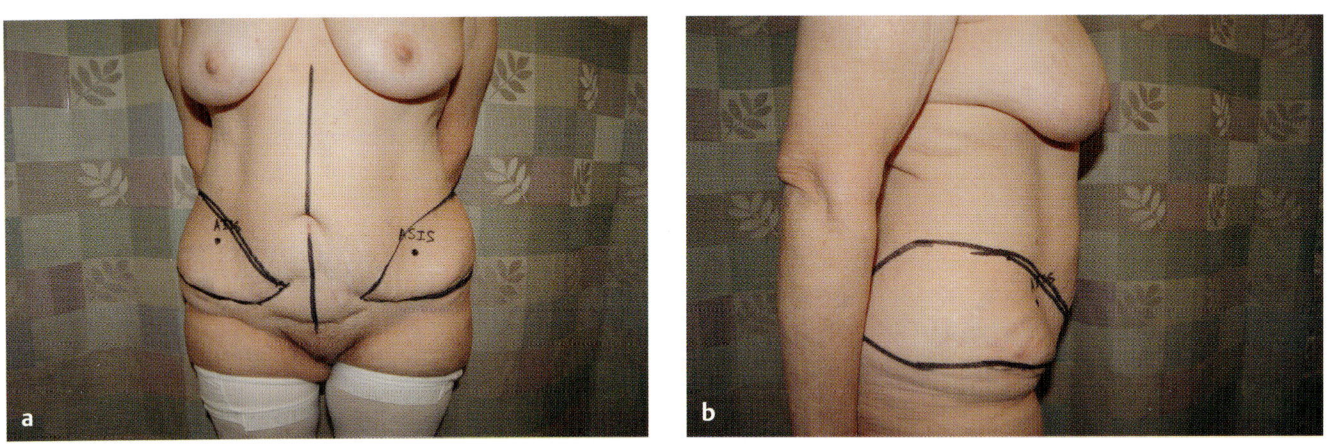

Fig. 15.2 (a) Markings designating tissue to be harvested. The *dot* shows the location of the DCIA. The excess tissue of the lateral abdomen is pinched to determine the amount of skin to be harvested. **(b)** DCIA markings: lateral view.

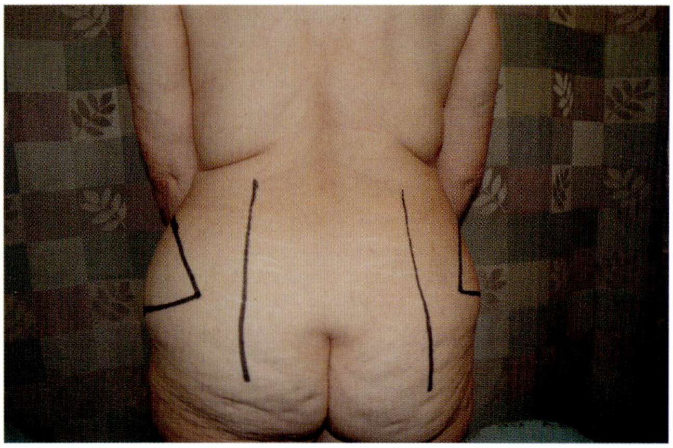

Fig. 15.3 Preoperative markings: posterior view. The posterior markings come together at a point just lateral to the mid-buttock line.

brought together posteriorly at a point just lateral to the mid-buttock line **(Fig. 15.3)**.

When harvesting a combined DCIA–DIEP or DCIA–SIEA flap, the markings for a standard DIEP or SIEA flap are done first. Then using these markings the DCIA flap markings are superimposed on them. As such the inferior markings of the DIEP–SIEA flap are treated as the prior abdominal wall scar as described above **(Fig. 15.4)**. Posterior markings are the same as for a single DCIA flap without the anterior abdominal included **(Fig. 15.5)**.

Harvest: Isolated DCIA and Combined DCIA–DIEP or DCIA–SIEA

The harvest of the isolated DICA flap starts at the most anterior/medial point of the flap. The skin and fat are elevated medial to lateral in an inferior to superior direction. Care is taken as the ASIS is approached. The perforator is usually found just superior and lateral to the ASIS. As with the DIEP dissection, the location of the associated skin Doppler signal directs the surgeon toward the location of the perforator vascular bundle. Typically there is a single dominant perforator vascular bundle, with two or three significantly smaller secondary bundles within a small area. Once the perforator vascular bundle is located, the flap is elevated from posterior to anterior. All secondary bundles are clamped temporarily and the flap perfusion characteristics are evaluated via flow through the dominant perforator bundle. Evaluation can also be done

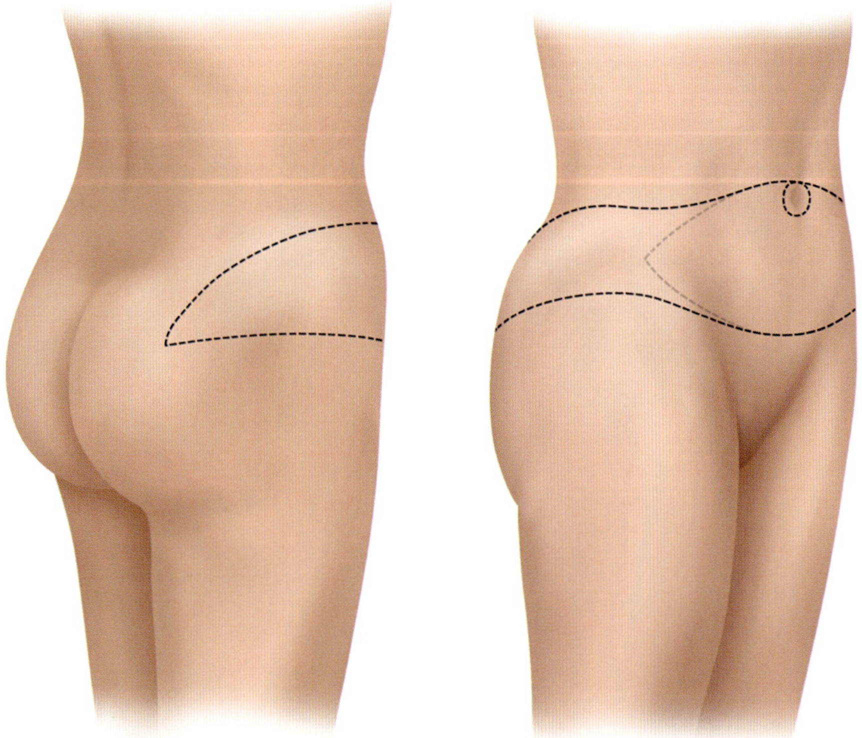

Fig. 15.4 Anterior markings for DICA superimposed on deep inferior epigastric perforator (DIEP) or superficial inferior epigastric artery (SIEA) markings in *light gray.*

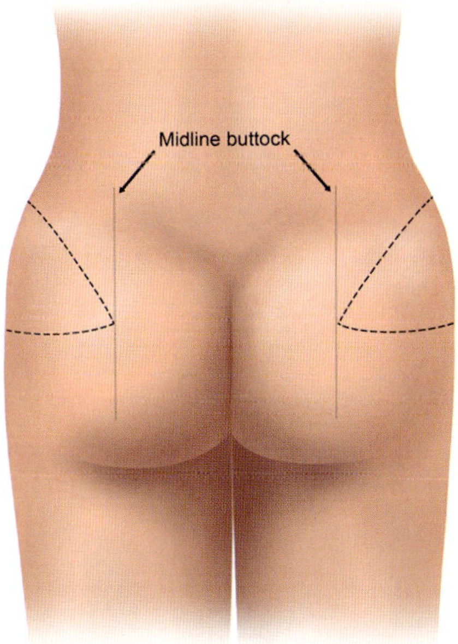

Fig. 15.5 Posterior markings. Midline buttock markings showing the limit of buttock dissection.

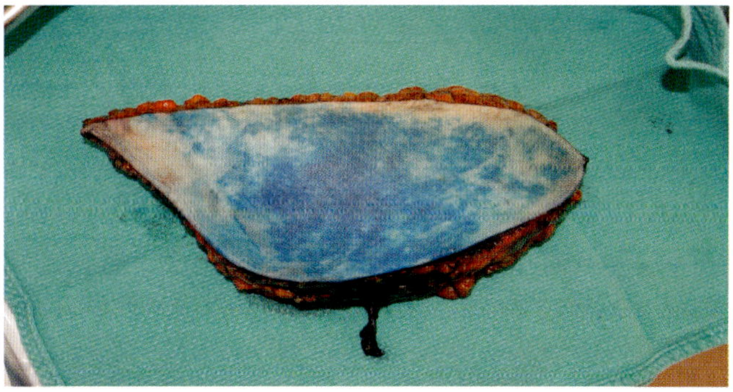

Fig. 15.6 Methylene blue injection in the DCIA flap.

clinically or through indocyanine green (ICG) angiography. Typically, the entire flank has adequate perfusion. Methylene blue injections and ICG angiography have repeatedly confirmed adequate perfusion characteristics of the harvested flap (Figs. 15.6 and 15.7). Once the perfusion of the marked skin territory is confirmed, the remaining superior skin marking is incised, and dissection is continued to the fascial level. The perforator bundles will now be the only connection of the body to the DCIA flap. The external oblique muscle fascial is now split along the direction of the fibers, extending superiorly and inferiorly from the point the perforator pierces the fascia (**Fig. 15.8**). The vessels are then dissected out for 1 to 3 cm until they pierce the underlying fascia of the internal oblique. Self-retaining retractors are valuable at this point to keep the external oblique fascia retracted (**Fig. 15.9**). The pedicle is followed through its course under the internal oblique until it pierces the transversalis muscle and runs along the medial border of the iliac crest. When harvesting the DCIA perforator flap, there is no indication to enter the

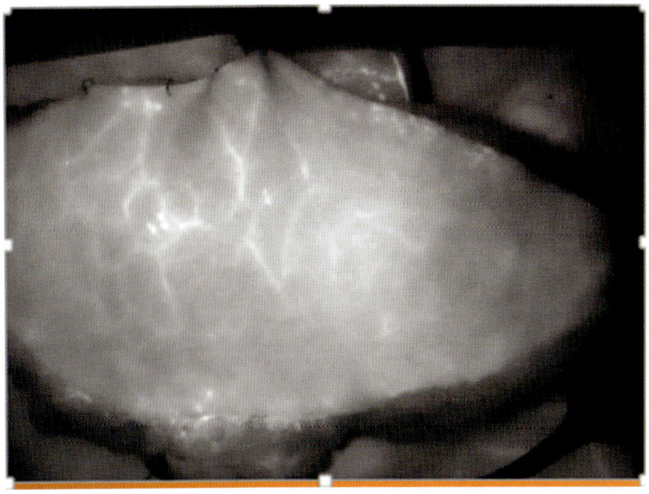

Fig. 15.7 Indocyanine green (ICG) angiography showing excellent perfusion of the DCIA flap.

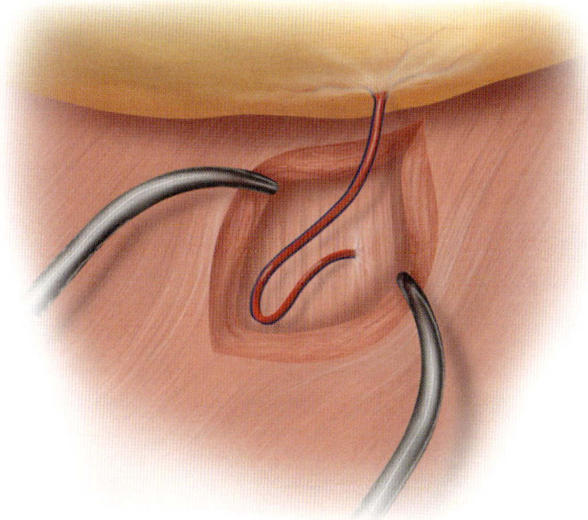

Fig. 15.8 DCIA perforator dissection through the external oblique fascia, which is split along the length of the fibers.

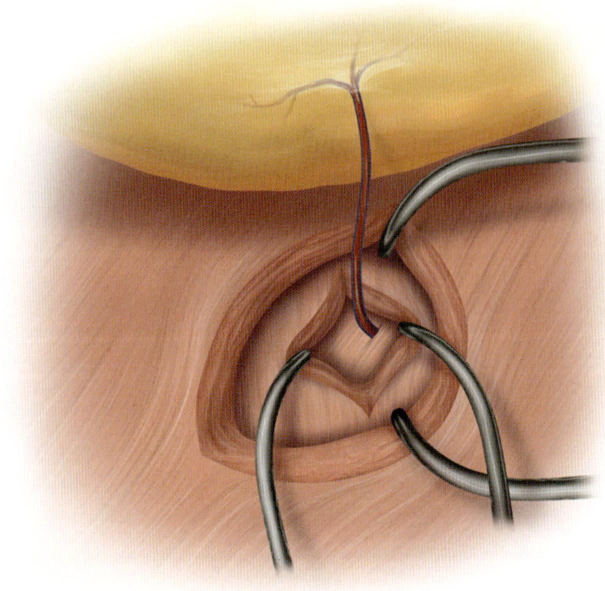

Fig. 15.9 Dissection through the external, internal, and transversus muscles with the aid of self-retaining retractors.

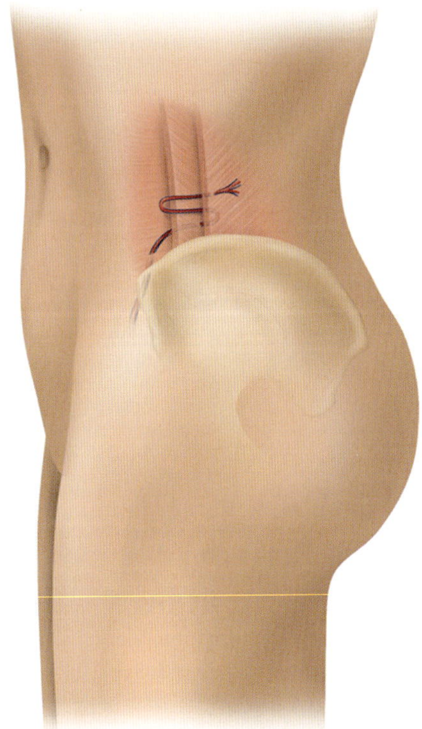

Fig. 15.10 DCIA perforator course: lateral view.

peritoneum. The length of the pedicle, from the base of the flap to the level of the transversalis muscle, has been greater than 6 cm in all cases and typically 6 to 8 cm. The arterial diameter at this point is greater than 1.5 mm, with the venae having a diameter of 1.5 to 2.5 mm.

There is limited reason to extend the dissection further into the pelvis. The pedicle length is typically longer than would be expected as the vessels travel back and forth between the layers of the abdominal wall muscles **(Figs. 15.10** to **15.12)**.

When the flap is designed as a DCIA–DIEP combined flap, the anterior abdominal wall (DIEP) component of the dissection is completed to the point of DIEP perforator

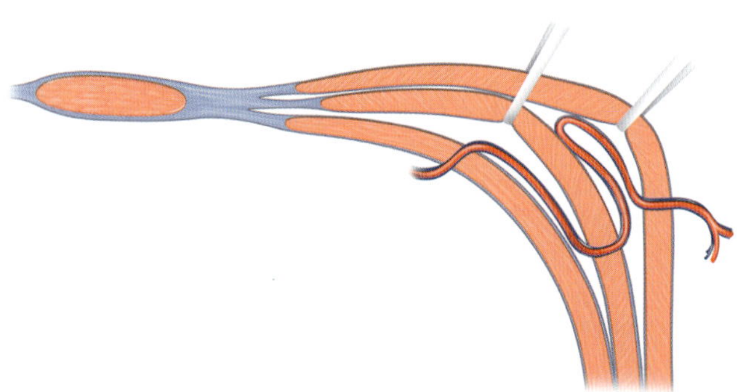

Fig. 15.11 DCIA perforator course through lateral abdominal wall muscles: coronal view.

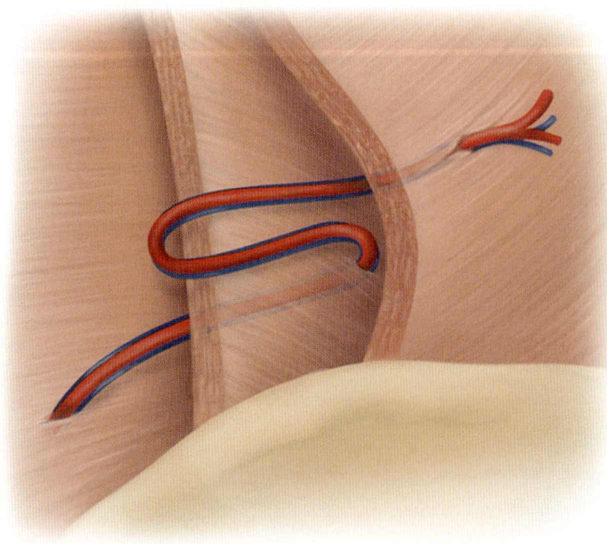

Fig. 15.12 DICA perforator path through lateral abdominal muscles: anterior view.

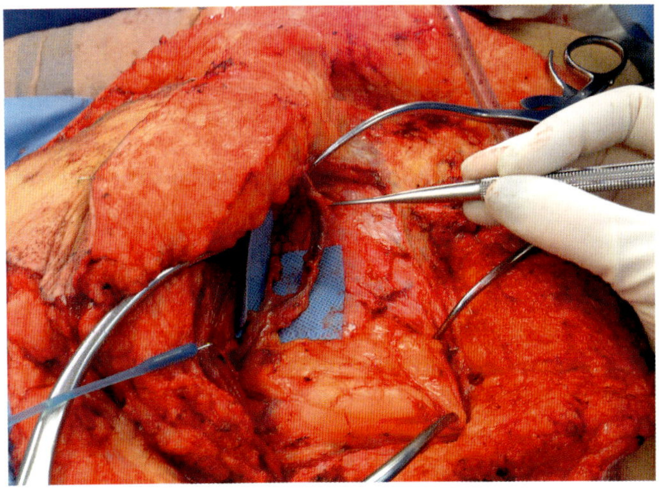

Fig. 15.13 Right DIEP dissected on a medial perforator (held in forceps), with extended harvest of lateral deep inferior epigastric vessels for anastomosis to the DCIA. (Courtesy of Joshua L. Levine, MD.)

vascular bundle isolation. The pedicles' perfusion to the designated DIEP tissue is clinically confirmed. Then the DICA dissection is done in a similar fashion as described above for the DCIA flap alone. The combined DCIA–DIEP flap can have each pedicle anastomosed separately to two separate donor vessels, or the DCIA pedicle can be anastomosed to the DIEP pedicle. When anastomosing the DCIA vessels and the DIEP vessels to two separate donor vessels, typically the internal mammary vessels are exposed in a way that enables antegrade and retrograde connection of the two flaps. Thus the flap can be folded with the vascular pedicle sandwiched on the inside, exiting the flaps on the medial side when anastomosed to the internal mammary vessels. The internal mammary vessels are our preferred donor vessels for all breast reconstruction and frequently are used simultaneously antegrade and retrograde, allowing for two sets of donor vessels in a similar location. Alternatively, the combined DCIA–DIEP can have the DCIA pedicle connected to the DIEP pedicle, and then the DIEP pedicle connected to the internal mammary vessels in the standard fashion. In this case, the side branch of the DIEP pedicle is dissected out and preserved when harvesting the DIEP flap **(Fig. 15.13).** This DICA to DIEP anastomosis can be done on the back table in order to maintain a stable controlled working environment **(Fig. 15.14)**. The flaps are sutured to each other and the deep flap is de-epithelialized prior to the DIEP pedicle anastomosis to the internal mammary vessels. The decision as to which method should be chosen is based on the length of the DCIA pedicle and the presence of a suitable side branch of the DIEP pedicle. If the DCIA pedicle is long (>8 cm), then there is the option of anastomosing it antegrade and retrograde to the internal mammary vessels. If the DCIA pedicle is short, a side branch anastomosis is the best choice, and a suitable side branch should be dissected out.

In either case the effective pedicle length is short after the completion of the internal mammary anastomosis. Care needs to be taken when insetting the flap through a skin-sparing mastectomy opening, as tension on the

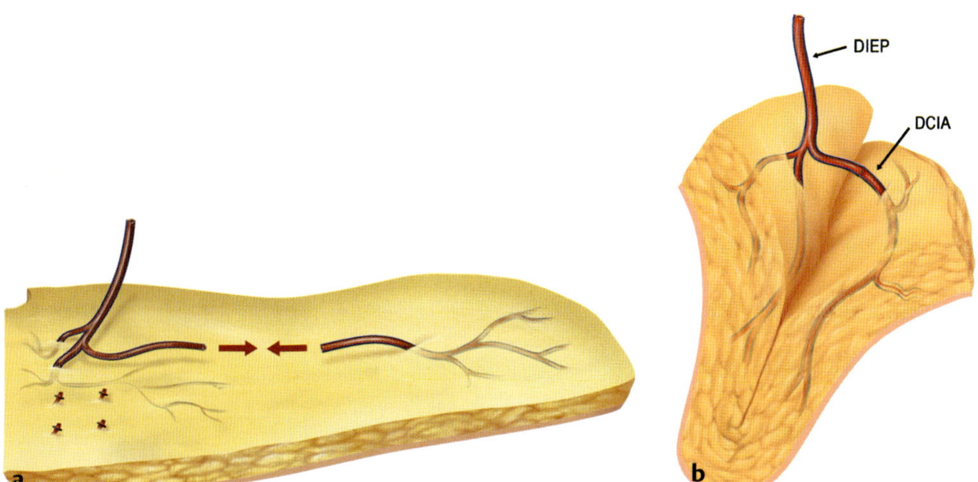

Fig. 15.14 **(a)** DIEP–DCIA flap internal flap connection: DIEP side branch to DCIA perforator pedicle. **(b)** DIEP–DCIA internal flap anastomosis completed with the DIEP pedicle prepared for anastomosis.

pedicle and potentially avulsion of the anastomosis could occur.

Closure

The closure of the anterior abdomen, medial to the ASIS, is similar to that done for the DIEP flaps. Closure of the DICA donor site has the internal and external oblique fibers approximated using permanent woven stiches in a figure-of-eight fashion. The direction of pull of each muscle is at right angles to the other, thus limiting the potential for hernia or bulging of the abdominal wall at the harvest site. The intercostal nerves travel along the direction for the muscle fibers, thus limiting the chance of inadvertent transection. In our series there has been no hernia or clinical bulging documented.

Once the fascia is closed, the patient's hips are slid toward the ipsilateral side of the operative table, thus facilitating closure of the ipsilateral posterior extent of the donor site. Posterior midline buttock closure becomes difficult without turning the patient, if the flap harvest extends medial to the midline of the buttock posteriorly. This is the main reason that the initial markings are limited to lateral to the midline of the buttock. Skin and fat are closed in three layers with absorbable sutures, as is the anterior abdominal wall donor site. Only two drains are placed, regardless of whether a DICA or a combined DCIA–DIEP flap was harvested.

Dressings typically consist of Steri-Strips, gauze, and an abdominal binder. The patient remains in a slightly flexed position postoperatively. The binders remain in place for 2 to 4 weeks.

Conclusion

The lateral flanks or "love handle" area of the trunk frequently has excess fat and adequate skin, which would be available for free autologous breast reconstruction. This area is valuable when the anterior abdominal wall has inadequate volume on its own or when the anterior abdominal wall has undergone prior resection. Thus the DCIA perforator flap can be used in combination with the DIEP or SIEA flap for increased volume or as a single flap when the anterior abdominal wall tissue is not available. In addition, harvesting bilateral flank tissue improves the aesthetic contours of the trunk in most patients. The DCIA perforator is predictably present with adequate vessel size to make the harvest and anastomosis safe and reliable. Although the length of the pedicle can be shorter than a DIEP or SIEA pedicle, there is sufficient length to complete an anastomosis to the internal mammary vessels. The DCIA perforator flap is a valuable secondary choice for autologous breast reconstruction that can be performed efficiently with limited donor-site complications.

References

1. Taylor GI, Townsend P, Corlett R. Superiority of the deep circumflex iliac vessels as the supply for free groin flaps. Clinical work. Plast Reconstr Surg 1979;64:745–759
2. Hendricks HP, Ingianni G, Bohm E, Schubert GE. A Microvascular peritoneal flap based on the deep circumflex iliac artery.—Ananatomic study. Eur J Plast Surg 1995;18:88–90
3. Bergeron L, Tang M, Morris SF. The anatomical basis of the deep circumflex iliac artery perforator flap with iliac crest. Plast Reconstr Surg 2007;120:252–258

16 Indocyanine Green/SPY Imaging in Perforator Flap Breast Reconstruction

Michael R. Zenn

Fluorescent angiography is a simple and effective tool for measurement of tissue perfusion both in and out of the operating room. This technology has been used clinically since the 1970s and is based on indocyanine green (ICG) dye that absorbs light in the near-infrared spectrum.[1–4] Since 2007, the technology has been used by plastic surgeons to assess the perfusion of tissues in real time in the operating room.[5–25] The technology can also be used multiple times throughout the same procedure as needs change. This ability of the surgeon to directly control the imaging of perforators and tissue perfusion in real time has been a game changer for the burgeoning field of perforator flap surgery.

The ICG dye is a water-soluble tricarbocyanine dye that was originally developed by Eastman Kodak for use in infrared photography. It was introduced into clinical use when, as a token of appreciation for his treatment at the Mayo Clinic, an executive at Eastman Kodak sent a variety of dyes to a clinician who was looking for suitable dyes that could be safely administered to patients and easily measured in blood. The clinically useful formulation of the dye, a stable lyophilized powder, was developed. For a time ICG was referred to as Fox Green after the cardiologist, Dr. Irwin Fox, who was responsible for its introduction into clinical practice. Initially, ICG was used to assess cardiac output by means of dye dilution technique.[26] The near-infrared absorption and emission of light by ICG makes it particularly well suited to visualizing small blood vessels. In the early 1970s, Flower[1] developed techniques for acquisition of fluorescence angiograms of the choroid utilizing ICG. Since that time, the basic technique has changed little other than improvement in near-infrared–sensitive cameras and light sources.

One of the biggest advantages of ICG over other dyes such as fluorescein is its rapid clearance from the tissues. Following intravascular administration, ICG is rapidly and extensively bound to plasma proteins, with α-lipoproteins being the major carrier in humans. The ICG is thus confined to the intravascular compartment with little leakage into the interstitium, making it an ideal tissue perfusion contrast agent compared with dyes such as fluorescein that remain in the interstitium, are not rapidly cleared, and therefore can only be used once.[27] Fluorescein, therefore, provides only a static picture of perfusion. The plasma half-life of ICG is very short, 3 to 5 minutes in humans, with the dye being taken up by the liver and being excreted into the bile without any further metabolism. There is no renal excretion of ICG, and so there is no contraindication for use in patients with renal insufficiency. Since its introduction into clinical practice, ICG has shown an excellent safety profile, with a low incidence of adverse events of 1 in 42,000 patients. Anaphylactic reactions are rare. ICG contains iodide, so patients sensitive to iodides should avoid this technology. Most reactions are usually mild in nature and entail a feeling of warmth or a sore throat.

A typical intraoperative imaging system comprises an imaging camera that houses an 806-nm diode laser to provide near-infrared illumination. This low-level laser does not require the use of protective goggles by the surgeon or the operating room staff. Optics within the camera can even provide near-infrared illumination over fields as large as 20 × 20 cm or as small as 1 cm in an operating microscope. Cameras have also been adopted for use in robotic surgery (e.g., the DaVinci, Intuitive Surgical, Sunnyvale, CA) and endoscopic surgery (e.g., Firefly, Intuitive Surgical). Image sequences are usually captured at 30 frames/second, and the image sequences are displayed on a monitor in real time for the surgeon to assess. Most systems have a computer for further analysis, review, and archiving of the data.

The SPY system (Novadaq/Lifecell, Bonita Springs, FL) is the most commonly used system in plastic and reconstructive surgery **(Fig. 16.1)**, although there are others.[28] It was originally developed for use in coronary artery bypass graft (CABG) surgery to confirm the patency of bypass grafts,[26] and was cleared for this indication in Canada, Europe, and Japan in 2001. The SPY system received regulatory clearance in 2005 from the U.S. Food and Drug Administration (FDA) for use in CABG procedures, and sub-

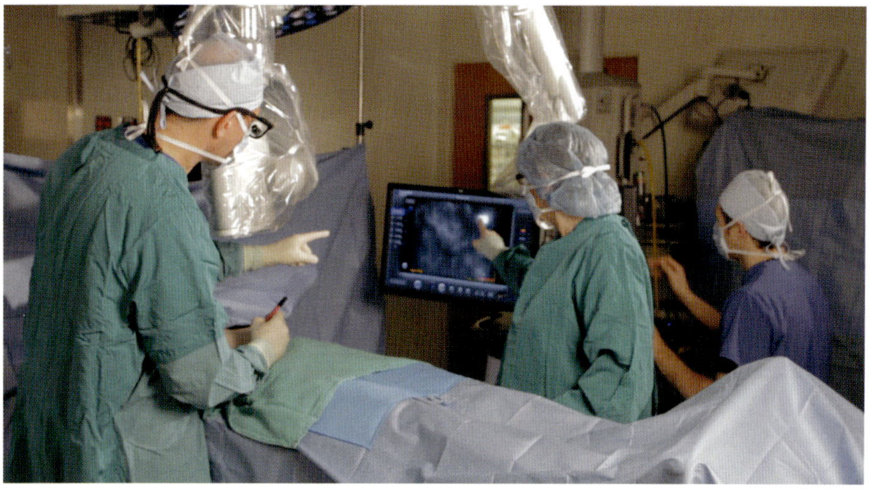

Fig. 16.1 Indocyanine green (ICG) imaging with the SPY Elite device. The infrared camera is draped and brought into the operative field whenever it is needed.

sequently clearance in 2007 for use in plastic and reconstructive and microsurgical procedures.

Technique

Once the surgeon is ready to perform the imaging, the camera is positioned and the anesthesiologist administers a 5-cc bolus containing 2.5 mg of ICG. No toxicity has been seen with total doses of 5 mg/kg (400 mg in an 80-kg patient). Typical acquisition times are about 1 minute. If one is attempting to visualize and localize perforating blood vessels, the camera is turned on immediately to record the first blush. If perfusion is the goal, the image is captured from the start of ICG injection to 1 to 3 minutes for full tissue evaluation. If a second scan is desired, the surgeon should wait 10 minutes to allow washout of the ICG for optimal scanning. Current software, such as the SPY-Q (Novadaq/Lifecell) enables the data to be seen with colormetric analysis for easier interpretation **(Fig. 16.2)**. This software can analyze data and plot the areas of maximal intensity that correlate with the best perfusion or perforator location, and can subtract any background ICG still present from a previous injection. This software has been used successfully to predict mastectomy skin and nipple necrosis in multiple studies.[29–32]

Applications

Indocyanine green imaging remains a superficial evaluation of tissue blood flow, which can limit its applicability. Despite this, the technology is highly useful when there is a need for perfusion assessment a few millimeters deep, and it can help the surgeon make clinical decisions. This is especially useful in perforator breast reconstruction where (1) evaluation of mastectomy skin flaps is critical, (2) localizing of perforators is desirable, and (3) definition of the angiosome/perforasome supplied by selected perforators can be visualized and marked directly. Postoperative monitoring with ICG is currently impractical but may have future applications.

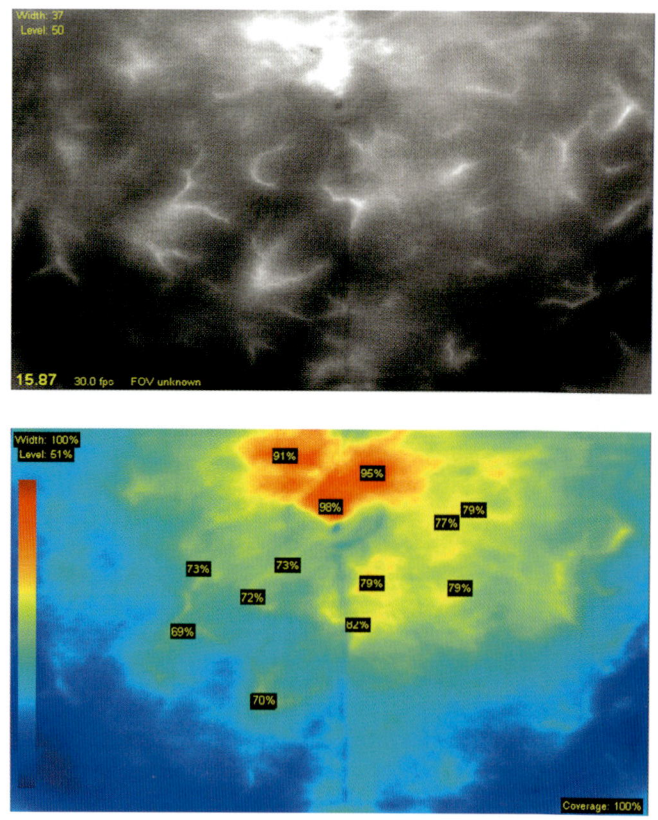

Fig. 16.2 The black and white ICG image is analyzed with the SPY-Q software package to colorize the image for easier interpretation of the perfusion detected.

Evaluation of Mastectomy Skin Flaps

As the mastectomy field has evolved to more nipple-sparing and skin-sparing mastectomies, the incidence of nipple and skin necrosis has increased, being as high as 40% in some studies.[27,29–32] Often, this is a result of over-dissection of the skin flaps and loss of axial blood flow within the flaps. These "random" skin flaps can be effectively evaluated by ICG **(Fig. 16.3)**. Areas within mastectomy skin or nipples that do not fluoresce are relatively ischemic and have an associated higher risk of necrosis. Software analysis can further define the at-risk areas. When confronted by such ischemia, often in the face of a normal clinical exam, the reconstructive surgeon should pay heed to it, and further surgical planning should account for it. In some cases this may mean skin resection and replacement with flap skin. In other cases, this may mean skin flap delay or delay of the entire surgical procedure until the skin declares itself **(Fig. 16.4)**.

Localization of Perforators

Indocyanine green laser angiography is often compared with computed tomography angiography (CTA) and magnetic resonance angiography (MRA) for perforator localization. Because ICG angiography is a superficial technology, it provides information on only the most superficial few millimeters of any surface examined. In flaps of this thickness (thin abdomen for the deep inferior epigastric perforator [DIEP], thin thighs for the profunda artery perforator [PAP]), ICG imaging compares favorably with CTA. It also has the advantage of being used in real time, and perforators can be marked directly onto the tissues as visualized.

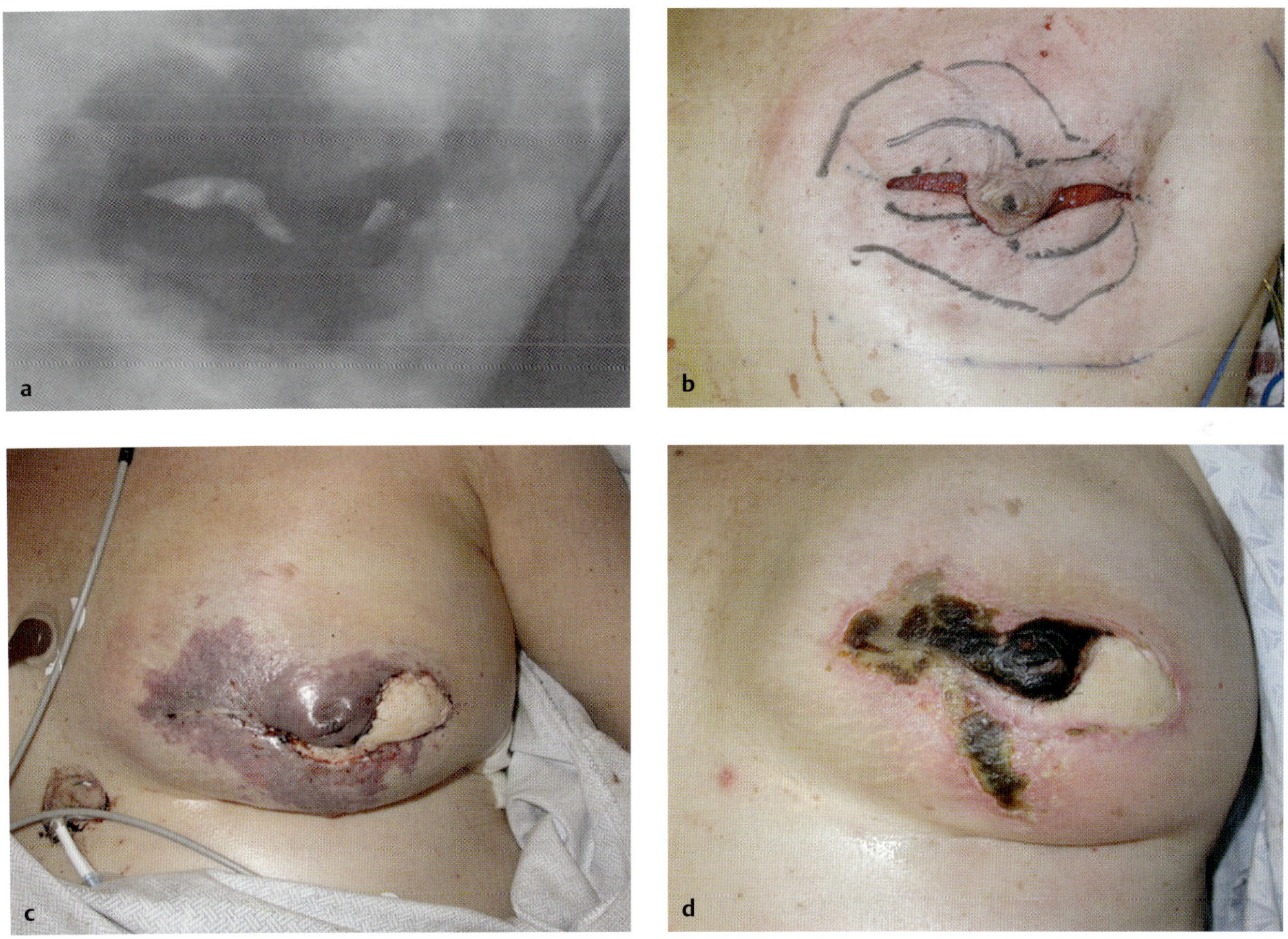

Fig. 16.3 (a) An ICG image of a nipple-sparing mastectomy showing the lack of fluorescence of the nipple-areolar complex. **(b)** Clinical photograph at the time of the ICG imaging showing a relatively normal-appearing nipple and mastectomy skin. The skin identified to be at risk by ICG imaging was not removed. **(c)** Photograph on postoperative day 1 showing ischemic changes closely correlating with the areas of poor fluorescence on ICG imaging. **(d)** Photograph 2 weeks postoperative showing full-thickness loss of mastectomy skin and the nipple-areolar complex.

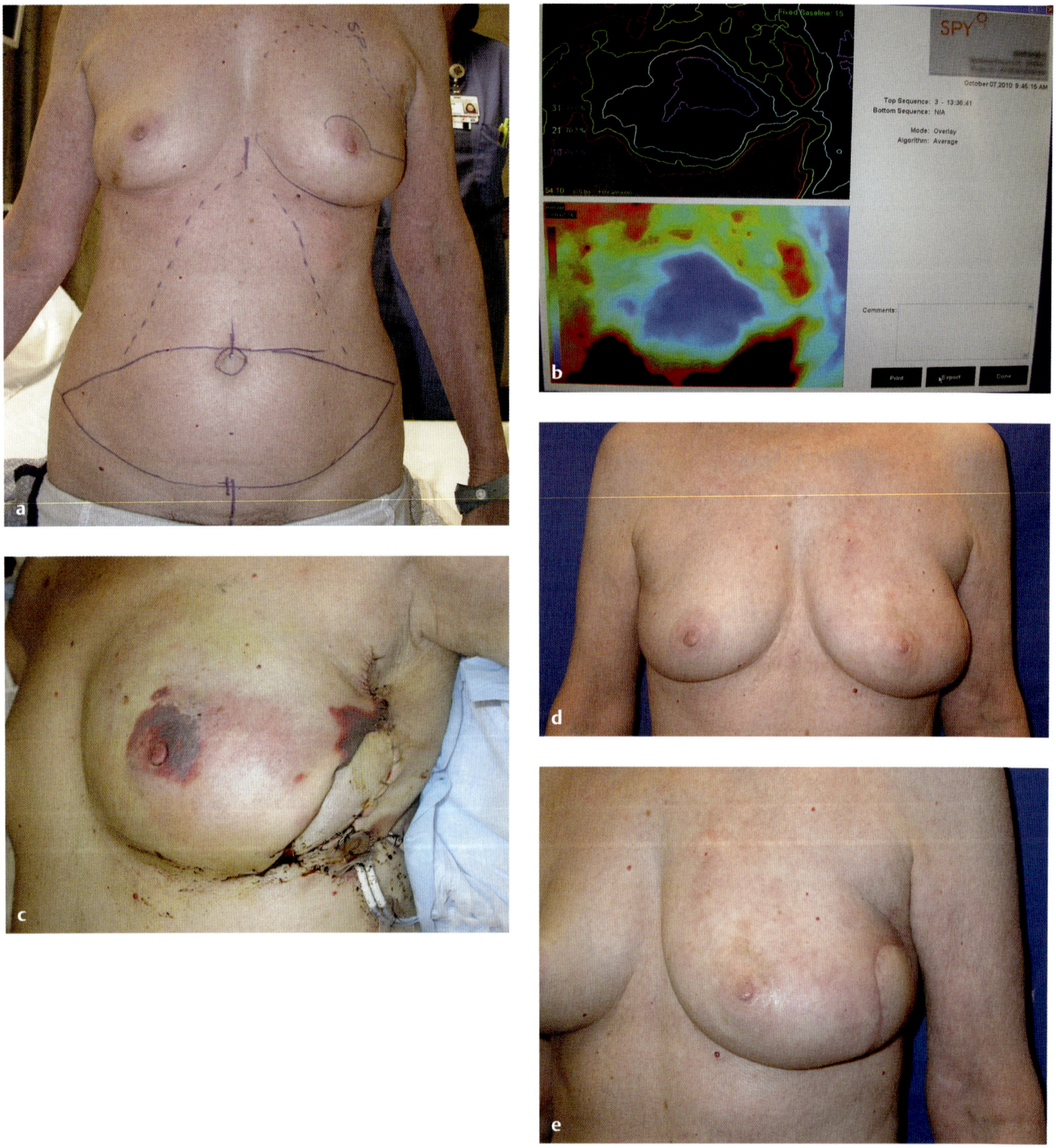

Fig. 16.4 (a) This 48-year-old patient presented for nipple-sparing mastectomy and deep inferior epigastric perforator (DIEP) flap reconstruction. A lateral approach was used instead of the marked periareolar incision to avoid ischemia to the nipple as seen in **Fig. 16.3**. **(b)** SPY-Q analysis of the ICG imaging after mastectomy consistent with ischemia of the periareolar area. Because of this finding, the DIEP flap was buried under the mastectomy skin to let the mastectomy skin and nipple demarcate. **(c)** Photograph postoperative day 4. Clinically, it appeared that except for the mastectomy skin laterally, the breast skin would survive, and the decreased nipple skin perfusion was superficial and not full thickness. Therefore, the lateral ischemic skin was resected, and the flap de-epithelialized except for a lateral monitoring skin paddle. **(d)** Photograph of patient 4 months postoperative showing good cosmesis. **(e)** Photograph of the skin paddle can be seen in the oblique view. The skin paddle was resected in a secondary procedure. ICG imaging enabled an informed conservative approach to successfully complete the nipple-sparing procedure.

For thicker tissues, greater than 1 cm, ICG imaging is less accurate for perforator localization.[21] As an analogy, with CTA and MRA one is looking at the trunk and the roots of a tree, but with ICG imaging one is looking only at the leaves of the tree. Decisions can still be made on first blush as to which tissues to include in flap design, but fascial location of the perforator is less certain as the distance from the skin to the fascia increases. Although the first blush of fluorescence is presumed to be the first and best perfused tissues, this has not been collaborated by clinical study. The same can be said of CTA and MRA, in that the largest noted perforator is presumed to have the best flow and distribution, although this has not been proven. CTA and MRA require a radiologist to measure perforator location in reference to a landmark. An advantage of ICG imaging is that a surgeon directly marks the area during the study.

Documenting Tissue Perfusion/ Angiosomes/Perforasomes

By far the greatest utility of fluorescent angiography is the capability of visualizing perfusion in real time. This is the vital information plastic surgeons require when evaluating tissues and creating flaps for reconstruction. The gold standard for evaluating perfusion is clinical judgment, and this judgment is acquired over a career. ICG imaging enables surgeons to see perfusion and ischemia in a way that is unobtainable by the unaided human eye. This information enhances the judgment of the expert and gives confidence and increases the learning curve of the novice.

An angiosome is a block of tissue that is supplied by a single blood vessel in isolation. When that supplying vessel is a perforator, the block of tissue is called a "perforasome."[33] The isolated vessel may also supply the neighboring, or "secondary," angiosome. Tissues separated by two angiosomes, also called "tertiary" angiosomes, are thought to be unreliable without a delay.[34] With ICG imaging, these angiosomes and perforasomes can be directly visualized in real time. As the ICG perfuses the tissues, the first blush corresponds with the primary angiosome. As this area begins to fade, the second angiosome lights up, somewhat fainter. Little or no fluorescence is seen in tertiary areas. Although this is obvious with the infrared camera, clinically the differences are subtle at best (**Fig. 16.5**). The degree of fluorescence can be influenced by the degree of spasm often present in dissected perforators, but the location and extent of angiosomes will not change without a surgical delay of a week or more. By identifying all significant perforators to a flap and selectively clamping vessels, one can test the degree of perfusion of tissues before committing to any one vessel. If there is not enough tissue perfusion, additional perforators can be carried with the flap. The ultimate goal of ICG imaging is to use only tissues in the marked zones of good perfusion for the reconstruction, thereby lowering the likelihood of postoperative complications such as fat necrosis and wound-healing problems.

Other Uses

Postoperative Monitoring

Indocyanine green imaging has a role in postoperative monitoring,[35] but its role is limited by the availability of ICG dye and the fluorescent angiography machines in the recovery room or the postoperative ward. In some

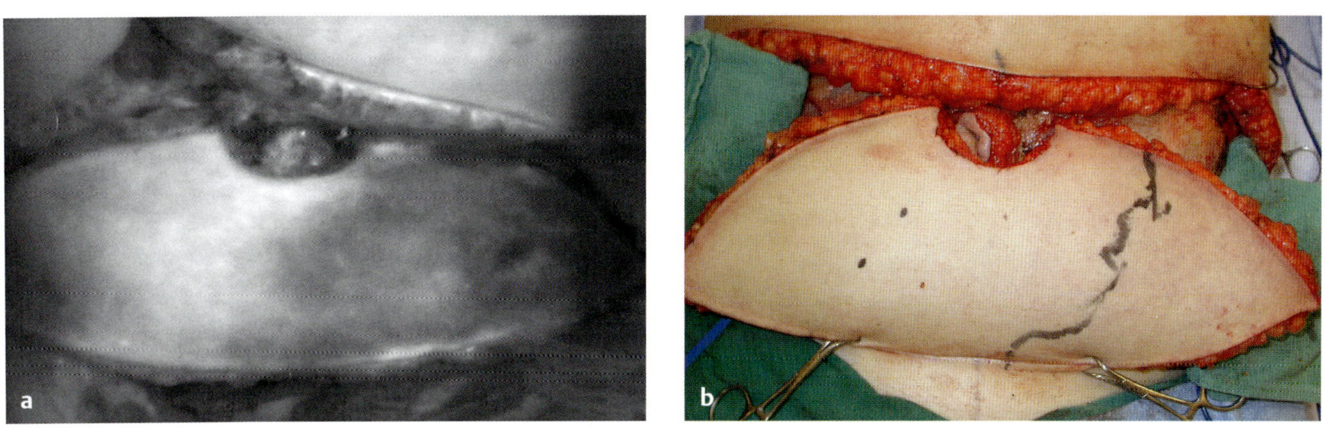

Fig. 16.5 (a) ICG imaging showing well-defined primary *(bright)*, secondary *(less bright)*, and tertiary *(dark)* areas of a muscle sparing TRAM flap. **(b)** Photograph of the TRAM flap at the time of ICG imaging. The zones of differential perfusion are not easily seen by the human eye alone.

perforator cases, the vessels are so small that implantable Doppler probes are problematic. In others, surface probes measuring oxygenation can be cumbersome. ICG imaging could be useful in such cases. Some centers are using ICG imaging routinely for monitoring postoperative digit replants.[36] As ICG imaging and infrared cameras become more widely available in hospitals, the use of this technology will increase for postoperative monitoring.

Evaluation of the Microscopic Anastomoses

One of the early and exciting uses of ICG imaging in plastic surgery was the evaluation of blood flow within arterial and venous conduits. ICG imaging can be visually impressive and reassuring as it shows blood entering and then leaving a flap. There are cases of low flow in some flaps with spasm where venous outflow is not always obvious and a Doppler signal is not obtainable even though the tissues are viable. This temporary phenomenon may last until spasm resolves or simply will improve over time due to reorganization of the blood supply within the tissue. ICG imaging can immediately confirm inflow and egress to allay fears and document patent anastomoses in the operating room, which eliminates the need to take down and evaluate an anastomosis. This has obvious time savings and prevents unnecessary surgery and tissue damage.

Documentation

In this era of protective medical documentation and malpractice liability, if an event is not documented in the record, it did not happen. ICG imaging can be helpful in certain cases where the physician appreciates the extra support of documentation of perfusion in tissues. It can be used to confirm or prove the existence of good perfusion during surgery or document poor perfusion as the basis for intraoperative decision making. This documentation can also be used in support of insurance or legal claims. Images may also be used to educate the patient and family about the procedure and to convey an idea of what things looked like during surgery or at the conclusion of the procedure.

Fluorescent Angiography in the Literature

In animal studies, infrared angiography with ICG has been used to assess the microcirculation of axial flaps,[2] to predict necrosis in axial flaps,[3] to visualize perforators for flap design,[5] and to quantitate arterial and venous compromise based on ICG fluorescence intensity.[4] This preliminary work confirmed the usefulness of the technology and built the foundation for further clinical study.

There have been many clinical studies of ICG imaging in reconstructive surgery.[7–25] The initial clinical studies focused on the utility of the technology in pedicled flaps. This experience was extended to free flap surgery. Studies have shown the utility of fluorescent angiography in flap design, postoperative monitoring, intraoperative anastomotic evaluation, and intraoperative decision making. Most studies have focused on breast reconstructive cases, and have reported the mapping of pedicle transverse rectus abdominis musculocutaneous (TRAM) flaps, deep inferior epigastric perforator (DIEP) flaps, and free superficial inferior epigastric artery (SIEA) flaps; the evaluation of mastectomy flaps; and the evaluation of flaps after inset. All of these factors may influence intraoperative decision making. Recent studies have highlighted the cost-effectiveness of ICG imaging as well.[37]

Future Directions

Indocyanine green imaging is an excellent and easy-to-use technology that is beneficial to plastic surgeons, and it reinforces their current concepts of blood supply and perfusion. This becomes more important with perforator flap surgery, in which the margins of adequate blood supply are pushed to their maximum extent: blood supply based on a single perforating artery and vein. When attempts are made to carry tissues on ever smaller blood vessels, circulation is compromised even more and the likelihood of ischemic complications such as fat necrosis certainly increases. What is currently not known is how the level of fluorescence and the study in general can predict future necrosis or flap survival. Only with increasing experience and prospective study can this be determined. One can imagine a future in which MRA and CTA images are integrated with ICG imaging data to help pick perforators by size, location, and angiosome distribution **(Fig. 16.6)**.

Although the focus continues to be on arterial inflow, clinically the concern is often more on the venous egress as the source of necrosis or failure in sugery.[4,38] ICG imaging holds the potential to assess venous egress by evaluating the disappearance of the ICG from the tissues. Venosomes and perforasomes do not always perfectly align, and this information would help raise perforator flaps with both adequate arterial perfusion and venous drainage.[33] A clinical standard for inflow and outflow would be invaluable for intraoperative decision making.

Another idiosyncrasy of ICG clearance and excretion enables the mapping of lymphatic systems. This is significant because total reconstruction of the breast should

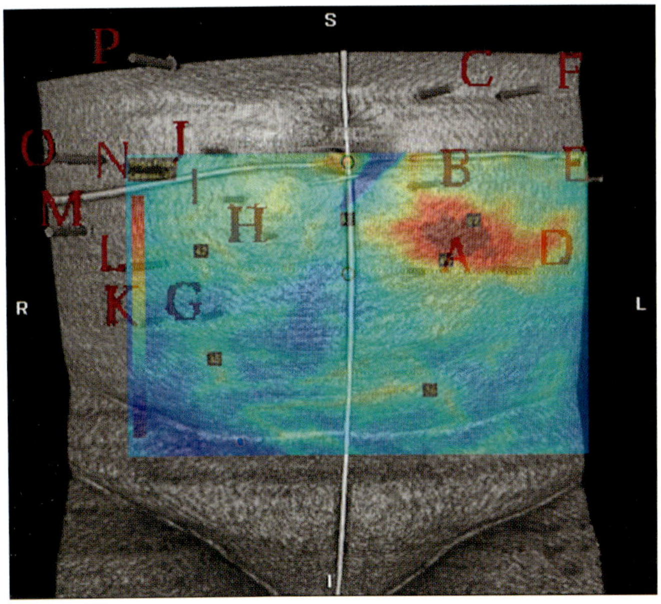

Fig. 16.6 A preoperative study superimposing computed tomography angiography (CTA) and ICG imaging data. CTA gives the location and size of perforators. ICG imaging shows areas of best perfusion.

include reestablishment of impaired lymphatics, and many authors have already documented success in this arena.[39–44] Further experience with ICG imaging in this arena will better delineate the optimal techniques for lymph node identification and harvest, and will facilitate care of the patient with potential or actual lymphatic impairment.

Conclusion

The old adage that there is no replacement for good clinical judgment is as true today as ever. No amount of technology can replace surgical experience. However, this does not mean that technology cannot aid us in surgical decision making and in improving our patient outcomes. ICG imaging puts valuable information about blood flow in the hands of the operating surgeon in real time so that decisions can be made at the time of surgery to optimize outcomes.

An ICG imaging study is only a snapshot in time, and thus its power to predict tissue survival will always have limits. Plastic surgeons know all too well that postoperative edema, dressings, blood pressure, nicotine use, patient activity, hematoma, seroma, infection, and countless other conditions can affect ultimate outcome. But knowledge is power. ICG imaging can assist in many aspects of the breast reconstruction endeavor: perforator selection, arterial perfusion and venous egress evaluation, mastectomy skin evaluation, lymphatic mapping and harvest, documentation of successful vascular and lymphatic reconnection, and postoperative monitoring. The future of ICG imaging certainly is bright.

References

1. Flower RW, Hochheimer BF. A clinical technique and apparatus for simultaneous angiography of the separate retinal and choroidal circulations. Invest Ophthalmol 1973;12:248–261
2. Eren S, Rübben A, Krein R, Larkin G, Hettich R. Assessment of microcirculation of an axial skin flap using indocyanine green fluorescence angiography. Plast Reconstr Surg 1995;96:1636–1649
3. Giunta RE, Holzbach T, Taskov C, et al. Prediction of flap necrosis with laser induced indocyanine green fluorescence in a rat model. Br J Plast Surg 2005;58:695–701
4. Krishnan KG, Schackert G, Steinmeier R. The role of near-infrared angiography in the assessment of post-operative venous congestion in random pattern, pedicled island and free flaps. Br J Plast Surg 2005;58:330–338
5. Lee BT, Matsui A, Hutteman M, et al. Intraoperative near-infrared fluorescence imaging in perforator flap reconstruction: current research and early clinical experience. J Reconstr Microsurg 2010;26(1):59–65
6. Matsui A, Lee BT, Winer JH, Vooght CS, Laurence RG, Frangioni JV. Real-time intraoperative near-infrared fluorescence angiography for perforator identification and flap design. Plast Reconstr Surg 2009;123:125e–127e
7. Still J, Law E, Dawson J, Bracci S, Island T, Holtz J. Evaluation of the circulation of reconstructive flaps using laser-induced fluorescence of indocyanine green. Ann Plast Surg 1999;42:266–274
8. Holm C, Mayr M, Höfter E, Becker A, Pfeiffer UJ, Mühlbauer W. Intraoperative evaluation of skin-flap viability using laser-induced fluorescence of indocyanine green. Br J Plast Surg 2002;55:635–644
9. Mothes H, Dönicke T, Friedel R, Simon M, Markgraf E, Bach O. Indocyanine-green fluorescence video angiography used clinically to evaluate tissue perfusion in microsurgery. J Trauma 2004;57:1018–1024
10. Holm C, Mayr M, Höfter E, Dornseifer U, Ninkovic M. Assessment of the patency of microvascular anastomoses using microscope-integrated near-infrared angiography: a preliminary study. Microsurgery 2009;29:509–514
11. Pestana IA, Coan B, Erdmann D, Marcus J, Levin LS, Zenn MR. Early experience with fluorescent angiography in free-tissue transfer reconstruction. Plast Reconstr Surg 2009;123:1239–1244
12. Yamaguchi S, De Lorenzi F, Petit JY, et al. The "perfusion map" of the unipedicled TRAM flap to reduce postoperative partial necrosis. Ann Plast Surg 2004;53:205–209
13. Holm C, Mayr M, Höfter E, Ninkovic M. Perfusion zones of the DIEP flap revisited: a clinical study. Plast Reconstr Surg 2006;117:37–43
14. Newman MI, Samson MC. The application of laser-assisted indocyanine green fluorescent dye angiography in microsurgical breast reconstruction. J Reconstr Microsurg 2009;25:21–26
15. Holm C, Mayr M, Höfter E, Raab N, Ninkovic M. Interindividual variability of the SIEA Angiosome: effects on operative strategies

in breast reconstruction. Plast Reconstr Surg 2008;122:1612–1620

16. Newman MI, Samson MC, Tamburrino JF, Swartz KA. Intraoperative laser-assisted indocyanine green angiography for the evaluation of mastectomy flaps in immediate breast reconstruction. J Reconstr Microsurg 2010;26:487–492
17. Singer R, Lewis CM, Franklin JD, Lynch JB. Fluorescein test for prediction of flap viability during breast reconstructions. Plast Reconstr Surg 1978;61:371–375
18. Losken A, Styblo TM, Schaefer TG, Carlson GW. The use of fluorescein dye as a predictor of mastectomy skin flap viability following autologous tissue reconstruction. Ann Plast Surg 2008;61:24–29
19. Komorowska-Timek E, Gurtner GC; Komorowska-TimekE. Intraoperative perfusion mapping with laser-assisted indocyanine green imaging can predict and prevent complications in immediate breast reconstruction. Plast Reconstr Surg 2010;125:1065–1073
20. Francisco BS, Kerr-Valentic MA, Agarwal JP. Laser-assisted indocyanine green angiography and DIEP breast reconstruction. Plast Reconstr Surg 2010;125:116e–118e
21. Azuma R, Morimoto Y, Masumoto K, et al. Detection of skin perforators by indocyanine green fluorescence nearly infrared angiography. Plast Reconstr Surg 2008;122:1062–1067
22. Liu DZ, Mathes DW, Zenn MR, Neligan PC. The application of indocyanine green fluorescence angiography in plastic surgery. J Reconstr Microsurg 2011;27:355–364
23. Matsui A, Lee BT, Winer JH, Laurence RG, Frangioni JV. Quantitative assessment of perfusion and vascular compromise in perforator flaps using a near-infrared fluorescence-guided imaging system. Plast Reconstr Surg 2009;124:451–460
24. Losken A, Zenn MR, Hammel JA, Walsh MW, Carlson GW. Assessment of zonal perfusion using intraoperative angiography during abdominal flap breast reconstruction. Plast Reconstr Surg 2012; 129:618e–624e
25. Mohebali J, Gottlieb LJ, Agarwal JP. Further validation for use of the retrograde limb of the internal mammary vein in deep inferior epigastric perforator flap breast reconstruction using laser-assisted indocyanine green angiography. J Reconstr Microsurg 2010;26:131–135
26. Desai ND, Miwa S, Kodama D, et al. A randomized comparison of intraoperative indocyanine green angiography and transit-time flow measurement to detect technical errors in coronary bypass grafts. J Thorac Cardiovasc Surg 2006;132:585–594
27. Phillips BT, Lanier ST, Conkling N, et al. Intraoperative perfusion techniques can accurately predict mastectomy skin flap necrosis in breast reconstruction: results of a prospective trial. Plast Reconstr Surg 2012;129:778e–788e
28. Lee BT, Hutteman M, Gioux S, et al. The FLARE intraoperative near-infrared fluorescence imaging system: a first-in-human clinical trial in perforator flap breast reconstruction. Plast Reconstr Surg 2010;126:1472–1481
29. Murray JD, Jones GE, Elwood ET, Whitty LA, Garcia C. Fluorescent intraoperative tissue angiography with indocyanine green: evaluation of nipple-areola vascularity during breast reduction surgery. Plast Reconstr Surg 2010;126:33e–34e
30. Moyer HR, Losken A. Predicting mastectomy skin flap necrosis with indocyanine green angiography: the gray area defined. Plast Reconstr Surg 2012;129:1043–1048
31. Kanuri A, Liu AS, Guo L. Whom should we SPY? A cost analysis of laser-assisted indocyanine green angiography in prevention of mastectomy skin flap necrosis during prosthesis-based breast reconstruction. Plast Reconstr Surg 2014;133:448e–454e
32. Munabi NC, Olorunnipa OB, Goltsman D, Rohde CH, Ascherman JA. The ability of intra-operative perfusion mapping with laser-assisted indocyanine green angiography to predict mastectomy flap necrosis in breast reconstruction: a prospective trial. J Plast Reconstr Aesthet Surg 2014;67:449–455
33. Saint-Cyr M, Schaverien M, Arbique G, Hatef D, Brown SA, Rohrich RJ. Three- and four-dimensional computed tomographic angiography and venography for the investigation of the vascular anatomy and perfusion of perforator flaps. Plast Reconstr Surg 2008;121: 772–780
34. Rozen WM, Phillips TJ, Ashton MW, Stella DL, Gibson RN, Taylor GI. Preoperative imaging for DIEA perforator flaps: a comparative study of computed tomographic angiography and Doppler ultrasound. Plast Reconstr Surg 2008;121(1, Suppl):1–8
35. Holm C, Tegeler J, Mayr M, Becker A, Pfeiffer UJ, Mühlbauer W. Monitoring free flaps using laser-induced fluorescence of indocyanine green: a preliminary experience. Microsurgery 2002;22:278–287
36. Buntic R. Personal communication with reconstructive surgeon, 2010.
37. Chatterjee A, Krishnan NM, Van Vliet MM, Powell SG, Rosen JM, Ridgway EB. A comparison of free autologous breast reconstruction with and without the use of laser-assisted indocyanine green angiography: a cost-effectiveness analysis. Plast Reconstr Surg 2013;131:693e–701e
38. Blondeel PN, Arnstein M, Verstraete K, et al. Venous congestion and blood flow in free transverse rectus abdominis myocutaneous and deep inferior epigastric perforator flaps. Plast Reconstr Surg 2000;106:1295–1299
39. Oshima A, Koshima I. Early diagnosis of lymphedema and indication of preventive lymphatic venous anastomosis. Plast Reconstr Surg 2011;128:100
40. Azuma S, Yamamoto T, Koshima I. Donor-site lymphatic function after microvascular lymph node transfer should be followed using indocyanine green lymphography. Plast Reconstr Surg 2013;131: 443e–444e
41. Hara H, Mihara M, Seki Y, Todokoro T, Iida T, Koshima I. Comparison of indocyanine green lymphographic findings with the conditions of collecting lymphatic vessels of limbs in patients with lymphedema. Plast Reconstr Surg 2013;132:1612–1618
42. Becker C, Assouad J, Riquet M, Hidden G. Postmastectomy lymphedema: long-term results following microsurgical lymph node transplantation. Ann Surg 2006;243:313–315
43. Dayan E, Mark SL, Mark S, Samson W, Dayan JH. Axillary lymph node transfer for the treatment of lymphedema: technique and case series. Plast Reconstr Surg 2013;132:86
44. Dayan E, Mark SL, Mark S, Samson W, Dayan JH. Performing vascularized groin lymph node transfer with confidence: the use of four anatomic and physiologic modalities for safe and effective flap harvest. Plast Reconstr Surg 2013;132:60

Index

Note: Page numbers followed by an *f* or *t* indicate a figure or table.